POLITICS, MEDICINE,
AND SOCIAL SCIENCE

POLITICS, MEDICINE, AND SOCIAL SCIENCE

DAVID MECHANIC

A WILEY-INTERSCIENCE PUBLICATION

JOHN WILEY & SONS
New York • London • Sydney • Toronto

4/28/75

Library of Congress Cataloging in Publication Data:
Mechanic, David, 1936–
    Politics, medicine, and social science.

    "A Wiley-Interscience publication."
    Includes bibliographical references.
    1. Medical care.   2. Social medicine.
3. Medical policy.   I. Title. [DNLM: 1. Social
medicine.   WA30 M486p 1973]
RA411.M38   362.1′042   73-14602
ISBN 0-471-59008-8

Printed in the United States of America

10 9 8 7 6 5 4 3 2 1

TO MY MOTHER AND FATHER
WITH LOVE

Preface

This volume includes some articles that I have published in recent years, with
several new ones, exploring the relationship between medicine, society, social
science, and the political process. Approximately half of these articles have
not been previously published; the other half have been published in journals and books in various fields. I have revised and modified some of the previously published articles to eliminate repetition and to weld the entire collection into a coherent theme. My purpose, here, is to identify the various points
at which the social and political context affect health and the practice of medicine, to examine social and organizational dilemmas in medical care, to
clarify the intimate relationship between medicine and psychiatric concerns,
and to specify how social-science analysis and behavioral perspectives can
contribute to the formulation of health policy in the future.

I am indebted to many colleagues who have taken time to read and comment
on various parts of the manuscript. Among those offering helpful comments
were Ralph Andreano, Alexander Brooks, Marshall Clinard, Jim and Diane
Greenley, Joel Handler, Robert Hauser, Bob Leonard and David Wiley.
Since the South African context was entirely new to me, I was particularly
careful about this chapter and solicited the reactions of a large number of
knowledgeable people in South Africa, in the United States, and elsewhere.
I am grateful for the assistance of John Cassel, Jack Geiger, Shula Marks,
Mervyn Susser, and Ralph Yodaiken; none of these persons are responsible
for errors or misplaced emphasis that may exist in the chapter. There are
many other South Africans I would like to thank but caution for their welfare in the face of repressive government tactics is prudent.

These articles—like much of my previous work—developed out of various
research projects on medical organizations and mental health services in the
United States, and in England and Wales. This work was supported in part
by the National Institute of Mental Health (Grants MH-8516, MH-14835,
and MH-07413) and by the National Center for Health Services Research
and Development (HS-00253 and HS-00091) for which I am grateful. I also
appreciate the generous assistance of the Robert Wood Johnson Foundation

which will allow us to continue our work in developing implications from social science research on ambulatory medical care for health policy.

I appreciate the willingness of each of the following journals and publishers to provide permission to reproduce previously published articles: *American Journal of Public Health, Society, Medical Care, New England Journal of Medicine, Journal of Health and Social Behavior,* and the *American Journal of Pharmaceutical Education.* Chapter XII was originally prepared for the National Institute of Mental Health task force, and is published with the Institute's consent. Small sections of this chapter previously appeared in *Psychological Medicine,* **3,** February 1973, pp. 1–4 and are reproduced with the permission of the British Medical Association. Chapter XI will also appear in a volume published by Basic Books and Chapter XIII appeared in a volume published by Charles Thomas. A small section of Chapter VIII was included in my paper "Hypochondriasis: A Sociological Perspective," which appeared in *Psychiatric Opinion,* **6,** August 1969.

I am also grateful to the following publishers who granted permission to quote relevant material: Doubleday and Company (excerpts from Erving Goffman's *Asylums*), Harcourt Brace Jovanovich (excerpts from Bruce Ennis', *Prisoners of Psychiatry*), and the *American Journal of Psychiatry* (statement of the Council of the American Psychiatric Association on the Right to Treatment).

I am particularly indebted to Donna Eder and Bruce Turetsky for the thankless job of putting footnotes into a standard form and assisting in proofreading, to Lorraine Borsuk for typing much of the manuscript, and to Abraham Yogev for assisting in data processing.

DAVID MECHANIC

University of Wisconsin, Madison
June 1973

Contents

POLITICS, MEDICINE,
AND SOCIAL SCIENCE

Politics, Medicine, and Social Science: Introduction

The character and distribution of health care, in many respects, reflect the ideological preferences of society. Although the nature of medical knowledge and technology limit the operation of ideological forces, the system of power and social stratification in society explains who receives care and under what conditions. In this sense, health-care delivery depends on the political process, since politics essentially determines how the resources of the community are to be distributed—how much and to whom.

It is becoming fashionable to think of health politics as the process of federal policy making. But the character of health care is molded, equally, by the clash of interests at the community level, the organization and promotion of particular structures of professional organization, and the continuing decisions made at the level of operating agencies of all sorts. Decisions about the character of health care are made at many points and by many individuals. This characteristic, particularly, gives the health context its complex diversity and uneven response to change.

This book is divided into five parts. Chapters I–III consider the relevance of health status and health care to the larger structure of society. Health care in South Africa is examined to illustrate the links between political policies generally and the health of the population. Then, having considered the influence of ideology and politics, I examine the limiting conditions of medical science and technology in order to explain the growing convergence of health practices in modern countries.

Part Two deals concretely with health politics and public policy in the United States. Current issues are reviewed with further consideration of the role of health-care research and social-science analysis on the development of health policy. The receptivity or resistance to social change among physicians is also examined on the basis of a survey of American general practitioners, internists, pediatricians, and obstetricians. Finally, confrontations between government and medical practitioners are explored by examining the clash in 1965 between British general practitioners and the English government.

1

Part Three explores the minipolitics of patient-practitioner systems. What patients seek from medical care is partly dependent on their cultural involvements and social networks, while the services that doctors are willing to provide are influenced by their prior orientations, their training, their professional attitudes and the conditions of practice. There may be a lack of congruence between what patients seek and what physicians provide. The management of patient-physician relationships is political, partly because it must confront the existing conflicts between the interests of patients and physicians and the possible social-control functions of physicians in society. Also it must, in some way, balance these competing needs.

In Part Four, I consider the problems of human adaptation in society and society's relationship to the health-services system. Since the problem of human adaptation within medicine is usually considered within the psychiatric context, this part focuses mainly on the administration of mental-health programs and needs. But I will also emphasize the importance of mental health problems in general medical settings. This section concludes with a discussion of the rights of the mentally ill in relation to the legal process and psychiatric institutions.

Finally, in Part Five, I analyze the possibilities for newly emerging roles in the health sector. Special attention is given to the tangential role of the pharmacist and the emerging interest in health education and maintenance. A plan to achieve a better geographic distribution of physicians is also discussed. I conclude with a consideration of the development of a viable national system of health care.

A health-care plan must encompass a particular political philosophy concerning both the patient's and the provider's roles and obligations. These philosophies usually arise from the political and economic orientations prevailing in the community. For example, in contrasting American and Soviet medicine, one can characterize American medical-care organization as a manifestation of a capitalistic entrepreneurial viewpoint emphasizing self-help, the maintenance of the private sector, and a pluralistic system. Barriers to access are prevalent and are legitimized on the basis that free goods are unappreciated and exploited; there is concern about the centralization of power. On the other hand, the Soviet system—influenced by Stalinist-Leninist perspectives—conceives of the health of workers as an important economic resource and the health system as an aspect of the government structure concerned with the public welfare.[1] Thus this system has a strong central direction; it gives emphasis to planning; it minimizes professional prerogatives and status; and it encourages the access and utilization of primary services.[2,3] Considerable emphasis is given to industrial medicine and preventive and environmental work, and services tend to be superior for segments of the work force that are vital to the economy. Also medicine is used, more obviously than in the United States, for political purposes and as a means of social control.[4]

The organization of medical practice, consistent with dominant political ideologies, is vividly illustrated by recent developments in China and Cuba. In China, the force of the cultural revolution and of Maoist thought has redirected medicine away from its urban, curative, and professional emphases toward a strong rural involvement, an impressive emphasis on public health, and a cooperative relationship between traditional and Western healing practices. The result is a vastly improved distribution of care and significant advances in coping with the problems of malnutrition, high fertility, and venereal disease.[5,6] Similarly, various informed reports of Cuban medicine [7,8] indicate an impressive redistribution of care to the countryside and productive efforts in dealing with preventable disease among the more deprived segments of the population.

Gains of this kind can be accomplished despite limited resources if there is a congruence between political and social ideals and the types of organization necessary to carry out health policies in an efficient and equitable fashion. A greater issue is whether such planned structures are possible in a context with more individualistic political and social ideologies. This concern has more relevance to the current scene in America.[9] Do we have to choose between our values and adequate health care? What are our options?

We must appreciate that bringing care to disenfranchised persons involves a redistribution of income in one form or another. If resources are reasonably stable and entitlement is extended, there will be greater competition among varying segments of the population for the use of the available services. Populations are always reluctant to yield benefits that they have enjoyed and, therefore, entitlement without an increase in service is likely to exacerbate social conflict. If there is sufficient economic growth, it becomes easier to disproportionately allocate newly acquired resources, but redistribution of what has been available in the past is, at best, difficult. In light of the realities, the trend is to emphasize efficiency and improvement in management practices. Although increased yields for our investments are possible and likely, the gains of improved management are exaggerated and are based on the translation of ideas from other sectors of the economy without serious appreciation of the special character and needs of medical institutions.

Most of the jockeying in health care at the federal level with respect to the development of some form of national entitlement involves three concerns: financing, coverage, and possible incentives for change in organizational practices. In legislative considerations, financing receives greatest attention because the necessary funds must be found to pay for any extension of entitlement in the population. Since there is a reluctance—in view of recent history with

Medicare and Medicaid—to allow open-ended expenditures in health care, control over expenditures is advocated by limiting coverage to particular populations or services and by imposing barriers to service through coinsurance and deductibles. The alternate option of universal entitlement, funded through a national allocation of specified health funds to various regions and localities, finds little favor in the current administration, although it constitutes the key mechanism in proposals for a national system of health care. In Part Five the implications of each of these approaches is explored.

A common way of circumscribing government responsibility is to limit the benefits that will be awarded and also the components of the population that will receive them. This has resulted in a pathology of categorical programs that are highly fragmented in terms of services offered and eligible populations. The most recent extension of Medicare benefits to patients with chronic kidney disease suggests the disorganized approach that is characteristic of such categorical extensions. Independent of political pressures, it is difficult to understand why a person who has one disease should have a lesser right to care and protection against financial disaster than a person who has another disease. Even the most liberal advocates for entitlement usually exclude or limit the extensions of psychiatric, optometric, and dental services on the basis that they are too costly, too unpredictable, and that national resources to meet the service demands are limited. Although dental services probably fit the case, I will later clarify the irrationality of excluding benefits such as psychiatric services from any major extension of entitlement.

In phasing entitlement or in limiting it, priorities must be established. Decisions must be made about the relative merit of financing preventive (as opposed to catastrophic) services, services for children in contrast to services for the middle-aged or the elderly, acute benefits versus chronic benefits, and the like. Similarly, it is necessary to establish the costs and advantages of freely allowing access to care and then limiting services, once persons have entered the health system, in contrast to developing a system of deductibles and coinsurance with the intention of limiting the flow of patients into the health system. Later I will explore the rhetoric and reality of these varying means of controlling the consumption of health services.

The extensions of federal financing in health care provide an opportunity to develop incentives to correct dysfunctional organizational practices and to attempt to direct practice priorities. Most proposals for universal entitlement make certain assumptions concerning the legislative effects on the organization and distribution of health services to the population. It is assumed that, by manipulating remuneration patterns, it is possible to provide incentives to redistribute resources and manpower, to insure peer review and greater efficiency, or to emphasize one pattern of practice instead of another. The indirect establishment of standards is always a tricky business, and government agencies are frequently unwilling to enforce them once they are in operation. This unwillingness is often related to political factors, but it also may result from the knowledge that the enforcement of standards may compel needed providers to withdraw from the program. Thus it is possible to make matters worse by attempting to enforce standards that depart too much from the state of things as they exist or that are impossible to meet.

Indirect incentives to change organizational practices have other difficulties as well. They frequently fail to achieve expected objectives, and organizations often find ways to meet the letter of the requirement without meeting its spirit. Although the standards may achieve little of substance, they may consume considerable resources within organizations to demonstrate compliance and within the government to insure enforcement. Thus, unrealistic and unenforceable standards may prove to be expensive as well as ineffectual. The indirect attempt to produce major organizational change in medicine through payment incentives is likely to produce less real change than a more direct attempt to establish a unified national health plan. It is precisely because a national health plan is more effective in directing the components of practice that it arouses such vigorous opposition. But we must, I believe, face the fact that reliance on uncoordinated incentives will not fundamentally alter the national problems of inequality in access, maldistribution of personnel and facilities, and uneven quality of care.

The health-care system of the United States is presently in a state of flux. Major legislative change is likely to come in the foreseeable future at both federal and state levels. In evaluating one program or another, it is useful to stand back and consider some of the larger and more basic issues concerning the function of health services in society, the relationship of health to other social institutions, and organizational and professional patterns. My purpose, here, is to explore part of this larger picture on the assumption that the enactment of effective specific legislation depends on understanding what it is one wants to achieve. Hopefully, this discussion will clarify the dialogue about the goals we seek and how to best implement them.

Notes

1. Field, M. (1967). *Soviet Socialized Medicine*. New York: Free Press.
2. Fry, J. (1969). *Medicine in Three Societies*. New York: American Elsevier.
3. Anderson, O. (1973). "Health Services in the USSR." *Selected Papers*, **42**, Graduate School of Business, University of Chicago.
4. Field, M. (1957). *Doctor and Patient in Soviet Russia*. New York: Free Press. More recently, there has been growing evidence of the use of psychiatry to control political dissenters in the Soviet Union.
5. Horn, J. (1969). *Away With All Pests*. New York: Monthly Review Press.

6. Sidel, V. (1971). "Medicine in the People's Republic of China." *Proceedings of the First Annual Meeting of the Institute of Medicine.* Washington, D.C.: National Academy of Sciences, November 17–18.
7. Navarro, V. (1972). "Health Services in Cuba: An Initial Appraisal." *New England Journal of Medicine,* **287**:954–959.
8. Stein, Z., and M. Susser (1972). "The Cuban Health System: A Trial of a Comprehensive Service in a Poor Country." *International Journal of Health Services,* **2**:551–566.
9. For an example of the view that this is unlikely in the United States, See E. Ginzberg, and Miriam Ostow (1969). *Men, Money, and Medicine.* New York: Columbia University Press.

PART ONE

THE CONTEXT OF HEALTH AND HEALTH CARE IN MODERN SOCIETY

CHAPTER I

Sociology and Public Health: Perspectives for Application*

Much of the content of sociology directly concerns man's adaptation to his changing environment and, thus, this field has important implications for public health practice. No short discussion can do justice to the variety of perspectives and recent research efforts that can be useful to the public health practitioner, but it is possible to review briefly some major perspectives and examples of research that illustrate how an appreciation of sociological variables can assist the public health practitioner.

First, we must observe how the perspectives of sociology and public health differ. Although public health is an applied endeavor that imposes normative criteria which it then attempts to implement, the sociologist's major concern is with understanding social phenomena independently of the immediate value of such understanding. This difference in perspective was made clear by Edward Rogers' challenge to sociology[1] to present its findings in a fashion that allows transformation in the form of public health programs. But if the sociologist restricted or even concentrated his efforts on the causes where intervention seems possible, his horizons would be limited, indeed. The pervasive belief that all public health problems are dysfunctions, which can and must be remedied, rather than part of a complex pattern of adaptation to changing life conditions and social patterns is in itself a value[2] that tells us more about the public health practitioner and his priorities than about the nature of social life.

The issue of values is fundamental to the entire question of sociological knowledge and application. As Elinson and Herr[3] suggested in their reply to Rogers' challenge, much of the difficulty in bringing sociological knowledge to bear in public health efforts may result from the limited way in which the practitioner poses the issue. It may be the practitioner himself who is part of

* Adapted from a paper in the *American Journal of Public Health*, **62**:146–151 (1972).

the problem—by defining certain relatively "benign" behaviors of others as problems, by projecting responsibility to clients rather than to the social institutions that serve them, or by allowing his values to limit the consideration of the real range of options for improving the life and health of people.

The general problem can be illustrated by reviewing the current ferment concerning abortion reform. In the state of Wisconsin, like elsewhere, sexual attitudes and patterns have radically changed over the generations, but the law continues to define contraceptives as lewd and indecent articles, and forbids physicians to prescribe contraceptives to unmarried women for the purpose of birth control. Many women who do not wish to bear a child become pregnant, yet find it difficult to obtain an abortion despite a recent ruling of the Federal District Court to the effect that forbidding an abortion is an abridgement of women's constitutional rights. The medical profession—including persons affiliated with public health—has, at best, sat on its hands, and some organized medical groups and hospitals have continued to resist change in traditional approaches to the problem.* Here one might see a variety of public health problems implicit in the situation depending on one's perspective. Is the problem one of promiscuity and a growing lack of responsibility among the young, or is it the intransigence of the State Medical Society and the physicians in the state? Should our major concern be the growing rate of illegitimacy and dependency, or the failure of the legislature and the system of medical care to respond more expeditiously to people's concerns and self-defined needs? The practice of public health embodies some system of morality, and part of the sociological effort must be devoted to examining the morality and its priorities relative to competing definitions. It may be that our concept of public health constitutes part of our problem.

Despite such issues, there are circumstances where considerable consensus exists as to the undesirability of particular conditions prevalent in the community. Although values come into play in a wide variety of ways, I shall assume here that there is substantial agreement on certain basic values relevant to problems of public health; and I shall develop particular themes that may help the practitioner.

Population Distribution and Selection

Basic to public health is an understanding of the significance of the distribution of populations over time and the various factors affecting fertility, mortality, migration, and social and genetic selection. Public health practitioners, however, sometimes seem less aware that social selectivity is a continuing and

---

* This was written before the Supreme Court decision on abortion, but the basic point remains valid.

persistent process that affects such varied matters as organizational participation, health maintenance behavior, utilization of medical and other institutional facilities, educational achievement, and almost every other aspect of social and community life. Any practitioner will tend to observe such selection processes from a particular vantage point, and he tends to form images of behavior that are constructions from a particular selected population.[4-6] By the nature of his position he is more likely to come into contact with people who take advantage of a particular program or people who seek a service, and such contacts are likely to influence his perceptions more than the actual patterns of behavior existing in the population at large. The constructions that the practitioner develops guide him in the options he adopts and in those he neglects, and profoundly influence his perceptions of situations.

The continuing awareness that one's own perceptions are molded by the context within which one works is nonspecific, but it nevertheless can be helpful because it alerts the practitioner to preventable errors and promotes continuing and serious scrutiny of the important forces in the environment affecting his work. In dealing with clients, such awareness facilitates considering not only the manifest issue, or the client's presenting complaint, but also the larger context within which the problem occurs and how it can be dealt with. This concern with populations and selectivity within populations has been basic to public health application, and the continuing development of this perspective will be examined in Part III.

Social and Cultural Aspects of Preventive Health and Illness Behavior

It is widely appreciated that there are cultural and social variations in the manner in which persons define health problems, participate in health maintenance programs, and utilize medical and other health services.[7] For example, there is considerable evidence that socioeconomic factors are related to knowledge about disease, use of medical and dental services, acceptance of preventive health practices, purchase of voluntary health insurance, delay in seeking treatment, and use of folk remedies and self-medications.[8-23] These socioeconomic variations encompass variations among populations in health values, understanding of disease processes, future and preventive planning, cultural expectations, and feelings of social distance between oneself and health practitioners.[24] The previously cited research also suggests that impoverished persons feel less at ease in medical settings than more affluent persons, that they have less understanding of how practitioners operate and that they are less willing to question their treatment.

Underlying these observed relationships are various social psychological processes that have yet to be fully examined. In recent years, various models have been suggested to explain processes underlying the relationship between socioeconomic factors and health and illness behavior. Rosenstock,[25] for example, giving emphasis to a motivational model, has argued that preventive health behavior relevant to a given problem is determined by the extent to which a person sees a problem as having both serious consequences and a high probability of occurrence. He also believes that such behavior emerges from conflicting goals and motives, and that actions will follow the motives that are most salient and the goals that are perceived as most valuable. Similarly, Zola,[26] approaching the problem from a somewhat different perspective, has delineated five timing "triggers" in patients' decisions to seek medical care. He calls the first pattern "interpersonal crisis," where the situation calls attention to the symptoms and causes the patient to dwell on them. The second trigger—social interference—comes into play when symptoms threaten a valued social activity. Similarly, he argues that action is precipitated by social pressures of others, perceived threat, and the nature and quality of the symptoms. Zola reports the impression that these triggers have different degrees of importance in varying social strata and ethnic groups.

Both of the above theories of health behavior focus exclusively on the client and give little attention to the manner in which characteristics of helping institutions affect the client's behavior and response. But the client's behavior may be strongly affected by the nature of services and how they are provided, and such factors as the availability and proximity of treatment resources, psychological and monetary costs of seeking treatment, stigma, social distance, and the like all may affect the client's orientation. Although it is true that people's responses to health and illness are often conditioned responses to prior background and experience, the health services system has the capacity to modify such behavior patterns. It can foster dependency or encourage self-reliance. It can respect and enhance the dignity of persons or contribute toward stigmatizing and humiliating them. As interesting as social and cultural precursors of health and illness behavior may be, we should not neglect the fact that considerable potential for making the delivery of services more congruent with need exists through the proper organization of health-care services.

Barriers to medical and health care that are a product of the way health professionals and health care services function are more amenable to change than client attitudes and behavior. There is evidence that when cost and other barriers are removed from access to medical care, and a valuable service is offered, differential utilization of medical services by social class largely disappears. For example, socioeconomic differences in the use of medical services comparable to those traditionally found in the United States do not exist in Great Britain, where services are provided without cost and on the basis of need.[27] It is significant that in the United States, when public health and research programs offer a free service to a particular population such as in the National Health Examination Survey[28] or in the Baltimore Morbidity Survey,[29-30] persons of lower socioeconomic status and nonwhites (the two groups with the lowest level of utilization of services on a national basis) are usually overrepresented in their participation as compared with other population groups. Finally, more recent data from the National Household Morbidity Survey shows that the unfavorable position of the lowest socioeconomic groups in respect to physician visits has improved.[31] These data suggest that government expenditures (particularly Medicare) have contributed toward closing the gap in the use of physicians' services. Moreover, experience with neighborhood health centers indicates that when valuable services were provided to poor black populations in both the North and the South—services that respected their dignity and integrity—there has been no difficulty in obtaining their responsiveness.

The importance of client response is evident, but such differential client response tends to operate within limits. Various studies show that social and cultural influences have a maximal impact on utilization behavior when the condition has a mild or moderate impact on the person and when the symptoms are identifiable, familiar, and easily explained. As the impact of the symptoms becomes more dramatic—and to the extent that the symptoms are unfamiliar, unpredictable, and threatening—the effect of social and cultural factors on help-seeking appears to be more limited.[32-34] Social and cultural patterns, as they affect health and illness behavior, are particularly important in the case of serious conditions that do not have a dramatic onset and have early symptoms that are common to a wide variety of more familiar and self-limited conditions.

Consequences of Medical Labeling and Response

Practitioners frequently think of their activities as purely medical and sometimes fail to consider the social and other practical consequences of medical decisions and clinical judgments. Although these risks have always been evident in the practitioner's work, they are very much exacerbated as medicine becomes a more highly organized activity under growing bureaucratic sponsorship.

Medical judgments and decisions affect the fate of people by influencing their social opportunities and potentialities.[35] Such influences occur in two ways: (1) through affecting the patient's attitudes, self-perceptions, confidence in his capacities and, therefore, his degree of activity; or (2) through defining the patient in such a fashion so that he is systematically discriminated against or excluded from various community opportunities. Obvious cases such as mental patients or epileptics immediately come to mind, but the relevant processes far transcend these particular groups of patients and have persistent effects on the rehabilitation and community functioning of many kinds of patients, including persons with heart disease, renal disease, cancer, and other conditions.

In situations where patients have had continuing relationships over time with a personal doctor, the patients were usually protected from obvious discrimination because of medical reasons, although they might have suffered iatrogenic disease as a consequence of the doctor's failure to consider social factors as part of his clinical assessment. But as medical contexts become more bureaucratic, and as knowledge of the patient's difficulties is shared by a variety of people, the possibilities and dangers of communication of medical judgments and their misuse increase, and the need to develop new protections grows.

It is essential to appreciate the extensive variation in disability and community adjustment among patients with comparable disease. The patient's definition of his condition and the social resources available to him affect the extent of his adjustment to work, his social relations, and his family life, and condition his productivity, life satisfaction, and the demands he makes on the health care system.[36,37]

The frequently heard lament of physicians that too many of their patients present trivial complaints or that they are hypochondriacs is partly a manifestation of the practice of medicine itself. Modern medical practice is characterized by growing demand on limited manpower and increasing specialization of medical functions. As doctors become more specialized, they are less interested in and less capable of meeting the more diffuse needs of patients, particularly patients suffering from psychological distress and physical conditions that are vastly complicated by psychological and social factors. These patients are difficult to treat under the best of conditions, but they might do well in a continuing supporting relationship with a physician who demonstrates concern and interest in their life situations.[38]

However, in accommodating to technological change and growing patient demand, medicine is increasingly more bureaucratized, resulting in greater frustration of such patients' needs. Bureaucratic organization of medicine is essential in insuring a high level of technical care that is distributed efficiently, but it is a poor instrument for dealing with the psychological needs of difficult patients. As doctors continue to become more specialized and more occupied by growing patient demand for services, they tend to insist more than ever that their patients' illnesses fall within the narrow limits of the medical disease model.[39]

These difficulties in medical care are frequently recognized, but one of the major problems is how to rationalize and organize medical services so that they are more efficiently distributed and, at the same time, responsive to the personal needs of particular groups of patients. Some health organizations have attempted to develop new roles for social workers and nurses who assume important responsibilities for various aspects of personal care.[40] Such mechanisms, thus far, have not been fully effective, since many people wish to have the doctor rather than other professionals deal with their problems.[41] It is likely that attacking this problem will involve not only the transfer of functions to well-trained workers with specific tasks but also concerted efforts to legitimize such role distributions from the perspective of clients. The latter task may be more difficult than the former.

Interactions, Communication, and Inducements

The suggestive powers of the physician are substantial, and doctors and other health workers are in a position to reduce the stress their patients experience by small gestures and behaviors that show an awareness and concern for the patient.[42-44]

Sympathy, support, and instruction can have great benefits. Frequently, persons who endorse the idea that the doctor should provide sympathy and support to the patient do so on the belief that this is a noble and human thing to do. It is rarely appreciated, however, that establishing such relationships with patients facilitates the informational process between doctor and patient, and contributes in an important way to the management of the patient and his progress toward recovery. To neglect, therefore, important facts that have bearing on these processes because they are of a social or psychological sort increases errors in prediction on the part of physician and inefficacy in the management of his patients.

Another aspect of the same problem concerns the inducements and encouragement provided by health workers and health institutions that facilitate patient activity and motivation for mastering their problems. Substantial literature documents the way that large impersonal hospitals allow inactivity, encourage dependency, and lead to various forms of skill deterioration and hopelessness.[45] The relationship between a health worker and patient is a powerful instrument to facilitate or retard the patient's social functioning, his sense of potency and potential, and his willingness to struggle against his illness. The failure to use these inducements and supports as a rehabilitative technique is as serious as the failure to prescribe necessary medication or to initiate other necessary medical procedures.

Influence of Professionalization and Professional Controls on Treatment Values

We usually think of professionalization as a vehicle for improving the quality of health services. We assume that, as the health worker incorporates the values of his professional group and subjects himself to the evaluation of his colleagues, he is directed toward worthy goals and is insulated from improprieties. One of the difficulties with this perspective is that professionals often become involved with their own subcultures which protect professional autonomy, define professional work in terms of the exercise of particular skills, and develop reward structures that tend to accord highest prestige and acclaim to persons who excel by professional criteria.[46] Since medicine as an activity tends to give high priority to technical and scientific skills, and defines tasks associated with such skills as most interesting, it is not surprising that doctors develop such orientations.

The development of technical skills is extremely valuable but, if overemphasized, it may lead to the neglect of more important social priorities, which doctors may recognize but define as uninteresting opportunities from a professional point of view. Doctors may objectively recognize that many of the efforts devoted to heroic efforts if rechanneled to other problems, such as differentials in infant mortality or child care, might yield large relative benefits. But the technical problems in such work as heart transplantation are defined as professionally exciting, while routine primary care is seen as mundane and uninteresting. Similarly, in psychiatry, rehabilitation is defined as intellectually unexciting and routine while psychotherapy, which is of questionable efficacy, is seen as interesting, thus justifying the tremendous imbalance of resources between these two fields.[47]

In view of the ways that doctors and other professionals are trained, it is not surprising that they seek opportunities that allow them to exercise and develop their technical skills and to avoid tasks, no matter how important, that are viewed as mundane and unchallenging.[48] This problem is particularly exacerbated where primary care functions are not structurally differentiated from more specialized medical activities. In countries where such separation is enforced by the nature of medical organization, persons performing what are viewed as lesser skills are often dissatisfied, in part, by their lower status, but the tasks are more likely to be met.[49] One way of approaching this problem is to functionally separate tasks requiring lower levels of skill and assign them to other health personnel, but this too raises problems of the segmentation of care, the acceptability of new health workers, coordination of services, licensing difficulties, and the like.

An important source of professional values is the training experience itself and the models of practice available to students within the training context. Practice consistent with values will depend, of course, on the situational aspects of the health worker's practice once his training is completed.[50] Medical education and the more professionalized nurses training programs emphasized the acquisition of technical skill and capacities in contrast to giving focus to meeting community needs and goals. It would be unrealistic to expect educational institutions, which have very special functions, to forego the development of their students' technical skills, but it is essential that these institutions provide realistic and acceptable models of practice as part of their training to allow their students to respond in meaningful ways to the health care needs of the community once they graduate.

The Influence of the Medical Care System on the Quality of Health

Every public health practitioner realizes that the medical-care system, as more narrowly defined, has only a limited role on the quality of health in populations. The quality of a population's health is a response to the overall nature of the environment, and medical care is only a part of the larger picture. Much of the vast progress in health status in the past century is a product of a higher standard of living, better sanitation, and improved nutrition; and many of the risks to health today are a product of man's constructed environments. Although good medical care—and in particular good preventive care—can be brought to bear at particular points in the life cycle so that it has impact, much of the necessary health action required involves larger social and political considerations and the development of new patterns of community behavior.

The system of medical care in any country reflects the tradition of the past and the social priorities for the future. Health care is a vast industry and subsumes many groups with conflicting perspectives and interests. How these interests are weighed, negotiated, and resolved determines, in part, the organization and provision of health services and the various priorities given to different aspects of health care. But certain limits on the nature of medical activity are also determined by the technical development of medicine and the character of population demands, and nations having vastly different political ideologies face many similar organizational problems in medical care. These problems are reviewed in Chapter 3.

Health and the Environment

In the final analysis, the health and vitality of populations are dependent on the ability to make successful adaptations to the environment within which man must survive. Man's ability to adapt depends on his capacities, skills, and psychological orientations. To a large extent, man constructs his own environment depending on the models and norms that his culture and society provide.[51] His skills and effectiveness depend on the preparatory institutions that his community provides for dealing with the problems he is likely to face as an individual and as a member of a group. His motivation and the direction of his

18   SOCIOLOGY AND PUBLIC HEALTH

interests and aspirations will depend on the incentives that the community promotes. His psychological capacities and strengths are influenced by the human resources and social supports that the environment can provide. Although men can do a great deal to promote their own health within rather narrow limits, in the larger context life and health are substantially dependent on community decisions and social forces, which are often outside of any single individual's control. The appreciation of these facts should direct the profession of public health as it faces the future.

Notes

1. Rogers, E. (1968). "Public Health Asks of Sociology...."*Science*, **159**:506–508.
2. Dubos, R. (1959).*Mirage of Health*. New York: Harper.
3. Elinson, J., and C. Herr (1969). "A Sociomedical Response to Edward S. Rogers: Public Health Asks of Sociology...." Paper presented at the Annual Meetings of the American Sociological Association, September 1, 1969.
4. Scheff, T. J. (1966). "Typification in the Diagnostic Practices of Rehabilitation Agencies." In M. Sussman (ed.), *Sociology and Rehabilitation*. Washington, D.C.: American Sociological Association.
5. Sudnow, D. (1965). "Normal Crimes: Sociological Features of the Penal Code in a Public Defender's Office." *Social Problems*, **12**:255–276.
6. Mechanic, D. (1963). "Some Implications of Illness Behavior for Medical Sampling." *New England Journal of Medicine*, **269**:244–247.
7. For a review of these studies, see D. Mechanic (1968). *Medical Sociology: A Selective View*. New York: Free Press, 115–157.
8. United States National Health Survey (1964). *Medical Care, Health Status, and Family Income*. PHS Series 10, No. 9. Washington D.C.: U.S. Government Printing Office.
9. Koos, E. (1954). *The Health of Regionsville: What the People Thought and Did About It*. New York: Columbia University Press.
10. Samora, J., *et al.* (1961). "Medical Vocabulary Knowledge Among Hospital Patients." *Journal of Health and Human Behavior*, **2**:83–92.
11. Pratt, L., *et al.* (1957). "Physicians' Views on the Level of Medical Information Among Patients." *American Journal of Public Health and the Nation's Health*, **47**:1277–1283.
12. Rosenstock, I. (1959). "Why People Fail to Seek Poliomyelitis Vaccination."*Public Health Reports*, **74**:98–103.
13. Deasy, L. (1956). "Socioeconomic Status and Participation in the Poliomyelitis Vaccine Trail." *American Sociological Review*, **21**:185–191.
14. Suchman, E. (1965). "Stages of Illness and Medical Care." *Journal of Health and Human Behavior*, **6**:114–128.
15. Cobb, B., et al. (1954). "Patient-Responsible Delay of Temperature in Cancer." *Cancer, 7*: 920–926.
16. Goldsen, R., et al. (1957). "Some Factors Related to Patient Delay in Seeking Diagnosis for Cancer Symptoms." *Cancer, 10*:1–7.
17. Blackwell, B. (1963). "The Literature on Delay in Seeking Medical Care for Chronic Illness." *Health Education Monographs*, Vol. 16, entire issue.

18. Kutner, B., and G. Gordon, (1961). "Seeking Care for Cancer." *Journal of Health and Human Behavior,* **2**:171–178.

19. Goldsen, R. (1963). "Patient Delay in Seeking Cancer Diagnosis: Behavioral Aspects." *Journal of Chronic Disease,* **17**:417–436.

20. Levine, G. (1962). "Anxiety About Illness: Psychological and Social Bases." *Journal of Health and Human Behavior,* **3**:30–34.

21. Brill, N., and H. Storrow (1960). "Social Class and Psychiatric Treatment." *Archives of General Psychiatry,* **3**:340–344.

22. Lewis, L., and J. Lopreato, (1962). "Arationality, Ignorance, and Perceived Danger in Medical Practices." *American Sociological Review,* **27**:514–523.

23. Cornely, P., and S. Bigman (1962). "Acquaintance with Municipal Government Health Services in a Low-Income Urban Population." *American Journal of Public Health and the Nation's Health,* **52**:1877–1886.

24. Mechanic, D. (1969). "Illness and Cure." In J. Kosa et al. (eds.), *Poverty and Health: A Sociological Analysis.* Cambridge: Harvard University Press.

25. Rosenstock, I. (1960). "What Research in Motivation Suggests for Public Health." *American Journal of Public Health and the Nation's Health,* **50**:295–302.

26. Zola, I. (1964). "Illness Behavior of the Working Class." In A. Shostak and W. Gomberg (eds.), *Blue Collar World: Studies of the American Worker,*Englewood Cliffs, N.J.: Prentice-Hall.

27. Cartwright, A. (1967). *Patients and Their Doctors: A Study of General Practice.* London: Routledge and Kegan Paul.

28. National Center for Health Statistics (1964). *Cycle 1 of the Health Examination Survey : Sample and Response,* PHS Series 11, No. 1. Washington, D.C.: U.S. Government Printing Office.

29. Roberts, D., and C. Wylie (1956). "Multiple Screening in the Baltimore Study of Chronic Illness." *Journal of the American Medical Association,* **161**:1442–1446.

30. Wylie, C. M. (1967). "Participation in a Multiple Screening Clinc with Five-Year Follow-up." *Public Health Reports,* **76**:596–602. D.C.: U.S. Government Printing Office.

31. National Center for Health Statistics (1968). *Volume of Physician Visits-United States— July 1966—June 1967.* PHS Series 10, No. 49. Washington, D.C.: U.S. Government Printing Office. Since this was written, further evidence has been presented suggesting that the gap in physician visits may not only have been closed, but the relationship to socioeconomic status may have actually been reversed. See Monteiro, L., (1973). "Expense is No Object—Income and Physician Visits Reconsidered." *Journal of Health and Social Behavior,* **14**:99–115; and Bice, T. W., *et al.* (1972). "Socioeconomic Status and Use of Physician Service: A Reconsideration." *Medical Care,* **10**:261–271.

32. Mechanic, D., and E. Volkart (1960). "Illness Behavior and Medical Diagnoses." *Journal of Health and Human Behavior* ,**1**:86–94.

33. Suchman, E. (1965). "Stages of Illness and Medical Care." *Journal of Health and Human Behavior,* **6**:114–128.

34. Dinitz, S.,*et al.* (1961). "The Posthospital Psychological Functioning of Former Mental Hospital Patients." *Mental Hygiene,* **45**:579–588.

35. Scheff, T. (1963). "Decision Rules, Types of Error, and Their Consequences in Medical Diagnosis." *Behavioral Science,* **8**:97–107.

36. For an example of an excellent study illustrating such processes as they occur through time, see F. Davis (1963). *Passage Through Crisis: Polio Victims and Their Families.* Indianapolis: Bobbs Merrill.

37. Imboden, J. B., et al. (1959). "Brucellosis: III Psychologic Aspects of Delayed Convalescence." *Archives of Internal Medicine,* **103:**406–414.

38. For a review of this issue in detail, see D. Mechanic (1969). "Hypochondriasis: A Sociological Perspective." *Psychiatric Opinion,* **6:**12–24.

39. Mechanic, D. (1970). "Correlates of Frustration Among British General Practitioners." *Journal of Health and Social Behavior,* **11:**87–104.

40. See, for example, G. Silver (1963). *Family Medical Care.* Cambridge, Mass.: Harvard University Press.

41. Freidson, E. (1959). "Specialties Without Roots: The Utilization of New Services." *Human Organization,* **18:**112–116.

42. Egbert, L. D., et al. (1964). "Reduction of Postoperative Pain by Encouragement and Instruction of Patients." *New England Journal of Medicine,* **270:**825–827.

43. Janis, I. (1958). *Psychological Stress.* New York: Wiley.

44. Skipper, J. Jr., and R. Leonard (1968). "Children, Stress, and Hospitalization: A Field Experiment." *Journal of Health and Social Behavior,* **9:**275–287.

45. For a review of this literature, see D. Mechanic (1968). *Medical Sociology: A Selected View.* New York: Free Press.

46. Freidson, E. (1970). *Profession of Medicine.* New York: Dodd, Mead.

47. Mechanic, D. (1969). *Mental Health and Social Policy.* Englewood Cliffs, N.J.: Prentice-Hall.

48. For an excellent discussion of these issues, see J. Richmond (1969). *Currents in American Medicine: A Developmental View of Medical Care and Education.* Cambridge, Mass.: Harvard University Press.

49. Fry, J. (1970). *Medicine in Three Societies.* New York: American Elsevier.

50. Becker, H., et al. (1963). *Boys in White: Student Culture in a Medical School.* Chicago: University of Chicago Press.

51. For an elaboration of this framework, see D. Mechanic (1970). "Some Problems in Developing a Social Psychology of Adaptation to Stress." In J. McGrath (ed.), *Social and Psychological Factors in Stress.* New York: Holt, Rinehart and Winston.

CHAPTER II

Health Status and Medical Care in the Republic of South Africa*

The Republic of South Africa is a country of great contradictions and striking contrasts. Although the total population is 21.5 million, approximately 4 million whites dominate every aspect of the social and economic life. The remaining population, consisting of about 15 million Africans, 2 million coloreds (mulattos), and more than one half million Asians, is by law and by social custom subjected to a variety of indignities and deprivations. While the Asians have the least deprived economic status among the nonwhites, and the coloreds hold an intermediate position, the great mass of Africans live under conditions of abject poverty.

Apartheid is the Republic of South Africa's official policy of segregation. It preserves and sustains the economic, political, and social domination of the white minority over all other groups.[1] This forced separation leaves the black majority with 14 percent of the land, gives the whites full control over the productive capacities of the nation, and results in enormous hardship and misery for the nonwhite population.

The patterns of disease and health care in the country reflect this social and economic organization. For example, in 1970 the number of white infant deaths per 1000 live births was 21.1. For Asian infants, the number was 37.1 and, for colored infants, it rose to 136.2.[2] Registration of births among Africans is incomplete and infant mortality is not reported, but a 1966 survey found that half of the children in a typical reserve die before reaching age five,[3] and doctors practicing among Africans in rural areas report that it is quite usual for African women to have lost half of their children.

In the summer of 1972 I was asked by the University of Witwatersrand in Johannesburg to be a visiting professor and to initiate a teaching program for medical students in the sociology of medicine. I visited South Africa for 25

* A modified version of this chapter appeared in *Society*, 10:36–44, 1973.

days, spending approximately half of my time in Johannesburg and surrounding areas and the remainder in visiting medical facilities and physicians in other parts of the country. If there are any biases in my observations, they result from having seen more urban than rural facilities and more prestigious than ordinary hospitals, and from having spent a disproportionate amount of time visiting "model" facilities. For example, I spent more time in the African township of Soweto than in other more impoverished townships and had an official tour of the "most progressive" of the reserves, medically speaking: the Tswana homeland in Hammanskraal. I made an effort to see medical facilities in different townships and reserves in varying parts of the country and visited several mission hospitals in rural areas. I saw white, colored, and African units in urban areas that were funded by the same authorities, and I had some opportunity to examine the degree of inequality in the provision of medical services.[4]

Twenty-five days gave me a very limited exposure, and I am aware of the difficulties in arriving at a balanced picture in so short a time. Thus I have made special effort to verify my personal observations by talking with knowledgeable physicians and medical scientists throughout South Africa and elsewhere and by consulting available publications on social and medical conditions in South Africa. I have stated my observations with care, and I am confident that they are valid.

Some Background on Social and Medical Organization in South Africa

The Republic of South Africa, according to the Minister of Health, has one doctor for every 450 whites and one for every 18,000 blacks.[5] There are relatively few nonwhite doctors in the country, with one colored doctor for every 6200 colored and one African doctor for every 44,400 Africans. South Africa has four medical schools for whites, which exclude Africans but which have a very limited number of colored and Asian medical students who are given special permission to attend. In 1971 the one black medical school at the University of Natal had 247 Indians, 172 Africans, and 38 coloreds.[6] Blacks have difficulty entering medical school because of deficiencies of prior education, lack of economic resources to support themselves, and limited access to medical education.

The legal exclusion of Africans and most other nonwhites from white medical schools relegates them to an inferior social and medical status, and those who become doctors receive lower wages by law than comparably trained whites.[7] Moreover, nonwhite doctors may never be in a position to give orders to whites, thus greatly affecting training opportunities and possibilities of occupational mobility, and they may not use white dining facilities at hospitals nor participate in other social activities.

The high doctor-patient ratio among whites makes white medical practice in South Africa highly competitive, and the white population receives exceedingly responsive care. Doctors are highly accessible; they make home calls and night calls; and their services are relatively inexpensive by American standards. The basic organization of services is private and on a fee-for-service basis; ordinarily, hospitalization is provided in nursing homes (somewhat akin to proprietary hospitals in the United States). Superspecialist hospital services are available in government-financed hospitals. Institutions such as Groote Schuur in Cape Town have medical capabilities comparable to those found anywhere in the world.

The vast majority of the white population of South Africa is affluent, well fed, well doctored, and suffers from disease patterns comparable to other affluent Western nations. Studies of peripubertal growth among Pretoria children show that nutritional status among whites is comparable or superior to the nutritional status of children anywhere else in the world, although blacks are clearly disadvantaged.[8] The existence of transplant teams and superspecialist care stands in stark contrast to the situation in African areas where starvation and malnutrition are pervasive medical problems. Problems such as schistosomiasis, trachoma, and idiopathic endomycardial fibrosis, which are extremely common in the black population, receive relatively little medical attention.

The organization of health care services in African areas varies: the services available in urban areas differ from the rudimentary services in some reserves and the nonexistent or inaccessible services for large parts of the population. To understand the differences in organization, it is necessary to consider the differences between the townships and the reserves.

Reserves (frequently called *Bantustans* and Homelands) are the land areas in which members of various tribes in South Africa have pseudoindependence and some citizen rights. Thus, in most of the country they are treated as "guest workers" and have no political rights. The reserves are not economically viable and are inadequate for separate development. The African townships, such as Soweto and Alexandra in Johannesburg, are defined as "legally" inside of white areas, and Africans require a permit to be there.[9] Access to these areas is controlled, maintaining the fiction that the urbanized African's home residence is in one or another of the reserves. Africans living in the townships are denied citizenship and property rights, and the government at its pleasure evicts populations from areas in which they have lived when it serves the political, economic, or social needs of the white population.

White society in South Africa depends on African labor, and the Africans depend on work in urban areas for their subsistence. The social and economic situation for Africans is sufficiently severe in the reserves to encourage large numbers to remain in urban areas without permits, despite harassment and a high risk of arrest. Such "illegal residence" is frequently encouraged by whites who desire access to cheap African labor. The police subject Africans to continual harassment, and they are required to produce passbooks on the demand of a police officer. Arrests for pass violations have been approximately 600,000 per year in recent years, and more than two-fifths of offenders serving less than four months in prison are incarcerated for pass offenses.[10]

In one township I observed large numbers of malnourished and neglected children near a day-care center. Personnel at the center—in telling me of their work—indicated that they had sufficient places for all of the children who wished to come. When I inquired about the children playing outside, I was informed that since their parents did not have residence permits, the day center was prohibited by the government from accepting the children despite available places. These children were just some of the many victims of brutal attempts to enforce apartheid.

Conditions in the townships are generally harsh and contribute in major ways to disease and social pathology. African men, coming to the townships to work in Johannesburg and other urban areas, cannot bring their wives and children with them; this causes long separations and family disruptions. Wages for Africans are extremely low—often below subsistence levels—with the result that there is widespread poverty and malnutrition not only in the native reserves but also in the townships. The family separations are harmful to all concerned. The wives, children, and elderly who are left in the reserves find it difficult to cope with existing economic, social, and physical conditions. More and more men in the townships live in hostels and bachelors' compounds. These men, separated from their families and knowing little about proper diet, often suffer from inadequate nutrition; and the conditions of life in the township breed alcoholism, violence, and crime. Although the police are ubiquitous in South Africa, policing is almost nonexistent in black areas, many areas have no lighting, and gangs prey on the residents—frequently robbing them of their hard-earned weekly wages.

Many of the disease problems arise from economic inadequacies. In the summer of 1972 the first national survey of African wages, made by the Productivity and Wages Association, was released.[11] The survey results came from 1086 companies, mainly in manufacturing, financial, and commercial sectors (excluding mining), involving more than 188,000 employees. The return rate among the firms surveyed was only 13 percent, and it is likely that the firms responding paid somewhat higher wages than the ones that did not participate. Moreover, since the survey was based on the amount firms paid instead of the amount Africans earned, it excluded the large number of unemployed Africans and those who do a variety of casual work and household work at even more exploitative wages.

Despite the conservative nature of the survey, it was found that 80 percent of Africans in the private sector earn less than 70 *Rand* a month (approximately $93 at current exchange rates, which constitutes the poverty line). The Johannesburg Chamber of Commerce has estimated that a family of five in Soweto requires at least a minimum of R82.19 a month to live acceptably. In 1970 the Human Sciences Research Council estimated that the minimum effective income level necessary for a white family of five in Pretoria was R158.90 per month; and if one takes into account the changes in the cost of living, R170 would be a more reasonable figures.[12]

The problem of low wages is compounded by discriminatory wage scales for white, colored, and African workers doing the same job, by the exclusion of Africans and coloreds from many jobs reserved for white labor, and by indentured service characteristic of mining and other aspects of the economy. In mining, Africans are paid 50 to 60 cents for a shift of eight hours. This is approximately one-seventeenth of what white miners earn.[13] The wage gap between white and black workers varies from one industry to another, but white earnings may exceed African earnings from five to twenty times.

The average social pension for an African is about R5.00 a month (approximately $7). He is expected to pay about half of that for housing in the township. The Reverend David Russell, in attempting to reveal the plight of the African, has tried to survive on R5.00 a month. I quote in detail from his letter of July 28, 1972 to the *Rand Daily Mail*:

I wish to emphasize that these conditions of tearing hardship do not only involve the so called "unproductive units." The situation is just as frustrating and harsh for the few able-bodied men "lucky" enough to be working as casual labourers for R20.00 per month. For this they must work a 46-hour week, starting at 7.30 am and finishing at 5.12 pm, Monday to Friday, with only half hour for lunch, and no tea break at all. . . . For a casual labourer with a wife and only four children there is a mere R3.34c a month per person for living. These wages and working conditions are shocking. For such a family the income per person is even less than the absurdly inadequate pension of R5.00 given to the aged and infirm. What a callous mockery for an able-bodied family man to be obliged to struggle to make ends meet on the basis of R3.34 per month per person. . . . The R5.00 per month I have been living on for the last three months leaves me significantly "better off" than most Dimbaza inhabitants [an African Resettlement Township near King William's Town]. Nevertheless I am feeling the strain. It is like serving a prison sentence—I hold on grimly counting the days. My life revolves around my stomach! Human joy is shrivelling up; my capacity for giving out is shrinking. My friends notice the difference in me.[14]

The common health problems of Africans are those generally found in the impoverished and underdeveloped world. The Africans are in a chronic state of malnutrition, and this contributes to a variety of disease problems and consequences. Protein-calorie deficiency disease is extremely common, and there is a considerable amount of pellagra and other nutritional diseases. Stunted physical and mental growth, often affected by chronic malnutrition, is also extremely common. There is a very high prevalence of gastroenteritis and pneumonia, diseases that are major causes of death among infants. Tuberculosis is rampant and so are its complications. Severe burns, resulting from falling into open fires that are used to keep dwelling units warm, are a common problem among children in winter. Because of the poor penetration of immunization and preventive medicine among Africans—particularly in the rural areas—measles, diphtheria, dysentery, and many other preventable diseases are quite common.

I was told over and over again that malnutrition was a product of the ignorance of the African, of his unwillingness to follow a healthy diet, and of his need for health education. This concerned note became the great rationalization used to explain the human deterioration so evident at every clinic and hospital. It is probably correct that Africans with a limited income could eke out a technically balanced diet if they adhered to a standard of austerity and self-denial that few whites could conform to. It is true that the African can eat what David Russell and other outraged people are attempting to eat as a means of protest: a daily food ration of 306 grams of mealie meal (ground maize), 125 grams of mealies, 75 grams of beans, 30 grams of skim milk, 15 grams of margarine, and 7 grams of salt. But to argue that the failure to follow this diet is primarily a product of ignorance is to engage in the worst type of sophistry. On October 14, 1972 *The New York Times* reported that the Reverend David Russell was at the point of collapse and was planning to end his ordeal. He was quoted as saying, "Trying to live on 5 *Rand* a month has been long and dreary. . . . I feel a great tiredness deep within me. I just do not know how Africans manage."

Mrs. Jean Sinclair, president of the Black Sash, who also attempted this diet described it as a "grim and devastating experience." She reported that she was "tired all the time, cold, irritable and very depressed. I found it difficult to concentrate and settle down to any particular task." She wrote to the Minister of Bantu Administration that:

The resettlement areas are soul-destroying, unproductive and isolated areas, where employment is almost impossible to find. Not only do these Africans have to live on a miserable diet, but they have no money for clothing, household equipment, fuel or for other necessities of life. This is ekeing out an existence. It cannot be described as living. Yet this is what the Government is doing to hundreds of thousands of voteless, voiceless citizens for whom it is responsible.[15]

Indeed, as one travels around the townships and the native reserves, and observes the conditions imposed on the people, it is a matter of wonderment that they have persevered so well and that they have not yet fallen into the depths of despair. In the resettlement areas, referred to by Mrs. Sinclair, the conditions are horrendous.[16] It is no credit to the Republic of South Africa, but it attests to the fortitude and capacities of the Africans to deal with adversity.

It is extremely difficult to obtain adequate figures on the scope of malnutrition in South Africa. At one time, kwashiorkor was a notifiable disease, but now notification has been discontinued; thus, the Minister of Health has remarked to Parliament that there is no malnutrition in South Africa. But a survey in Pretoria suggested that half of the Urban African school children studied in the age group 7-11 are adapted to a suboptimal protein intake, although the basis of the estimate may not be fully valid.[17] Dr. Neser of the National Nutrition Research Institute has written, on the basis of her survey, that "at least 80 percent of school-going children from Bantu households in Pretoria suffer from malnutrition and under-nutrition." These estimates are conservatively based, since rural children are obviously more malnourished than children from urban areas, and children most malnourished are less likely to be in school.

Identified malnutrition is only a small proportion of the cases existing in the population. One estimate suggests eight or nine additional potential cases for every one recognized, and an assessment made at the University of Cape Town suggests that for every case of kwashiorkor seen by doctors at clinics, there are 40 undefined cases of malnutrition. Similarly, it is well known that the occurrence of tuberculosis is related to nutrition, and this may serve as a proxy for estimates of malnutrition. As in the United States, tuberculosis is relatively uncommon among the white population of South Africa. In some African areas, as much as one-fifth of the population may have tuberculosis.[18]

Care in Hospitals and Clinics

Soweto, the major African township in Johannesburg, is served by a large provincial hospital, Baragwanath, which occupies the physical facilities of a restored army barracks. It is a teaching institution of the University of Witwatersrand Medical School. The medical and nursing staff is well trained. It is concerned about the health status of the Africans and copes admirably with an unending flow of pathology within considerable budgetary constraints. Despite an enormous number of beds (approximately 2200), the needs are so great that only the very sickest patients are admitted, and they are released sooner than desirable. Particularly impressive is the pediatrics unit, which is especially dedicated and is doing extraordinary work despite the severe limitation of funds and space.

In the townships, medical responsibility is highly fragmented between curative hospital medicine, preventive and curative clinics, and the social services.

They are each under different authorities, making it extremely difficult to develop or coordinate a wholistic approach to the problems of the Africans in the townships. The hospital has no authority or funding for preventive work and must deal with an unending flow of pathology with few tools to alter the conditions producing pathology in the community. Physicians often find their efforts futile; patients return time and time again for the same difficulties that recur on return to noxious community conditions.

The curative clinics in the townships are crowded dispensaries providing limited and superficial care. Waiting periods to see a doctor are long—with patients queuing up early in the morning—and the number of patients processed by each doctor is extremely large. Dental and ophthamological services are virtually nonexistent. Even though I made special efforts to visit pediatric services, day care centers, and preventive clinics, I did not see a black child in the Republic of South Africa with eyeglasses.

The preventive clinics are worthy institutions, but they have inadequate financing and manpower to cope with the existing difficulties in the community. They provide immunizations, prenatal and postnatal care, health education, and birth control services. Staffed by nurse-midwives and health visitors, they make considerable effort to improve prevention, but the inadequacy of financing and staffing makes community penetration difficult. The government subsidizes the availability of skimmed milk powder, which can be obtained at the preventive clinics for young underweight children. More subsidy is approved than is utilized, indicating a clear inability to reach much of the population in need.

Birth control programs are probably more enthusiastically implemented by the authorities than any other program, and wherever I went, this facet of prevention was emphasized. This is not surprising, since the white community fears the growing black population and would like to limit its fertility. Although many black women are amenable to birth control, the existing conditions make others in the black community skeptical. The main strength of the blacks in South Africa, they maintain, is in their numbers, and they are reluctant to support efforts to control their population. Similarly, women are frequently skeptical about limiting their fertility when so many of their youngsters die. Children not only are culturally valued but also provide some security in old age, since social services are almost nonexistent. It is my impression that birth control, without associated efforts to limit infant mortality in the black community and to improve the social situation of the blacks, will be a futile effort. The authorities have not yet been willing to confront these issues.

In the reserves, medical care is within the jurisdiction of the Department of Bantu Administration, and it is possible to develop an integrated approach to preventive and curative medicine. I was taken to part of the Tswana homeland near Hammanskraal—by the Secretary of Health and three of his major assistants heading up various aspects of the health department in Pretoria—to see the evolving plan for heath services in the homelands which, in their view, was well developed in this specific area. I was told that the population of that particular area was approximately a quarter of a million and that it was fairly widely dispersed with limited access to transportation. All of the hospital services for the population are provided by the mission hospital, having a staff of five physicians.

The rural African population has depended heavily on the various mission hospitals for the limited medical services available to them.[19] These hospitals are frequently staffed by mission doctors from abroad and vary in their orientations—some mixing religion with medicine as a condition of service, others with a much more secular attitude. The mission hospitals that I visited were staffed by physicians with dedication and concern. Some hospitals limit the patients they serve in terms of available space and resource; others never turn away a patient in need, keeping beds in every available place—indoors and on outdoor porches. These hospitals obviously have made (and continue to make) an important contribution and, without them, the health status of the African would be even more dismal.

Mission hospitals sometimes hospitalize young infants with their sick mothers, since the infants' survival is often precarious when the mother goes to the hospital. A common practice in both urban and mission hospitals is to have mothers stay in the hospital with their dehydrated infants, assuming part of their care and having some exposure to health education concerning nutrition and child care. This was one of the few practices I saw in South Africa that we should follow.

The most impressive mission hospital that I visited was the Charles Johnson Memorial Hospital in Nqutu, KwaZulu. It has about 338 beds with an average daily case load of approximately 650 people. It administers clinics in outlying areas, has its own school for training African nurses, and deals impressively with an unending flow of pathology and disease. The hospital personnel, understanding the basic plight of the region they serve, do what they can to assist in preventive and community matters, but the task is immense and resources extremely limited. Although the hospital has made important contributions to the region, it is clear that no hospital or clinic has the means to intervene effectively in the conditions causing disease.

Not far from the Johnson Memorial Hospital there is a settlement of about 500 people, uprooted from white farms and forced to resettle elsewhere. Officially their presence in the area is illegal and, sooner or later, they will be moved on again. Food is difficult to scrape together and water is scarce. The people dig holes in the dry earth, hoping that they will collect some underground water and, since their presence in the area is "temporary" (they have been there two years already), the authorities will take no measures to provide a decent and safe water source. *The Guardian* of September 23, 1972 reported that when the director of the hospital discussed the issue with the authorities and tried to do something to improve the situation, he was told to mind his own business and that he was interfering with the Bantu. It may be a coincidence that at the same time an official telephoned the hospital questioning the permit of its welfare officer to enter the reserve.

The mission hospitals now receive financial support from the government, although they are underfinanced to meet the needs of the regions they serve. The existing plan is to provide primary medical care and preventive services from satellite clinics dispersed throughout the region, but it has not yet been made operational in most areas. In the Hammanskraal area, where the plan was said to be in practice, I visited satellite clinics staffed by nurse-midwives who provide other than hospital services, and the clinics are visited occasionally by physicians from the hospital. I was told that there was approximately one session every two weeks. These clinics give considerable attention to family planning and immunizations, prenatal care and midwifery, and they are the primary site for milk-powder distribution. There are no dental or ophthamological services at these clinics, and the basic medical care is rudimentary. Staffing is far too inadequate to reach many people in need in the population. Although these clinics provide sites of care that are of value, the character, scope, and quality of service would be totally unacceptable to the white population of South Africa.

To get an idea of the extent of inequality of medical care, I visited white, colored, and African pediatric units in the same evening—all funded by the same governmental authority. In the African hospital, the wards were extremely crowded with very limited staffing. In one of the infant units I saw two nurses attempting to feed, change, and generally cope with 37 very sick children. I then went to the comparable white hospital where two nurses were caring for five white children who were less ill. The comparable unit for coloreds in the same hospital was somewhere between these two extremes. Generally, the physical facilities and amenities followed the same pattern.

I also visited the major hospital serving the colored community in Johannesburg—Coronation Hospital—and the various areas in which these persons live. Although conditions are not quite as harsh as in the African community, they are generally comparable. Housing is inadequate and frequently unavailable, community conditions are poor, and malnutrition and preventable diseases are common. Medical services cannot cope with the magnitude of disease and pathology created by community conditions. From many of the colored areas, transportation is especially difficult to Coronation Hospital, and medical services in the community are rudimentary. As "separate development" proceeds, persons and communities are evicted from their homes and involuntarily relocated, producing profound social and family problems.

Few medical facilities are available in the African and colored communities after dark. If problems should develop, it is frequently difficult to get to the hospitals serving these areas. In both Johannesburg and Capetown, there are projects carried out by medical and law students, which provide some health and legal services to a colored community. These projects are carried out by volunteers and deserve to be commended, but the type of patchwork service provided by a number of volunteers—each contributing a little time—does not provide first-rate care, nor is it an ideal educational experience. The clinics tend to be erratic, depending on the academic schedule, and supervision is spotty. The medical schools involved have a responsibility to make such community services part of the overall approach to medical education and to provide the resources and supervision that guarantee a more adequate service. The practice of community medical care should be as much a part of medical education as work in the teaching hospital, and it should be more than a volunteer effort among the students who feel a sense of social responsibility. It must be clear, however, that the medical schools also are a reflection of South African society and are largely meeting the needs of its white elite. The basic problem is much deeper than the social responsibilities of medical education, since the health of the African population is determined primarily by social and political policies, and these policies affect the performance of medical education and all other human services.

Appearances and Realities: An Experience in Cultural Contrasts

It is well known that the assumptions and conditions under which people live have a pervasive effect on their perceptions and behavior, regardless of their particular ideologies. Social structures have the capacity to accent the best or worst in people and, under some conditions, even well-meaning and idealistic persons take for granted behavior that they would not condone if they lived in a different social context. In this regard, I often had the impression that people thought they were showing me one thing, but that I was seeing quite another.

My visit to a model prison was the most dramatic of my experiences. Prisons are not particularly well regarded in South Africa, and some of them have notorious reputations. The daily prison population is 417 per 100,000 in contrast to a comparable rate of 72.5 in Great Britain.[20] When I first asked to see a prison, someone responded that it is quite easy to get into one but difficult to visit one. However, a visit was arranged at the Leeuwkop Prison, a farm complex housing about 5500 African prisoners outside of Johannesburg. Many guests from around the world come to Leeuwkop and, in comparing notes with a colleague—a well-known criminologist who visited South Africa

—it was apparent that we had pretty much the same tour. I am not an authority on prisons, but I have seen some and, as prisons go, this one, although crowded, was not too bad. Indeed, the only time I ever heard the United Nations mentioned in South Africa was when I first appeared at the prison and was promptly informed that the institution adhered to United Nations' standards. This struck me as being incongruous, since the South African government is not exactly a booster of the international body. It was not the only thing I found incongruous at Leeuwkop.

I was shown everything I asked to see in the prison by a personable officer who was conversant with modern rehabilitation concepts. Although I was told various things that were inconsistent with the facts as I understood them—for example, that the pass laws were only intended to control foreign labor*—the gentleman was sincere. Indeed, he informed me that he had studied sociology, and on the first page of the official brochure of the prison there was a quotation from Edwin Sutherland (an important figure in the history of Chicago sociology). One of the units that I asked to see was ultramaximum security, and I was particularly interested in seeing its hospital. It was clear that each unit was informed of my impending visit, because, when we appeared, no beds were occupied; the patients who were inside were standing against the far wall awaiting "the visitor," I assume. I was taken past the patients in isolation who were suspected of some infectious disease; they stood in line at attention, holding their medical records in front of them for my scrutiny. Perhaps the most incongruous of all was leaving ultramaximum security and being awaited at the gate by a chorus of black prisoners who, we were told, wished to sing for us. Even the selection was propitious:"Ain't going to study war no more." Unfortunately, I saw little in South Africa for Africans to sing about!

At one point I visited a landscaped park in Soweto, which is a stopping point for the visitors' bus tour. Sitting on a hill overlooking the township, there is an elegant tearoom pleasantly surrounded by flowers and plants. Since I had noticed no parks, playgrounds, or green areas in Soweto, I asked whether Soweto residents used the park. My escort, somewhat embarrassed by the inquiry, indicated that it was off limits; as an afterthought she indicated that the purpose was to protect against vandalism.

I had similar experiences in my visits to various hospitals. Even among persons of conscience and commitment, a certain callousness and disregard of human factors were frequently evident. This was apparent in many little ways. Some doctors who were obviously persons of integrity and compassion would lecture me loudly on the ignorance and superstitiousness of the African as we went from bed to bed. Few thought it necessary to explain to patients,

---

* As a South African historian later pointed out to me, the officer was technically correct. Under South African law, all blacks are foreign, since their technical home is the designated reserves.

whose treatment was being disrupted by my visit, who I was or why they were being disturbed. When I embarrassedly requested that a patient be asked to give me permission to take his picture, I was assured over and over that I could take pictures of anybody or anything and that I did not need permission. Perhaps this was just courtesy to a foreign visitor.

A disregard for human dignity is found in hospitals, the world over; it is not unique to South Africa. But in South Africa it would take saintly qualities to be anything but paternalistic and hardened under the social and political conditions that prevail. One falls in with the culture and the persons with whom one must cooperate in assumptions and behavior. Even in my short stay I could observe the process occurring in myself; by the time I left I was beginning, unconsciously, to accept conditions that I found shocking when I first saw them. Human survival depends on steady concessions to the social and cultural milieu. Thus I have gained the greatest respect for the South Africans in all walks of life who speak out loudly against the brutalities and indignities of their social structure. And if they sound paternalistic from time to time, it is not too difficult to understand why. Already Africans are rejecting their more paternalistic white advocates and, indeed, the time may be coming when they reject all whites. This reaction is also clearly understandable, although discouraging; it is a product of the limited options available.

These economic, social, and medical inequalities are already known to informed physicians, government officials, and the involved public in South Africa. But existing conditions make it difficult for many concerned persons to speak out without personal risk. Yet, throughout my visit I was impressed by the concern of many South Africans who were struggling to do what little they could within the constraints imposed on them. There were many concerned physicians in the hospitals; but curative medicine, no matter how important, is somewhat of a smoke screen if it is not complemented by better preventive efforts and improved conditions in the community. Moreover, it is obvious that progress and decency in South Africa must involve more than good will and concern of individuals; it must be embedded in the social structure and social conditions that are the primary determinants of health and illness in society. Social policies that divide men, disrupt communities, separate family members against their wishes, and breed distrust and hate cannot be conducive to a healthy society.

Some South Africans maintain that theirs is a poor country, and that it is inappropriate to impose the kind of standard I have imposed in my observations. They point to poverty elsewhere in Africa and to the fact that there are other starving Africans. I would be less likely to regard this as a grand rationalization if the country were not so rich in natural resources, if the white population did not dominate so much of the country's resources, and if it did not live in ostentatious affluence in the midst of such great poverty. South Africa has had an enormous rate of economic growth, but it has not shared its growing affluence with its black population. The only relevant comparison is an internal one that takes into account the economic resources and capacities of the country and compares the differences in how the white and black populations live and the impact of social policies on maintaining or closing these differences.

Similarly, I would be more impressed with concerns about the ignorance of the African if education among Africans were encouraged, if they were not legally excluded from white schools and universities, and if they did not have to pay from their meager wages for education that is freely available to whites. The fact is that many of the Africans in the Republic of South Africa are highly urbanized, and their disabilities arise not from ignorance or ineptitude but from systematic exclusion from social and economic opportunities enforced by apartheid policies. South Africa persists in plundering its greatest resource: the capacities, labor, and potentialities of its people.

Notes

1. See L. Marquard (1969). *The Peoples and Policies of South Africa*. London: Oxford University Press (fourth edition); also see H. Adams (1971). *Modernizing Racial Domination: The Dynamics of South African Politics*. Berkeley: University of California Press; and B. Higgs "The Group Areas Act and Its Effects." United Nations Unit of Apartheid, Department of Political and Security Council Affairs.

2. South African Institute of Race Relations (1972). *A Survey of Race Relations in South Africa, 1971*. Johannesburg, January 1972.

3. *The Star*, Johannesburg, May 10, 1969.

4. Also see R. Hoffenberg (1970). "Inequality in Health Care in South Africa." United Nations Unit on Apartheid, Department of Political and Security Council Affairs, December 1970.

5. Minister of Health, Assembly Hansard 15, Col. 7263, May 26, 1972.

6. South African Institute of Race Relations (1972). op. cit., p. 308.

7. *Ibid.*

8. Tobias, P. V. (1970). "Puberty, Growth, Malnutrition and the Weaker Sex—And Two New Measures of Environmental Betterment." *The Leech*, 40:101–107; and "Growth and Stature in Southern African Populations." In D. Vorster (ed.), *Proceedings of the International Biological Programme: Human Adaptability Section*. Blantyre, Malawi, April 1971, pp. 96–104.

9. Hellmann, E. (1971). *Soweto:Johannesburg's African City*. South African Institute for Race Relations.

10. South African Institute of Race Relations (1972). op. cit., p. 142; also see A. S. Mathews (1972). *Law, Order and Liberty in South Africa*. Berkeley: University of California Press.

11. South African Institute of Race Relations (1973). *A Survey of Race Relations in South Africa, 1972*. Johannesburg, January 1973, p. 235.

12. South African Institute of Race Relations (1972), op. cit., p. 176.

13. *Ibid.*, p. 229; also see F. Wilson (1972). *Labor in the South African Goldmines, 1911–1969*. London: Cambridge University Press.

14. *Rand Daily Mail,* Johannesburg, July 28, 1972.

15. Hyman, J.)1972). "Living on 16 Cents a Day." *Rand Daily Mail,* Johannesburg, July 28, 1972.

16. For a description of a personal survey of such areas, see C. Desmond (1972). *The Discarded People.* Baltimore: Penguin.

17. Reid, J. V. O. (1971). *Malnutrition.* South African Institute of Race Relations, p. 13.

18. *Ibid.*

19. To grasp the conditions of medical practice among the Africans in rural areas, a vivid description is provided by A. Barker (1959). *The Man Next to Me: An Adventure in African Medical Practice.* New York: Harper; see also S. L. Kark and G. W. Steuart (1962). *A Practice of Social Medicine.* Edinburgh: E. and S. Livingstone.

20. *The Star,* Johannesburg, March 25, 1972.

CHAPTER III

Ideology, Medical Technology, and Health-Care Organization in Modern Nations*

Despite varying political and ideological orientations, there is a growing convergence in medical-care organization in modern nations. This convergence is the result of the growth and elaboration of medical technology and the rising aspirations and expectations of populations for accessible, comprehensive, and effective medical care. Wherever I go—in the United States, in Canada, in Scandinavia, in England—medical-care institutions are faced with comparable dilemmas and are moving toward similar solutions. Moreover, the literature from countries such as the Soviet Union and China and the literature on the developing nations suggests that they are not exceptions to this rule. All medical-care systems, like other social institutions, develop within their own historical circumstances and forms of professional organization, and thus the hypothesis of convergence does not imply that they develop identical patterns of organization. The hypothesis does argue, however, that they all strive to deal with certain common problems and that, in coping with these in the most effective way, the problems become more similar.

In recent decades the growth of medical technology and advances in the medical sciences have caused a growing emphasis on medical specialization and subspecialization and on curative work in hospitals. With the vast increases in basic medical knowledge and growing dependence on hospital facilities, diagnostic and laboratory aids, and a vast array of paraprofessional health workers, physicians are trained to require these supports and find it difficult to practice without them. Moreover, with the proliferation of knowledge and technology, emerging physicians have become more and more discouraged about mastering the whole of medicine. Despite their intentions to

* Adapted from a paper published in the *American Journal of Public Health*, January, 1974.

practice as generalists on entering medical school, most of them have decided on a specialty by graduation time. To some extent, this emphasis has been encouraged by medical educators, who are themselves specialists and superspecialists and who strive to interest students in their particular field. In the United States this trend has been particularly marked, and the growing emphasis on specialist services relative to generalist care is incongruent with the population's needs and expectations. Although reasonable practices suggest that perhaps one-fifth of all physicians should be in the consulting specialties, approximately four-fifths of American physicians practice as specialists.[1] Most numerous of all practitioners are the ones in the surgical specialties, and many observers believe that these practitioners are responsible for the fact that the rate of surgical operations in the United States is double the per-capita rate in England and Wales.[2] To some extent, each type of physician that we train approaches problems from his own perspective. Thus a primary practitioner, a medical specialist, or a surgical specialist may view the same case from different vantage points.

Although this trend toward specialization is most exaggerated in the United States, it is also evident in medical systems such as the National Health Service in England and Wales, where concerted attempts have been made as a matter of government policy to retain a balance between generalists and specialists. And despite government decisions it has been a difficult process. It has been hard to get physicians who were trained in hospital-based medical schools to accept roles as general practitioners, and the number of general practitioners has lagged while the rates of utilization and the size of the population have increased.[3] From 1964 to 1966, for example, the actual number of doctors in general practice decreased by 505. During 1966 there were 183 fewer doctors than in the previous year, although the population increased by 300,000. In 1965 and 1966 the increasing work load and other factors contributed to a threat by 18,000 general practitioners to withdraw from the National Health Service. An agreement was reached that prevented a more destructive clash, but there are even less general practitioners now, relative to the population, than there were during the crisis of 1965 and 1966.[4] Therefore, despite concerted efforts on the part of government to maintain a balance, it has been an uphill battle against the forces of technology and specialization. In Sweden, where medicine is heavily based in hospitals, there has been a persistent shortage of general practitioners, and the government has vastly increased the number of doctors to try to remedy the situation.[5] Even in countries such as the Soviet Union and China, where there is greater control over the allocation of manpower and resources, it has been necessary to utilize a variety of paraprofessional workers to provide basic services to the population.

Physicians who become dependent on hospital facilities, colleagues in related specialties, and a variety of health workers, and who are trained to practice a curative, hospital-based medicine, are becoming more and more unwilling to distribute themselves in rural areas or locations without supporting facilities. Every modern nation with a developed medical technology has difficult problems in distributing medical personnel in rural areas or in areas that offer less personal middle-class amenities. One generally finds a maldistribution of physicians who cluster in and around the major urban and suburban areas. In the United States, where we have approximately 132 physicians per 100,000 persons delivering patient care, we find 320 nonfederal physicians per 100,000 persons in Washington, D.C., 203 in New York State, 69 in Mississippi, and 75 in Alabama. Within each state we find large variations from urban to rural areas, and many counties have no doctors at all. In England and Wales, where the government makes a direct attempt to redistribute doctors and where the country is relatively small and highly urbanized, there is still a maldistribution of doctors with a concentration in London and Southern England and shortages in the Midlands and Northern England. This is reflected in the size of the average list of general practitioners, which may vary from 1800 or 1900 patients for each doctor in some areas to more than 3000 in other areas.[6] Even such countries as the Soviet Union, which has 240 physicians per 100,000 inhabitants (double the rate of England and Wales), have had difficulty in serving rural areas and have used paraprofessionals to meet rural needs.[7] China, in initiating great changes in medical organization, has developed ancillaries called "barefoot doctors" who provide first-line care in smaller agricultural communities.[8]

The growth and complexity of knowledge and technology have brought into question the individual entrepreneurial tradition in medical care, and all systems of care are moving toward greater organization of health-care efforts. Specialization, in the absence of aggregation of personnel and integration of services, has resulted in a growing fragmentation of care and in poor medical care from a community viewpoint. Functions such as preventive care, follow-up care, health education, and wise management of patients' difficulties within the context of family and community conditions have been difficult to maintain in systems of fragmented services where no person or agency has responsibility for the whole individual. In the United States, Britain, and Sweden, for instance, greater attention is being given to the aggregation of fragmented services by developing such new specialties as family medicine, by encouraging the growth of health centers and polyclinics, and by attempts to better integrate preventive, curative, and rehabilitative medicine.

Finally, the character of developing medical technology has confronted all modern medical systems with profound human dilemmas. These dilemmas have vastly increased the financial burden of medical care and have raised difficult legal and ethical issues. With modern medical technology it has become possible to maintain the life of hopeless patients for months, while patients who could benefit have difficulty in obtaining adequate care. The development of transplantation and other life sustaining measures has raised expectations and resulted in enormous financial costs. In the United States it is estimated that maintaining a patient on renal dialysis in a hospital unit varies from $15,000 to $30,000 a year, and many of the heroic efforts that sustain life among older people for short periods of time consume enormous financial resources. This does not mean that these problems are easy, that they are amenable to simple answers, or that expensive ventures in care (as in the transplantation of kidneys) are not a worthy endeavor. But in America and elsewhere there is a growing appreciation that medical resources are not un-limited, and that the consummation of resources in one situation may limit resources in other situations of greater need. If money is alternatively invested in improving the nutrition of the poor or in reducing infant mortality by better prenatal and postnatal care, an investment comparable to that made to keep the hopeless alive would reap enormous social and personal benefits. The technical problem of establishing decision rules for defining hopeless patients has many difficulties, and raises profound ethical issues. However, we must still establish priorities and, I believe, medical services must be distributed in terms of some concept of need—not in terms of the ability to economically command them.

Physicians working in the field of curative medicine learn to adopt what economist Victor Fuchs[9] calls the "technologic imperative." If the technology is available, it must be used to guarantee to the individual patient all of the possibilities that medicine can command. But as Fuchs points out, there are serious consequences in this orientation. The guarantee of all that is possible to some parts of the population insures that other parts of the population will receive less than a minimal standard. More and more, all nations must face the issue of planning the distribution of health services in some reasonable relationship to needs and overall benefits because, if they do not, they will exacerbate social divisions and bitterness among men.

These trends in medical knowledge and technology (as well as other changes) have caused common problems to medical-care planners throughout the world. We have found that, with increased education and affluence, people desire more—not less—services and, as they become better educated, they demand services of greater sophistication and responsiveness. As the overall burden of medical care costs has risen—and medical care costs are rising every-where in the world—government is assuming a larger part of the financial cost, and health care costs are consuming a larger proportion of the gross national product. In the United States, where we have the largest per-capita health expenditures in the world, we presently spend $83 billion a year on the health sector, and health consumes 7.6 per cent of our gross national product. It is estimated that in the near future we will be spending more than $100 billion on health, and that the proportion of the gross national product will continue to increase. Similar trends are evident in Sweden, Canada, the Soviet Union, and even in England, despite the fact that the central government has made serious efforts to contain expenditures for health care.

In the United States, with the enactment of medical care programs for the aged and for the medically indigent, the proportion of total health expenditures paid by the government has increased since 1967 from 22 per cent to almost 40 per cent. No serious observer doubts that the government will assume responsibility for a larger proportion of the total health costs in the foreseeable future, and competing programs of national health insurance are now under active discussion.

The United States has been slow to assume this responsibility, although in other developed nations, government has assumed the major obligation for health care. For all practical purposes, all expenditures in the Soviet Union for health are paid by the government, and approximately 85 per cent of all expenditures are assumed by government in Britain and Sweden. Although countries may differ in the degree of government financing, there are growing demands for all governments to underwrite the costs of medical care as a social and political right.

There are five major points of convergence: (1) greater emphasis in all countries on insuring a minimal level of services to all and in decreasing inequalities in the availability of health care; (2) greater emphasis on linking the organization and distribution of services to defined populations; (3) developing new forms of delivering primary medical care; (4) attempting to integrate the fragmented parts of health services; and (5) improving the efficiency and effective operation of the health services system. These points are discussed below.

An Increasing Tendency to Diminish Inequalities in Health Care

As populations have become more sophisticated about health care, they have demanded greater equity in the provision of services—between rich and poor, black and white, old and young, city, suburb and town. In the United States this has resulted, partly, in making health a political issue, in initiating a program of health centers for poverty areas, in the development of Medicare and Medicaid, and in our movement toward some system of national health insurance. The basic principle of equity in the provision of health care has been accepted and implemented in Canada, Britain, Scandinavia, the Soviet Union, China, and in most other parts of the developed world. It is becoming rare to hear the argument that health is a privilege to be purchased like other consumer goods rather than a right for all people in civilized societies.

A Tendency to Link the Provision of Health-Care Services to the Needs of Defined Communities for which Providers of Health Care are Held Responsible

There has been an increasing emphasis on health planning and regional organization of services in most modern nations. It has become apparent that when services are provided by multiple units without responsibility to a particular defined population, it is impossible to assess the problems that must be dealt with. It is also impossible to develop an organized and effective means to deal with the problems and to monitor the performance of health providers. If the provision of services is not linked to defined populations, accountability is difficult to achieve. In this area the United States has been slow to develop. But there is a growing appreciation that such organization is necessary, and various bills before the Congress are attempting to develop systems that hold particular providers responsible for comprehensive services to defined populations. Senator Edward M. Kennedy's Health Security Program, constructed on a regional system, and the Nixon administration's flirtation with "Health Maintenance Organizations" are attempts—even though inadequate—to encourage the responsibility of providers for the overall welfare of patients.

Integrating the Fragmented Components of the Health Services

The proposals in the United States encompass this concern and encourage providers, through incentives, to take total responsibility for the preventive, curative, and rehabilitative needs of patients. In England and Wales the traditional separation of the services offered by general practitioners, hospitals, and the local authorities is an issue of grave concern. Proposals to achieve a better integration of these services are receiving discussion and consideration.[10]

Certainly, these are not easy problems to overcome. The patterns are well entrenched, there are strong special interests in preserving existing practices, and no group likes to give up its power or autonomy. But the effort is serious, and ferment is evident. It is reasonable to anticipate that there will be some improvement in the existing situation, if for no other reason than that attention is being drawn to it.

A Common Desire of All Countries to Deal with the Growing Difficulty of Maintaining Primary Medical Services

Throughout the world the viability of the role of the general practitioner is being questioned, and fewer physicians are willing to undertake this function. In attempts to reestablish the role, American medical schools are developing specialty programs in family medicine. In Britain the Royal Commission on Medical Education has suggested that general practice be elevated to a specialty with training periods comparable to other specialties.[11] These attempts and suggestions are not particularly realistic, and the answer to this problem probably will require other types of solutions.

Throughout the world there is a growing emphasis on the establishment of health centers that will aggregate physicians so that they can provide patient care in a comprehensive way, utilizing the gains in medical technology and diagnostic aids and a variety of affiliated health workers. The aggregation of physicians and facilities makes possible an economy of scale not only in the use of the laboratory and special services but also in the use of outreach workers, home visitors, social workers, nutritionists, pharmacists, and the like. In Britain, health centers were recommended as early as 1920 by the Dawson Committee, and they were to be the key feature of the health service established in 1948. For a variety of reasons this idea was not implemented until recently.[12] But health centers were supported by the Royal Commission on Medical Education and are now receiving more encouragement from the government.

Similarly, health centers have been established in the United States, Scandinavia, Canada, and many other countries. Although physicians resist group organization, there is a growing trend toward group practice and the training of a variety of personnel that facilitates a more comprehensive service. In the United States we are experimenting with physician assistants, nurse practitioners, outreach workers, and health educators. In poverty areas we have been using persons hired from the area to undertake outreach work within the community as part of the overall health service. The National Institute of Mental Health has even subsidized the training of Navajo medicine men for dealing with emotional disturbances, since the people believe in medicine men and they appear to have success in dealing with some life problems. We are learning to utilize the ideas people believe in to encourage their participation in the health system, instead of rejecting their ideas as being ignorant and irrelevant. We must remember that medical care is basically a human endeavor and that what people think and feel is important. The fact that particular beliefs and practices may not contribute toward improved health as measured by usual indices is not crucial, since consequences flow from what men define as reality and not from reality itself. The acceptance of another person's beliefs as being as important as our own provides a context for acceptance and influence. It increases the potentiality of truly making a difference.

Modern Medical Systems, Faced with the Escalation of Medical-Care Costs, Are Seeking to Improve the Efficiency and Effectiveness of the Health-Care System

In examining the practices from one geographic area to another, it becomes clear that many medical-care practices are arbitrary and unrelated to a rational basis. Such matters as the number of beds provided, the number of patients admitted to hospitals, their average length of stay, and the prevalence of certain surgical procedures vary enormously from one area to another in a fashion unrelated to the population's needs or the prevalence of morbidity. There is a growing emphasis on health services research for establishing more rational criteria for medical-care practices.

In short, the economics of medical care and its technical development are beginning to require responsible medical-care agencies, in all countries, to reassess their practices and priorities. This will not take place overnight, but the emerging pattern is discernible. In the following chapters, some of these issues that bear on government policy and practice organization will be explored.

Notes

1. Stevens, R. (1971). *American Medicine and the Public Interest.* New Haven: Yale University Press.

2. Bunker, J.P. (1970). "Surgical Manpower: A Comparison of Operations and Surgeons in the United States and England and Wales," *New England Journal of Medicine,* **282**: 135–144.

3. Great Britain Ministry of Health (1964–1966). *Annual Report,* Cmnd. 2688, 1964, Cmnd. 3039, 1965, Cmnd. 3326, 1966. London: Her Majesty's Stationery Office.

4. Mechanic, D. (1972). "Rhetoric and Reality in Health Services Research." *Health Services Research,* 7:61–65.

5. Anderson, O. (1972). *Health Care: Can There Be Equity: The United States, Sweden, and England.* New York: Wiley-Interscience.

6. Department of Health and Social Security (1972). *Annual Report--1971.* London: Her Majesty's Stationery Office.

7. Field, M. (1967). *Soviet Socialized Medicine.* New York: Free Press.

8. Sidel, V. (1972). "The Barefoot Doctors of the People's Republic of China," *New England Journal of Medicine,* **286**:1292–1300.

9. Fuchs, V. (1968). "The Growing Demand for Medical Care." *New England Journal of Medicine,* **279**:190–195.

10. Great Britain (1972). *National Health Service Reorganization: England,* Cmnd. 5055. London: Her Majesty's Stationery Office.

11. Great Britain (1968). *Royal Commission on Medical Education, 1965–68, Report,* Cmnd. 3569. London: Her Majesty's Stationery Office.

12. Mechanic, D. (1968). "General Medical Practice in England and Wales: Its Organization and Future." *New England Journal of Medicine,* **279**:680–689.

PART TWO

POLITICS, PUBLIC POLICY, AND THE DELIVERY OF HEALTH CARE

CHAPTER IV

Politics, Social Science, and Health Policy in the United States*

It is one thing to enunciate lofty goals and quite another to implement them. A growing national consensus is emerging in support of the idea that every American should have accessible to him necessary medical care of high quality and at reasonable cost. This consensus can be maintained as long as the discussion proceeds at a high level of generality, but it becomes more tenuous as we deal with such issues as defining needs, developing appropriate organizational means to meet them, and agreeing on acceptable and effective financing mechanisms.

The fact is that the distribution of health care services—like most other products or services in our society—is dependent on the economic and social abilities to command them;[1] and general goals, when translated to more specific policies, make conflicting interests more apparent. An increase in the accessibility, the quantity, and the efficiency of services is unlikely to enhance the quality of individual patient care without an increase in its basic component resources. The most effective health system for the nation as a whole does not necessarily insure optimal care for each individual patient, or optimum satisfaction for health professionals, and it is at the point that competing interests become evident that greatest acrimony is likely to develop.

The problem of accessibility is particularly acute, and the average person feels strongly about it. Perhaps the most frequent complaint concerning health services is that a doctor or source of care is not readily available when needed. This is reflected in the growing demand for ordinary ambulatory services from hospital emergency departments. Increasing accessibility requires more than

* Paper presented at Boston University, Conference on America's Health System in the 1970's, May 1972.

47

expanding the volume of services, since the capability of physicians and other facilities to generate demand for their services precludes the need to redistribute themselves in order to earn adequate income,[2] except perhaps under circumstances of a large surplus.

The problem of accessibility is related to three aspects of the organization of physician services: the total number of physicians and their social and geographic distribution; the degree of specialization and distribution of functions among physicians; and the nonphysician manpower pool and the allocation of functions between such manpower and physicians. Each of these areas has been widely recognized and publicized in recent years under the general headings of the physician shortage, the absence of sufficient primary care physicians, and the need for new health manpower (particularly physician assistants). Although a great deal has been said about each of these issues, much of it has been misleading and contradictory.

Even though increasing the number of physicians does not make likely adequate distribution, it does not follow that it is unnecessary to do so. Assume that the present availability of physicians theoretically might be adequate under more optimal conditions of distribution, efficiency, and use of new manpower. Nevertheless, we must seriously weigh the likelihood of achieving optimal situations where the health care system is highly pluralistic and complex, where government (for the most part) does not own and operate facilities but only exercises control indirectly through incentives and modest regulation, where the providers are not held accountable for meeting the needs of specifically defined populations, and where policies tend to be the product of mediating involved interest groups. Since physician services constitute a relatively scarce commodity, the use of whatever incentives we are willing to impose to achieve redistribution will be more likely to be effective in a situation of greater abundance. As the potentiality to deliver more service grows, the extension of services to needy groups is less likely to be felt as a deprivation by persons who are presently satisfied. Obviously, it is much more difficult to redistribute what people have come to take for granted than it is to differentially increase new forms of availability.

The most difficult problem in increasing accessibility to basic health-care services is the existing irrationality in the distribution of medical functions. Although a relatively small proportion of physicians would be required to satisfy the needs for consulting specialties—perhaps 15 or 20 per cent of all physicians—specialists have proliferated by establishing monopolies of work relative to different age groups, parts of the body, and routinized technical functions. As Rosemary Stevens effectively points out in her history of the development of medical specialization in the United States,[3] its character has been molded more by professional and economic interests than by a rational approach to postgraduate medical education or the delivery of health-care services.

More recently the mythology has developed that the internist and pediatrician—and even to some extent the obstetrician—function as a reasonable substitute for the general practitioner of the past; but in a recent national survey, examining the scope and character of their work, I found their efforts much more restricted than the replacement notion implies.[4] The overelaboration of specialties, beyond the need for consultation or special skills, has resulted in a fragmented pattern of care and one not particularly responsive to the human problems motivating much patient concern.[5]

The imbalance in the division of medical functions has important consequences for the work performed, since physicians to some extent tend to generate work consistent with their interests and orientations. The more surgeons we have, the more surgery will be performed,[6] for example, and the absence of primary-care physicians results in neglecting many important problems. Certainly a rational system of health care should attempt to allocate manpower in some meaningful relationship to the prevalence of varying problems and needs in the population.

In light of the many points at which decisions are made pertinent to such matters as accessibility, there is little likelihood of a monolithic solution to this problem, nor is one necessarily desirable. The pattern of clearly stratifying the medical profession by organizationally requiring approximately half of the available physicians to provide general medical services, such as in the British system, is one alien to our history and one that carries costs of some magnitude.[7] The attempt to redevelop a commitment to family medicine by defining this too as a specialty has advantages, but to some extent the perspective of family medicine is one looking backwards; and there is little evidence that it can combat existing trends.

The attempt to reestablish a practitioner who has a wide scope of practice makes clear the basic tension between specialization, on the one hand, and the need for generalists, on the other. To many internists and other specialists, the family practitioner appears to have a wide scope of practice and interest but less detailed knowledge and sophistication than the appropriately trained specialist; and thus he is seen to practice a lower level of medicine than is possible. Since family medicine, as it is taught and practiced both in the United States and abroad, is based on the same fundamental assumptions and perspectives as other types of practice, it often seems no more than a poor substitute for more sophisticated services. Its main advantage, as presently envisioned, is its scope and continuity, not a fundamentally different approach to medical needs.

Part of the justification of family medicine is that the physician of first contact spends a great deal of his time managing problems that are either not medical in the traditional sense or are highly complicated by social, psychological, and environmental factors. These problems include depression, psychophysiological disorders, drug problems and alcoholism, sexual difficulties, and a variety of mild and self-limited complaints compounded by anxiety. It is my experience that most physicians conceive of managing such problems as providing "tender loving care," and the use of the term often carries some derision. The image of the family physician that results is something of a high-minded and good-natured fellow who has limited grasp of the fundamentals of medicine, who operates under great uncertainty, and who basically does not practice as a scientist-physician. Although physicians committed to family medicine have a more flattering image of themselves, it is not really an image based on a new perspective.

If family medicine is to be a specialty in a meaningful sense, it must develop unique knowledge and skills on a scientific basis that enhance the management of problems highly prevalent in general practice; and this is where its status is most uncertain. It is not generally the view that family medicine has a distinctive scientific role and that the special problems it faces require careful scientific investigation. Admittedly, scientific knowledge is relatively limited in understanding alcoholism, drug abuse, difficulties in sexual development, failure to conform to medical regimen, and the like, but a viable discipline of family medicine would require a scientific and investigatory stance toward these problems. I contend that there are few medical schools in the United States, if any, prepared to do this at the present time, and many of the new programs in family medicine lack this capability. Although I believe that the family-medicine movement is a useful one, it seems to me that as medical knowledge continues to develop, it will seem more and more unreasonable to provide a highly complex and differentiated set of services through a generalist in contrast to a highly coordinated and sophisticated team that is held accountable for the necessary services to the client.

If one of the functions of the family-medicine movement is to enlarge the comprehensiveness of services offered by a physician, then it is clear that it is compatible but also in competition with the use of physician extenders. Physician extenders have been described as having three types of functions: (1) to offer primary care in a limited form where medical manpower is unavailable or inaccessible; (2) to increase the efficiency and productivity of the individual physician by assuming simple and repetitive tasks associated with his practice so that he can see more patients; and (3) to offer services and to exercise skills that physicians are unwilling to take on or to offer entirely new services. While family medicine assumes that the physician must take on broader functions and exercise these functions as efficiently as he can with appropriate ancillary assistance, much of the emphasis on extenders is based on a search for new alternatives to physician services. Within the context of professional interests and medical politics, extenders will probably come to be used primarily as adjuncts to physicians. Although much discussion has been given to the notion of primary care extenders, the most likely use of extenders is to perform delimited technical tasks, and a certain scale of operations will be necessary to use such persons effectively. As for primary care, the distinction between such primary-care extenders and registered nurses is hard to sustain with any clarity; and it is not evident that this phase of the movement is anything more than a symbolic crusade, designed more to change attitudes and legal requirements than to develop new forms of health manpower. Even, if possible, I doubt whether developing entirely new primary-care personnel is a responsible course for the nation to follow, and I suggest that a more fundamental reconsideration of the allocation of physicians among medical functions is required.

The most effective way to assure accessibility to adequate primary care is to develop systems that hold providers accountable for delivering specified comprehensive healtl. services to defined populations and that pose minimal barriers to seeing a physician. These units, thus, are held responsible for providing or coordinating the necessary services, and this burden is not left with the consumer. To get involved here in the overall merits and disadvantages of prepaid group practice would take us too far afield; as I see it, the question is not so much how medical practice is specifically organized as whether we can hold health units accountable for performing specified functions at some established price and whether it is possible to monitor performance.

Financial incentives for the provision of more comprehensive services does not necessarily lead to increased accessibility and, indeed, bureaucratized organizations have a reputation for developing new barriers to use as financial barriers are removed. In such circumstances the more knowledgeable and aggressive patient is more likely to receive service, and less-skilled or more intimidated patients may experience greater difficulties. I believe that it is important and feasible to make physicians readily accessible to the population. A mythology has developed that when economic barriers and deductibles and coinsurance are removed, there is an uncontrolled flow of trivial and unnecessary complaints. I have carefully attempted to examine existing data on this matter in the United States and elsewhere, and I find little basis for the conclusion that there is excessive increased use of physician services when economic barriers are removed. Many of the complaints defined as inappropriate or trivial tend to be problems that worry the patient; while they might not be technically exciting to the physician, they certainly fall within his responsibilities. Let me emphasize that the extension of primary care services is not particularly expensive, relative to other components of cost. Most of the total cost of medical care is a product of the choices and decisions physicians make, once patients enter care, and not a product of access.

Although new models of care may provide incentives for greater attention to primary care services, it is not evident that sufficient incentives will exist for any fundamental redistribution of medical manpower from one area to another. How, then, might we move toward a more balanced distribution of health-care resources? One possibility is a national system of financing health care where allocation of funds is relatively centralized and distribution occurs on the basis of population and need. As federal financing of health-care services reaches a certain level, the control over resources and guidelines for reimbursement offer a powerful if not perfect mode of redistribution of facilities and manpower. I doubt that such a system would work as frequently visualized, and people with power and sophistication would continue to command disproportionate resources; but I do not doubt that such a system, if politically acceptable, could achieve significant redistribution.

Since the immediate likelihood of such change in modes of financing is dubious, other alternatives for insuring more adequate distribution should be considered. The field is not fertile with possibilities, and there is a general acceptance that the problem of physician distribution is relatively intractable. Although there is much talk about physician extenders and the use of new technology, these suggestions reveal the inability of the system to exercise the political leverage necessary to fundamentally change the forces affecting the distribution of medical manpower.

I suggest that there is a major alternative that is not at odds with political realities, which has been overlooked. Today, the number of qualified students who wish to enter the nation's medical schools far exceeds the available places. The extent of public financing of medical education makes it possible to insist that medical schools give emphasis to public needs in contrast to private goals, and it would not be difficult to allocate a fixed percentage of available medical school places to qualified students who are willing to commit themselves to practice, at least for a time, in areas designated as being medically needy. Unlike other proposals, this one ties the availability of a medical school place, not solely student financing, to a public commitment. Schools can be readily encouraged to designate medical school places for such a program through financing mechanisms established by the federal government. No single mechanism, of course, is likely to develop the conditions conducive to effective health care delivery. Also needed is a careful development of the facilities, resources, and manpower to practice good medical care in underdoctored areas, as well as adequate educational models for such care, and sufficient financing of medical education to attract qualified students from a wide range of social, economic, and geographic backgrounds. This plan is discussed in greater detail in Chapter 17.

The Role of Social Science in Health Care Planning

Let us shift emphasis and consider how the social sciences can contribute to more effective health policy in the future and how they can assist in translating goals into effective program planning. I doubt whether our record has been particularly good so far, and it is important to consider how social science might make a more significant contribution in the future. Social science research, I believe, has relatively little direct effect on policy decisions that are visibly political in nature and that involve the clash of important interest groups. We deceive ourselves if we fail to take into account the fact that policy decisions are part of a political process, and social science studies usually involve only limited considerations relevant to such decisions. The impact of social science on policy is probably in inverse relation to the extent to which decisions involve a major shift in resources from one interest group to another, and it is naive to anticipate that social science—no matter how relevant or elegantly performed—will necessarily result in specific policy modifications.

In my view, social science affects policy most substantially by enlarging the social and intellectual climate within which policy-making discussions take place and by affecting the types of information considered relevant to social policy decisions. Climate refers not only to the specific awareness those making policy have of social science thinking and research, but to the extent to which their thinking and the media to which they are exposed have been influenced by social science perspectives.

As government assumes greater responsibility for health policy generally, and as greater aggregation and coordination of health facilities and services develop, the potentialities to use social science techniques and analysis as instruments of policy increase. At the present time the persons responsible for policy must deal with a highly pluralistic and vastly complex system of facilities and services that cannot be held accountable for meeting the health needs of specifically defined populations. Since it is enormously difficult to gauge levels of performance, policy makers cannot readily ascertain the effects of alternative policy interventions. Also, in view of the character of the public-private mix in health affairs, the heterogeneity from one area to another, and the nature of medical politics, the realistic alternatives available for policy implementation are frequently restricted. Furthermore, the volatile nature of health politics makes it difficult to anticipate the issues that will surface at a particular time and to be prepared with the necessary information and alternative policies to respond effectively.

As the policy maker comes to view health care as a system of services planned in relation to defined populations and their needs, a social science capability can effectively serve the policy-making process.[8] Although such a capability will not necessarily insure effective policy implementation, it promotes the conditions necessary for the development of an informed and coherent approach to utilizing opportunities for change as they develop.

The development of long-range policy options requires an appreciation of the political and social context of health care; historical and social experience with varying types of incentives, legislative innovations, and organizational

modifications; and the ability to estimate or assess the impact and consequences of one or another policy alternative. These functions cannot reasonably be performed without an ability to quickly retrieve relevant data that are
sufficiently current and facilitate estimates of cost, demand, effectiveness, distribution of services, and the like. This requires a sophisticated data system
that combines various types of surveys, special studies, and data aggregation
from ongoing operations that allow estimates for different levels of service,
varying regions of the country, and particular subgroups of the population. To
be effective, these data systems must be reasonably simple and parsimonious,
comparable from one part to another, and relatively rapid in their ability to
turn over data. I am not confident that we quite know how to achieve these
goals, although I am reasonably sure that we can do a great deal better than at
present. It is striking to observe the tremendous disparity between the requirements for data specified in various recent health-care legislation and our present ability to generate such estimates. To some extent this disparity reflects the
unrealistic view taken by legislators of the requirements for obtaining adequate population data; to some extent it reflects the chaotic character of our
health-care system; and partly it reflects our failure to use what we know in
developing a more adequate description of what is truly happening in the
organization and delivery of health-care services. There are, of course, a variety of methodological and conceptual problems in the development of an adequate information system, which are not easily solved, but regardless of the
limitations, these data will facilitate a clearer concept of important issues and
more realistic estimates than are now available.

Although such descriptive data assist in locating problems and indicating
the existing conditions, they do not necessarily provide an understanding of
how to correct deficiencies nor do they allow specification of the program
components responsible for varying impacts. Information systems can vary in
effectiveness depending on the extent to which they are constructed around
evaluating the implementation of specific goals, the extent to which responsibility for varying functions and services is clear, and the extent to which the
definitions of morbidity, services, and cost are conceptually adequate and
comparable from one part of the data system to another. But in the long run,
health policy planning also requires a vital research and development program, which defines new goals, and more sophisticated technologies and interventions than the ones available.

Although monitoring, evaluation, and development are easily understood,
there tends to be increased emphasis on instant relevance and a growing skepticism of more fundamental research efforts. We should remember that, in
emphasizing delivery of services, we had better continue to be concerned with
what it is we are delivering. Many of the fundamental issues relevant to illness, disorder, and disability remain unresolved and, in our search for instant

solutions, we are in danger of deprecating important efforts for the long range. Not all of these efforts are fruitful, and some may even appear trivial and absurd, but it is such efforts—both in the biomedical and behavioral sciences —that will determine the vitality of health care in the future.

When problems are pressing, there is a tendency to adopt instant solutions; and it is proper that efforts be made to relieve suffering, regardless of the level of knowledge and technology. But we should be aware that this is what we are doing, and our attempts to meet current problems should not deflect continuing long-range efforts to develop more adequate approaches to difficult and complicated problems. My assertions may appear obvious, but we presently face a growing tendency to neglect and even to deprecate the longer-range issues, not only in government but also in the universities.

Equity and the Organization of Health Care Services

I conclude with a general discussion of the issue of equity in the provision of health-care services. What is fair and proper is not self-evident, and experience in a variety of domestic spheres illustrates how divergent concepts of equity can be. For example, does the availability of financing meet the goal of equity if efforts are not made to insure a more reasonable distribution of facilities and manpower? Is equity achieved by extending opportunities to previously disenfranchised groups, or does it also require that special efforts be made to see that they make use of such opportunities? If the risks of death, disease, and disability are disproportionately distributed in the population, does equity also require that service availability be fitted to differential risk? In short, does equity encompass access to a minimal level of care or to equal opportunities to care, or does it also encompass efforts toward the achievement of equal health status and function? The distribution of resources might vary quite radically, depending on how these questions are answered.

Not only are groups in the population subject to varying risks of disease and disability but the manner in which health care is defined and organized involves different gains and costs for varying groups. The social and medical values that emphasize some diseases and functions rather than others tend to place a disproportionate burden on the poor and unfortunate, since the maladies that are more likely to affect them are problems that are given lower priority within the context of our health care system. The list is long but well known; psychoses, drug addiction, alcoholism, abortion, retardation, and the like have been the wasteland of the health care system, and there has been no great receptivity toward meeting the needs in these areas. The neglect of such problems is often a product of the uncertainty of knowledge and the absence of clear interventions, but not exclusively so. Many of the priorities of medical care reflect professional and middle-class values and orientations as much as they do an objective stance toward meeting health-care needs.

One of the functions of social science research is to make salient the perspectives that are not evident to the practitioner or policy maker. Both come to observe the delivery of health services from a particular vantage point. The perspectives they adopt and the images of behavior and problems they have are constructions that derive from their work and its special problems, and their particular location in the health-care structure. The policy maker frequently comes to think in administrative terms and is often unappreciative of the profound human consequences of one or another administrative solution. The practitioner also comes to view the problem from his experiences and his particular needs and not from a larger view of the problems as they occur in the community as a whole. We all adopt stereotypes based on our own experiences that facilitate making sense of our world and performing our duties, but when applied to new situations they can be faulty and maladaptive. Social science can assist in avoiding such errors which, when they occur as part of a nationwide policy, cause great mischief.

In the larger context of the development of social policies in health, some issues achieve public visibility, but most do not. When visibility is low, then special interests with more knowledge, resources, and greater accessibility to government come to dominate the way that problems are defined and resolved. Frequently, other possible definitions of the problem are not represented and are not considered, not because they would be unsuitable or politically unacceptable, but because there is no one available to present them. Social science can serve as a form of community representation by proxy, attempting to put forth in the most reliable and objective way the likely repercussions of one or another policy on varying groups in the community.

Finally, I believe that a well-developed and honest social science can enhance the democratic process and retard the dominance of special-interest perspectives. It can, through its analyses, represent and bring into consideration the needs of affected groups outside the mainstream of government decision making. I am not naive about the political difficulties of such a role or the danger that social science (which has its own needs and vantage points) will, itself, become a special interest or serve the interests that presently prevail. Therefore, the responsibility for objectivity, openness, and accessibility to criticism and review is very great. The task is hard and the prospects uncertain, but I have faith that it is one worthy of our dedication.

Notes

1. Ginzberg, E., and M. Ostow (1969). *Men, Money, and Medicine*. New York: Columbia University Press.

2. Fuchs, V., and M. Kramer (1972). *Expenditures for Physicians' Services in the United*

States, 1948–68. Washington, D.C.: National Center for Health Services Research and Development, D.H.E.W. Publication No. HSM 73–3013.

3. Stevens, R. (1971). *American Medicine and the Public Interest.* New Haven: Yale University Press.

4. Mechanic, D. (1973). "General Medical Practice: Some Comparisons Between the Work of Primary Care Physicians in the United States and England and Wales." *Medical Care,* **10:** 402–420.

5. Mechanic, D. (1972). "Human Problems and the Organization of Health Care." *Annals of the American Academy of Political and Social Science,* **399:**1–11.

6. Bunker, J. (1970). "Surgical Manpower: A Comparison of Operations and Surgeons in the United States and in England and Wales." *New England Journal of Medicine,* **283:** 135–144.

7. Mechanic, D. (1968). "General Medical Practice in England and Wales: Its Organization and Future." *New England Journal of Medicine,* **279:**680–689.

8. Fourteenth Report of the WHO Expert Committee on Health Statistics (1971). *Statistical Indicators for the Planning and Evaluation of Health Programmes,* Geneva, World Health Organization Technical Report Series, No. 472.

CHAPTER V

Policy Studies and Medical-Care Research*

Medical-care or health-services research, in contrast to biomedical research, has had little discernible impact on public policy, the behavior of health professionals, or the organization of health facilities. Although there are instances where persons with official responsibilities justify particular policies through references to specific research, there is little evidence that the initiation of policy flows directly from research findings. As mentioned in the previous chapter, however, research may, in the long run, help to shape the climate within which decisions are made.

Part of the difficulty in discerning the impact of research on policy reflects the vagueness of the concept of policy itself. If by policy we mean legislative and governmental administrative actions, then it is obvious that research is only one of many relevant factors that are taken into account. At this level, it is clear that the range of variables that are amenable to manipulation is limited at any particular time, and political feasibility is an important consideration. If we think of policy in terms of administrative actions at a variety of levels of organizational functioning, then we face a problem of diffusion of results. In a pluralistic system where there is a multitude of decision points, we would not expect that a solution demonstrated in one context would necessarily be viewed as relevant or adaptable to another. Thus, solutions affecting smaller units of organization often diffuse very slowly, if at all. In considering the impact on policy, it is not apparent what criteria are reasonable to impose or what constitutes an appropriate span of time for diffusion to take place.

Yet, even in considering the diffusion process, it is clear that some findings diffuse rapidly while others have little success. Findings in the area of biomedical technology and science have greater effectiveness than most health-services research. This results partly from the fact that biomedical research tends to

* Paper presented at the NIMH-ASA Conference on Sociological Research, December, 1972.

shape technology without intruding in major ways on the interests or life styles of professionals, while health-care research poses a greater threat to professional autonomy, work priorities, and control over work. Here, I will discuss the difficulties in implementing health-care research by focusing on studies dealing with social and psychological factors in the treatment of hospital patients and with the failure of physicians and medical facilities to give adequate attention to such concerns.

I will examine two studies carried out at Yale-New Haven (a Yale University teaching hospital): one, a very specific experimental study of the role of communication in patient care; and the other, a general investigation of the quality of patient care. The first study,[1] rigorously performed and yielding specific results and implications for intervention, has been generally ignored. The second,[2] a provocative descriptive study, with important implications but serious methodological problems, resulted in a vigorous counterattack by elite members of the academic medical establishment.[3] I will discuss these works as part of a larger line of inquiry, since findings documenting the failure to give adequate attention to social and psychological factors are common in the literature.[4,5] I think that the rejection of the second study would have occurred regardless of its methodological rigor because similar findings have been reported, based on a variety of methodologies, and these, too, have been generally ignored.

In the first study (reported by Skipper and Leonard), children admitted to a hospital for tonsillectomy were randomized into experimental and control groups. In the control group, patients received the usual care, while in the experimental situation, mothers were admitted to the hospital by a specially trained nurse who tried to facilitate communication and to maximize the mothers' opportunities to express their anxiety and to ask questions. An attempt was made to give the mother an accurate picture of the realities, and mothers were told what routine events to expect and when they were likely to occur. Mothers in the experimental group experienced less stress, and their children experienced smaller changes in blood pressure, temperature, and other physiological measures; they were less likely to suffer from posthospital emesis and made a better adaptation to the hospital; and they made a more rapid recovery following hospitalization, displaying less fears, less crying, and less disturbed sleep than children in the control group. In considering this study, notice that tonsillectomy is one of the most frequent surgical procedures performed in the United States and the main cause of hospitalization of children.[6] Controlled prospective studies demonstrate that tonsillectomy is a dubious surgical procedure in the great majority of cases, and psychological problems are a major adverse effect of the procedure, especially in young children. Thus, the importance of alleviating the distress of the mother and child when the procedure is performed should not be minimized.

I have discussed this study with the investigators and various other persons associated with the hospital in which the study was carried out. There is consensus that the study had very little impact on the delivery of services. The innovation was not continued beyond the study period, and it had no observable effect on the general philosophy of patient care. Very likely, the results of the study at the hospital are not widely known, and there is agreement that the medical and surgical staff have little interest in such studies. One of the investigators told me that a high-ranking physician on the staff asked him why he was wasting his time with such trivial problems.

The second study (carried out by Duff and Hollingshead) describes in detail the general problems and complexity of a major teaching hospital, but focuses on a sample of 161 patients who received care on medical and surgical services in the private and ward facilities of the hospital. The investigators extensively interviewed patients, doctors, nurses, families, and other hospital personnel; they examined medical records, observed patient care, and made follow-up visits to the patients when they returned home. Many of the findings are based on Duff and Hollingshead's global appraisal of each case and, except for anecdote, it is difficult to assess specifically how they made various judgments. Yet two major findings emerge from the study, which I believe are unchallengeable and do not rest on the fragility of methodological approach. First, it is clear that a very different style of patient care prevails on the public in contrast to the private services, and that patients on the public wards were more likely to be taken for granted. Second, this study dramatically illustrates the failure of physicians treating the patients' illnesses to become sufficiently aware of their social and psychological circumstances and to take these circumstances into consideration in the total management of the patient. Without accepting Duff and Hollingshead's specific evaluations of the adequacy of diagnosis, the mental status or adjustments of individual patients, or on many other technical matters, it is difficult for me to see how an impartial reader can reject the more general conclusion that there was a consistent failure to give adequate attention to the life circumstances of patients in relation to their illnesses. Nor is this observation inconsistent with observations elsewhere. The recommendations by Duff and Hollingshead are rather modest in relation to the magnitude of the issues they raise, but include such suggestions as that "health professionals be trained to deal systematically with the personal and social factors which affect the diagnosis and treatment of patients."

Unlike many other investigators in the area, Duff and Hollingshead published their findings as a "trade" book, and its publication was accompanied by considerable newspaper publicity, including an article in *McCall's Magazine*. Perhaps because of its public visibility, it brought forth criticism for failure to publish "results via accepted channels for scholarly communication" and also a public rebuttal in *Harper's Magazine*.

The counterattack on Duff and Hollingshead came from two elite members of the academic establishment. A lengthy review appearing in the *Yale Journal of Biology and Medicine* was published by Paul Beeson of Oxford University, who had been chief of the Yale University Medical Service during the study period. A second review by Franz Ingelfinger, editor of the *New England Journal of Medicine*, appeared in *Harper's*. Both men, usually described as enlightened and progressive forces in medical care, offer a detailed rejoiner that, at times, borders on the petty. Both make an issue, for example, of the fact that Dr. Duff, an associate professor of pediatrics at Yale, described his interests in the preface of the book as "not exactly medicine and not necessarily sociology."

I do not believe that the methodological problems in the Duff-Hollingshead study were key issues in the rejection of the study, since research findings on behavioral factors in disease have been generally ignored regardless of results, the type of study, or the rigors of methodology. Rigor and methodological adequacy are obviously important considerations, but it is striking how frequently weak and uncertain results in support of one or another position are cited when they support the viewpoint of the advocate.[7] Two standards seem to be imposed: one for studies whose findings you like, and another for studies whose findings appear less attractive. This is particularly true when policy positions are advocated, and it supports the earlier observation that research results are used more frequently to justify policies than to suggest new approaches.

Although Duff and Hollingshead's attempt to make the issues public through the popular presentation and promotion of their book was bitterly criticized, they at least were able to elicit a hearing. Even though the powers that be at Yale-New Haven probably were sufficiently angry with the results of the study to facilitate its rejection, and even though the study had no apparent effect on the organization of services at the hospital, it has contributed importantly to a discussion of the issues raised in the larger society and among younger health professionals. Thus, although the study had no demonstrable impact directly, it probably has contributed to a climate of concern. It is difficult to evaluate the effect of a "trade" book in contrast to journal articles in a particular case, but if *Science Citation Index* is any indication of the extent to which a particular project arouses interest in the scientific community, then it is clear that the Duff-Hollingshead study was considerably more successful than the Skipper-Leonard investigation. As one of the authors of the latter study wrote me in a response to an earlier draft of this chapter, "accepted channels" may be a way of simply burying a study.

In considering why the Duff-Hollingshead study had little effect on the functioning of Yale-New Haven and why it would be unlikely to have effect regardless of its level of methodological elegance, I suggest that the implications of the findings are simply too radical. Such studies have little effect because, if taken seriously, they would require a fundamental reorganization of how medical services are delivered and how health personnel are trained. In this regard, Duff and Hollingshead do not show sufficient appreciation of the fundamental reorganization of medical education and practice necessary to achieve what they would like. In contrast, the limited specific recommendations, if implemented, would have very little effect in the face of the existing pattern of medical and hospital work. It is instructive to consider the larger criticisms of the Duff-Hollingshead study that are not specifically directed to their methodology or their motives. These criticisms basically fall into two groups.

1. Both critics make the point that hospitals deal with serious organic disease and thus must establish priorities in terms of known interventions. They argue that since time and energy is limited, you do what you know how to do. As Ingelfinger puts it: " 'I rob banks,' said Willie Sutton, 'because that's where the money is.' "

2. Both critics deeply resent the unveiling of the "mystique of medicine." Both take bitter exception to what, as far as I can tell, is an accurate account of the process of obtaining autopsy permissions and of the methods used. This criticism tends to be an attack on sociology itself, since both critics imply that it was irresponsible to unmask the process. Ingelfinger describes this as "preoccupation with learning in its most ghoulish aspects" and Beeson makes the hysterical statement that "I'm sure that no lay person who has read their book will ever grant this permission after the death of a relative." I cite this because both reviews, by men of unquestionable repute, display considerable paternalism in their discussions of patient care. They imply that patients have no right to know about the more ghoulish aspects of hospital care, since the mystique of medicine is truly in their interests.

Perhaps because Ingelfinger was less personally involved, he expresses greater ambivalence in his review and is more willing to concede that Duff and Hollingshead have raised real issues, although he expresses criticism of their one-sided presentation of them. In respect to the difficult problem of weighing the need for further diagnostic search against the possibility that psychogenic factors are the cause of the patient's difficulty, he notes that:

There is no easy solution to the philosophical and moral problem, but to use this dilemma to "prove" the narrow focus of the physician's interest or his lack of diagnostic drive verges on demagoguery.

Although Ingelfinger has probably overstated his point, he does raise a serious problem with the Duff-Hollingshead work and many other sociological studies in the "debunking" tradition. The study is presented in terms of patient advocacy, and Duff and Hollingshead do not present the issues as seen by each of the major participants. In depicting the process of obtaining an autopsy and in its implications of disapproval of the means, it does not give attention to the high-minded ends that have produced such adaptations. And this is the crux of the issue. Both Ingelfinger and Beeson frequently point out the noble ends that have their associated seamy aspects, but Duff and Hollingshead emphasized the seamy aspects and gave little attention to the goals and needs that inspired them. As Beeson notes in exasperation, "The authors' combination of smugness and naivete is hard to bear by someone who has been dealing with the realities."

I find the issue of autopsy a particularly interesting one because both Duff and Hollingshead and their critics miss what I regard as the crucial point. Clearly, autopsies are important for evaluation of work, continuing education, and improved performance; and a teaching hospital, worthy of the name, will attempt to obtain permissions to perform autopsies. In their zealousness, physicians sometimes commit the types of excesses described vividly in the Duff-Hollingshead volume and may even cajole and trick persons into providing the necessary permission. While Beeson and Ingelfinger focus on the noble functions of the autopsy, Duff and Hollingshead focus on the excesses. Neither study examines the way to balance the needs of the teaching hospital with the rights of patients and their families to be treated with dignity and to be given an opportunity to truly consent to requests. Achieving this is, of course, a complex and time-consuming process, and teaching hospitals are busy places. But when ends come to justify contemptible methods, we pay a price, irrespective of the technical gains. Physicians also come to pay a price, for we are what we do, and the doctor who comes to adapt functional "tricks" loses some of his humanity.

In Beeson's view, "A low-keyed, well-documented report, aimed at professionals and written for professionals, could have immense and lasting value. After all, doctors and nurses are the only people who possibly can alter the conditions of patient care." This is in sharp contrast to the Duff-Hollingshead view that "*The answer is basically a society-wide issue rather than a problem for medical professionals alone*. Sickness is inextricably linked with society and society will have to look at itself for the solution." It is within these two contrasting views that the positions on both sides can be understood.

Beeson sees the solution to problems largely in terms of the efforts and good will of individual actors. He contends that since physicians and nurses provide care, change must come through influencing them to view some forms of professional behavior as desirable in relation to others. He appears to see sociological research in medicine as ancillary to the medical function, as one more aid to assist the physician and nurse to do a better job. In this light he views the Duff-Hollingshead book as a bitter and unjustified attack on medicine itself or, as Ingelfinger puts it, opening "new veins of muck for those who make it their business to rake the medical profession." In contrast, Duff and

Hollingshead are indicting the structure of medical care itself and the societal pressures and values that sustain it in its present form. Although this attack on the basic structure of medical care in America is never fully or adequately developed, it seems apparent—but not to the physicians involved—that it is not a personal indictment. This is reflected in the following way. Duff and Hollingshead frequently quoted young physicians who from time to time used expressions among colleagues that they would be unlikely to use elsewhere; this is, of course, typical in the back regions of all occupations and may even be seen as a way of adapting to the stresses of work and uncertainty. Beeson, however, takes these anecdotes personally and views them as degrading:

> The criticism of the house staff extended even to attributing phrases to them which to me have a phoney ring, and perhaps merely represent what Duff and Hollingshead thought such characters ought to say! For example, I never heard the wards of the hospital referred to as "the zoo," nor do I think that the Emergency Admission Room was commonly referred to as "the pit," . . . I knew these young people well, far better than the writers of this book. I regarded them as able, likeable, dedicated and hard working—on the way to becoming outstandingly good physicians and surgeons.

The basic issues of how to effectively utilize knowledge of patients' life situations in diagnosis, patient care, and rehabilitation and how to weigh more elaborate attempts at physical diagnosis in contrast to considering other approaches to the patients' problems are difficult issues. We lack clear-cut concepts of how to appraise such difficulties or to effectively intervene, and it is natural that medical efforts should emphasize scientific medical orientations to care. The fact is, however, in focusing on such problems there is a tendency to develop callousness and to lose a sense of medicine as a human enterprise as well as a science. Moreover, the teaching hospital is the training ground not only for physicians who care for the desperately ill but for all physicians, and its emphases and orientations may not be well suited for much of the care physicians are called on to provide. However, even in the care of the seriously ill patient, social and psychological factors are of major importance, but the teaching hospitals have largely ignored them and served as a model encouraging future generations of physicians to give them low priority.

And now a concluding question: What might we learn from such controversies that might be helpful in making future efforts more effective? It is clear that if the intent of such studies is to bring about change in the contexts studied, rather than to add to knowledge or to inform the climate of general opinion, it is necessary to involve more intimately in such investigations the persons who have operational authority for the programs studied. In examining medical services, the persons concerned should be intimately involved in the design and progress of the study, and the investigation should require "informed consent" not only for patients but also for the professionals involved.

As a sociologist who works in medical contexts I can attest to how difficult this can be and, like the physician who fails to tell the patient everything in order to facilitate his management of the patient, the sociologist is also frequently tempted to say less than necessary in order to protect his access to the situation. I have come to believe that sociologists ought not to work on units in which the medical leadership will not accept them with a *realistic* understanding of the advantages and risks of sociological research. I emphasize the word "realistic" because it has been my experience that physicians who expect too much from behavioral science are as difficult to cooperate with as those who expect too little. It is crucial that physicians involved with behavioral-science research programs in medicine have a reasonable concept of the likely product and the strengths and weaknesses of behavioral studies. It may be necessary in some contexts, such as in custodial institutions, to keep research concerns more covert, but it is unlikely to stimulate change from within. To the extent that the physicians are themselves involved in medical-care research and are committed to it, it is more likely that significant findings will be implemented.

It is also likely that research resulting in recommendations for fundamental restructuring of activities is unlikely to yield significant change. If Duff and Hollingshead were more analytic in their book, it would be clear that the failures of the teaching hospital cannot be resolved by simple changes here and there, but will require substantial restructuring of health care financing, medical education, and medical practice. Professionals must work within the context of real constraints, and thus global recommendations for restructuring the overall approach leave helpless the people who are urged to make the adaptations. In this sense, Duff and Hollingshead were basically correct that the issues at stake are issues for the larger society and not only for the health professionals involved. In this sense the authors were using their observations at Yale-New Haven for a larger purpose, and their results have limited implications for reform of Yale-New Haven outside of more extensive reforms of the health care system as a whole. It is unfortunate that the study alienated some people whose support will be needed in implementing the changes necessary to integrate social and psychological considerations in medical education and medical care. These differences partly represent conflicts of perspective that, to some extent, are inevitable; but they also suggest the importance of careful planning, not only of the research effort but also of the relationship of the researcher to the institutions studied.

Notes

1. Skipper, J. Jr., and R. Leonard (1968). "Children, Stress, and Hospitalization: A Field Experiment." *Journal of Health and Social Behavior*, **9**:275–287.
2. Duff, R. S., and A. B. Hollingshead (1968). *Sickness and Society*. New York: Harpers.

3. Beeson, P. B. (1968). "Special Book Review of Sickness and Society." *Yale Journal of Biology and Medicine*, **41**:226–240; and F. J. Ingelfinger (1968). "The Arch-Hospital: An Ailing Monopoly." *Harper's Magazine,* **237**:82–87.

4. Cartwright, A. (1964). *Human Relations and Hospital Care.* Boston: Routledge and Kegan Paul.

5. Ley, P. and M. S. Spelman (1967). *Communicating with the Patient.* London: Trinity Press.

6. National Center for Health Statistics (1971). *Surgical Operations in Short-Stay Hospitals for Discharged Patients: United States—1965.* PHS Series 13, No. 7, Washington; U.S. Government Printing Office.

7. See, for example, the discussion of Health Maintenance Organizations in U.S. Department of Health, Education and Welfare (1971). *Toward a Comprehensive Health Policy for the 1970's: A White Paper.* Washington D.C.: U.S. Government Printing Office. For a review of some of the issues, see D. Mechanic (1972). *Public Expectations and Health Care.* New York: Wiley-Interscience, pp. 102–111.

CHAPTER VI

Factors Affecting Receptivity to Innovations in Health-Care Delivery among Primary-Care Physicians

Today, there is considerable ferment in the organization of health-care services and a growing emphasis on modified forms of organizational arrangements, such as prepaid group practice, community health centers, medical foundations, salaried practice, systematic peer review, the use of physician extenders, and increased government financing of health-care costs. As the debate continues, many voices are heard about the consequences or advisability of one or another organizational arrangement. This chapter examines the factors that affect physicians' attitudes to these innovations and the forces that influence receptivity to organizational change.

As the existing literature on attitudes and actions illustrates, attitudes are only one of many factors affecting how persons respond to social change. Persons frequently adapt to social change regardless of their prior attitudes, and modified attitudes may follow rather than precede organizational modifications. Colombotos,[1] for example, found that although physicians in New York state were relatively hostile to the impending Medicare program, the vast majority of them participated in it within a short time after its enactment. In this case, more favorable attitudes were a result of participation. The evidence that physician cooperation was more difficult to obtain following the enactment of the Medicaid program in New York state suggests that the consequences of program components for the physician are an important aspect of its acceptability.

The attitudes of physicians toward innovations in medical-care delivery stem from a variety of factors, including their prior training and experiences, and the effects of varying organizational arrangements on their conditions of work and remuneration, for instance. Generally, we know that many physicians are extremely skeptical of organizational modifications and tend to oppose them. Much of the rhetoric of opposition is voiced as professional opinions rather than as statements of self-interest or philosophical or political perspectives. To the extent that this opposition reflects philosophical or political viewpoints, it must be given no more credence than other political and social viewpoints. To the extent that discussions of organizational change reflect scientific determinations of effectiveness and professional experience, it must be taken more seriously. The hypothesis to be examined here is that support for (or opposition to) many new organizational modifications in health-care delivery is affected more by the physician's political-philosophical orientation than by objective factors characterizing his training, practice structure, or modes of professional behavior. Following a study by Pastore,[2] which found that scientists' preferences for hereditary as compared to environmental interpretations were reflections of their political and social attitudes, it was anticipated that how a physician sees the debate on organizational change is a reflection of his overall political philosophy more than his assessment of relevant facts or professional experience.

Procedures

The data reported here are from a random sample of office-based general practitioners, internists, pediatricians, and obstetricians, selected with different sampling ratios among group and nongroup practitioners classified by their primary activity code. The population from which the sample was drawn included 82,271 nongroup practitioners and 12,772 group practitioners. Among the nongroup population, 56 percent were general practitioners, 21 percent internists, 14 percent pediatricians, and 9 percent obstetricians. Among group practitioners, 37 percent were general practitioners, 32 percent internists, 15 percent pediatricians, and 16 percent obstetricians. A questionnaire was sent to each member of our sample between the period of October, 1970 to March, 1971. After five approaches, 1458 physicians (66 percent of our sample) returned completed questionnaires.

The American Medical Association provided the investigator with a tape containing information on the entire sample from their Physicians' Records Information System. Comparing the data describing physicians who responded to our survey with the total sample on such attributes as year of graduation, sex, state within which the doctor practices, birthdate, license year, National Board year, amount of postgraduate education, source of professional income, present employment, government service, specialty boards, and memberships in specialty societies, no differences of note were found. In no case did any category vary by more than a few percent in comparing the persons who responded with the entire sample. It seems clear, at least in respect to these limited characteristics, that respondents were representative of the entire sample.

A somewhat sharper picture of possible biases emerges in comparing the minority who did not respond to the survey with those who did. Here we find that nonrespondents include a higher proportion of older doctors (23 percent, 61 years or older), those who graduated from medical school in 1935 or earlier (20 percent), and those who were licensed to practice in 1940 or before (23 percent). The comparable figures among respondents were 16 percent, 13 percent, and 18 percent. Nonrespondents were more likely to be in individual fee-for-service practice (53 percent) than respondents (44 percent) and also were more likely to be on full-time salaries (4 percent versus 2 percent). Nonrespondents were also less likely to have their specialty boards (23 percent) than respondents (33 percent) and were less likely to belong to at least one specialty society (34 percent versus 49 percent). This selective tendency relative to specialty boards and specialty societies is most pronounced among pediatricians. In sum, although the respondents are characteristic of the entire sample in respect to the information available, there was some selective response to the survey.

Indicators of Receptivity to Organizational Change

Receptivity to organizational change depends, of course, on the specific changes under consideration. Although there may be a general trait of receptivity or nonreceptivity among individuals, responses are likely to be dependent on how individuals perceive specific changes affecting them and their usual modes of activity. In our survey we asked physicians to what extent they approved or disapproved of various modifications in the organization of health-care services. Our analysis here deals with four dimensions of change based on ten questions in our survey: (1) federal government financing of health-care services; (2) more organized or salaried practice; (3) more intensive peer review; and (4) use of physician extenders. Since responses to all ten indicators were positively associated, we also built one grand index that we call receptivity to organizational change, which is a simple additive scale based on the ten individual items. This scale only measures receptivity to certain types of changes and not necessarily to change in general. The responses to various items used in this analysis are shown in Table 1.

Table 1 Attitudes of American Primary Care Physicians toward New Features of the Organization of Medical Care

Proportion responding that they strongly approve or moderately approve	*General Practitioners* Nongroup N = 599 (per cent)	Group N = 111	*Internists* Nongroup N = 231 (per cent)	Group N = 91	*Pediatricians* Nongroup N = 136 (per cent)	Group N = 43	*Obstetricians* Nongroup N = 150 (per cent)	Group N = 58
Financing								
Concept of government financing of medical care as in the Medicaid Program in your state	38	44	44	57	45	51	39	51
Federal financing of medical care through some system of National Health Insurance	32	44	41	51	43	54	39	41
Practice organization and innovations								
Community health centers such as those established by the Office of Economic Opportunity	52	59	69	78	68	80	60	66
Prepaid group practice such as the Kaiser-Permanente Plan or the Health Insurance Plan of New York	40	61	54	65	61	86	45	76
Doctors working on a salaried basis	37	54	50	57	54	68	39	66

Controls over medical work

Peer review of medical work in the hospital	83	90	88	96	93	100	85	90
Peer review of medical work in the doctor's office	44	57	67	77	69	78	54	64
Review of hospital work by physicians from outside one's community	35	44	54	57	51	60	44	34
New practitioners								
The use of specially trained physician's assistants who work under the doctor's supervision in his practice	78	85	79	87	82	93	74	88
The training of non-M.D. associates who work independently to some extent in underdoctored areas	51	72	62	75	63	68	55	65

Results

Table 2 presents the zero-order correlations among the individual items for both group and nongroup practitioners. In general, the ten items are correlated moderately in a positive direction with some clustering that is consistent with expectations. For example, the two items dealing with financing, the three items with peer review, and the two items with physician extenders are more closely correlated with one another than with the other items. Although the items dealing with prepaid practice, salaried practice, and community health centers make up a less clear-cut cluster, their similarity makes it reasonable to combine them in a single measure; the average intercorrelation among these three items is .35 among group practitioners and .34 among nongroup practitioners.

In our analysis, we have examined a large number of independent variables as predictors of receptivity to various organizational changes. We began with more than 100 variables but, after excluding those that were obviously redundant or theoretically uninteresting, we carried out our basic analysis using 38 predictor variables. These were grouped by type: (1) *Political Orientation* (self-description as liberal or conservative, political party identification); (2) *Social Background, Experience, and Life Style* (religion, father's education, father's occupational prestige, government service, years in practice, sex); (3) *Community and Practice Structure* (geographic region, specialty, number of affiliated physicians, major source of income, community size); (4) *Practice Pressures* (number of patient consultations, hourly and weekly efforts); (5) *Medical Training and Practice Behavior* (amount of post-graduate training, continuing education, specialty boards, range of practice, use of diagnostic procedures, scope of treatment procedures used); (6) *Doctors' Satisfactions and Attitudinal Orientations* (measures of receptivity to social aspects of practice, physician satisfaction, attitudes toward sacrifice, perception of uncertainty in general practice); and (7) *Professional Affiliations* (membership in local medical society and specialty societies).

In attempting to predict receptivity to organizational change, we took as our working hypothesis that the doctor's political-philosophical orientation would be most important in predicting attitudes toward organizational innovations. Furthermore, we expected that receptivity to organizational innovations would, to some extent, reflect experience with such organizational arrangements, and thus physicians who were working within the types of arrangements involved in our dependent measures would be more favorable to them. This type of finding, of course, could reflect the selection of those more favorable toward organizational innovations into such work arrangements. Working with these general ideas, we examined the correlates of (1) overall receptivity to organizational change (all 10 items); (2) receptivity to government financ-

Table 2 Correlations among Indicators of Receptivity to Organizational Change among Nongroup and Group Physicians (Decimal Points Excluded)[a]

	1	2	3	4	5	6	7	8	9	10
1. Government financing of medical care as in Medicaid Program in your state[b]		41	35	27	29	12	17	13	11	09
2. Federal financing of medical care through some system of national health insurance	38		36	33	34	16	22	22	19	21
3. Prepaid group practice such as Kaiser-Permanente or HIP	31	39		34	35	24	27	24	24	24
4. Doctors working on salaried basis	23	22	44		33	13	13	13	14	18
5. Community health centers such as those established by OEO	36	28	25	35		21	20	19	26	29
6. Peer review of medical work in hospital	22	19	33	14	29		58	32	22	20
7. Peer review of medical work in the doctor's office	20	23	33	20	23	63		43	22	21
8. Review of hospital work by physicians from outside one's community	12	24	25	09	18	25	39		20	17
9. Use of specially trained PA's who work under doctor's supervision in his practice	19	23	29	23	26	26	27	12		56
10. The training of non-MD associates who work independently to some extent in underdoctored areas	17	26	23	25	26	19	22	13	47	

[a] Correlations for nongroup physicians above diagonal; correlations for group physicians below diagonal.
[b] Physicians were asked to "indicate the extent to which you approve or disapprove of each of the following practices" and were given four response categories: strongly approve, moderately approve, moderately disapprove, or strongly disapprove.

ing (items 1 and 2); (3) receptivity to more organized practice (items 3, 4, and 5); (4) receptivity to peer review (items 6, 7, and 8); and (5) receptivity to use of physician extenders (items 9 and 10).

Table 3 gives the zero-order correlations between our 38 predictors* and our five measures of receptivity to organizational change. At the zero-order level, the doctor's description of himself as liberal or conservative is clearly the most consistent and strongest predictor of his receptivity to organizational change.† Political party identification follows a similar pattern, but it is generally weaker, particularly in respect to receptivity to peer review and receptivity to physician extenders. In respect to most of the other predictors, the size of zero-order correlations are either small or inconsistent across the five receptivity measures. Since the predictors are substantially intercorrelated, there is limited value in attempting to examine these relationships prior to applying a multiple regression approach.

In Table 4 the coefficients of determination for varying sets of predictors are presented relative to each of our five dependent variables separately for group and nongroup practitioners. Models 1 to 6 use as predictors the six sets of independent variables shown in Table 3 (A-F), and in each case the variables within the set are introduced in order of the magnitude of their contribution to the coefficient of determination. The coefficients shown in Table 4 include only variables that account for significant changes in the coefficient of determination at the .05 level.

In Model 1 all of the explained variance is attributed to the single measure of the physician's estimate of his own liberal-conservative outlook. Once this variable is taken account of, political party affiliation does not significantly contribute to the coefficient of determination. As Table 4 shows, political orientation is a more powerful predictor of overall receptivity and receptivity to federal financing and organized practice than it is of attitudes toward peer review or physician extenders. But in each case, political affiliation alone can account for a significant proportion of the variance explainable using all 38 predictors (see the results for Model 8). For example, introducing all 38 variables, using the .05 level as a criterion for inclusion, explains 36.5 percent of the variance in overall receptivity among group practitioners; political orientation alone explains 18.9 percent of the variance. Although political orientation only explains 2.5 percent of the variance in receptivity to peer review among nongroup physicians, the total explainable variance, using all 38 predictors, is less than 14 percent.

---

* Several of the independent variables involving nominal categories are handled as dummy variables: for example, subspecialty and region of practice.

† The question was worded: "Which one of the following best describes your present political views?" Alternative responses were very liberal, somewhat liberal, somewhat conservative, and very conservative.

Table 3 Zero-Order Correlations between Various Independent Variables and Measures of Receptivity to Organizational Change

	Overall Receptivity		Financing		Organized Practice		Peer Review		Physician Extenders	
Independent Predictors[a]	Group	Non-group	Group	Non-group	Group	Non-group	Group	Non-group	Group	Non-group
A. Political Orientation										
1. Describes oneself as liberal	43	38	35	36	36	35	24	16	24	22
2. Describes oneself as a Democrat	25	20	22	24	24	20	11	07	11	08
3. Describes oneself as a Republican	-28	-19	-26	-22	-24	-20	-15	-08	-15	-06
Social Background, Experience, and Life Style										
4. Reported income (high)	-27	03	-21	-03	-28	-07	-10	08	-10	08
5. Years in practice (high)	-15	-17	-02	-00	-13	-13	-09	-20	-09	-12
6. Father's education (high)	06	-08	03	-01	03	-08	07	-08	07	-05
7. Sex—male	-13	02	-05	02	-16	00	-03	00	-14	01
8. Father's occupational prestige (high)	-01	07	-01	-00	03	06	-04	06	-04	05
9. Protestant	-23	-11	-18	-16	-17	-11	-19	-05	-19	-01
10. Catholic	03	-03	-02	-00	-05	-03	11	-00	11	-05

Table 3 (Continued)

Independent Predictors[a]	Measures of Receptivity									
	Overall Receptivity		Financing		Organized Practice		Peer Review		Physician Extenders	
	Group	Non-group	Group	Non-group	Group	Non-group	Group	Non-group	Group	Non-group
11. Jewish	15	10	14	13	21	11	01	02	01	04
12. Has had government service	05	14	−02	04	09	07	02	16	08	10
B. *Community and Practice Structure*										
13. Northeast	14	08	12	10	12	11	10	02	03	−02
14. North Central	−04	−05	05	−06	05	−05	−04	−05	−08	03
15. South	−15	−12	−15	−10	−15	−10	−09	−07	−06	−06
16. West	07	11	−02	09	−02	06	05	11	11	04
17. General Practitioner	−16	−22	−06	−10	−16	−18	−13	−20	−06	−09
18. Internist	15	14	09	06	08	11	16	12	08	08
19. Pediatrician	10	16	02	09	11	15	10	11	02	09
20. High number of other doctors in practice	36	12	15	05	39	11	26	10	17	05
21. Size of community (large)	10	11	−03	08	12	14	07	03	07	05
22. Major source of income—fee-for-service versus other	−28	−15	−13	−13	−39	−15	−05	−08	−21	−05

C. *Practice Pressures*

23. High number of total patient consultations—previous day	−32	−07	−16	−07	−27	−11	−23	−02	−23	01
24. High number of patients seen at office on previous day	−14	−04	−14	−08	−11	−07	−03	02	−03	01
25. High number of office patients on a busy day	−24	−09	−14	−09	−18	−14	−15	−03	−15	02
26. Total hours—typical week	−20	−08	−15	−08	−17	−17	−13	05	−13	−02

D. *Medical Training and Practice Behavior*

27. High number of diagnostic procedures used	−09	−00	−07	−03	−14	−04	03	04	03	04
28. More organized course work taken	−04	03	−10	01	−05	02	−04	05	03	03
29. Amount of postgraduate training (high)	08	06	−02	03	11	09	06	03	07	00
30. Specialty boards membership	17	−01	07	12	18	18	09	20	11	14
31. Broad range of practice activities	07	10	−02	05	06	12	05	10	11	−01
32. High number of particular medical procedures performed	31	17	13	12	13	18	21	10	25	04

E. *Doctors' Satisfaction and Attitudinal Orientations*

33. Positive attitudes toward social aspects of practice	07	14	02	06	07	09	07	14	07	10
34. High general satisfaction	−07	−08	−04	−09	−09	−14	01	00	01	00

79

Table 3 (Continued)

Independent Predictors[a]	Measures of Receptivity									
	Overall Receptivity		Financing		Organized Practice		Peer Review		Physician Extenders	
	Group	Non-group	Group	Non-group	Group	Non-group	Group	Non-group	Group	Non-group
35. Positive attitude toward sacrifice	-12	-05	-03	02	-10	-05	-12	-07	-12	00
36. Agrees there is uncertainty in general practice	19	15	16	16	18	15	08	05	08	06
F. *Professional Affiliations*										
37. Membership in local medical society	-30	-12	-09	-12	-31	-12	-23	-04	-23	-07
38. Membership in specialty societies	-12	-03	-12	00	-15	-01	01	02	-06	02

[a] Positive correlation indicates that the predictor variable is associated with higher receptivity.

For each of our five dependent variables there are two comparisons, one for group practitioners and one for nongroup practitioners. In seven of the ten possible comparisons among the models, the single political orientation measure is the most powerful predictor. Model 3, including community and practice structure variables, is most influential in explaining overall receptivity among group practitioners. Five variables contribute to the coefficient of determination of 19.7 percent: number of other doctors in practice (12.7 percent), major source of income other than fee for service (2.9 percent), practice located in the Northeast (1.6 percent), internist (1.1 percent), and pediatrician (1.4 percent). Similarly, Model 3 is most influential in explaining receptivity to organized practice among group practitioners. Four variables in this model account for the coefficient of determination of 25.3 percent; major source of income other than fee for service (15.3 percent); number of other doctors in practice (7.4 percent), practice located in Northeast (1.2 percent), and pediatrician (1 percent). Model 3 also is the most influential model in accounting for receptivity to peer review, although the total coefficients of determination obtained were small. In the case of group practice, three predictors explained 9.7 percent of the variance: number of other doctors in group (6.5 percent), internist (2 percent), and pediatricians (1.2 percent). Among nongroup practitioners, three variables accounted for 5.7 percent of the variance: less years in practice (3.9 percent), government service (1.5 percent), and lower income (.3 percent). Table 3 also presents Models 9 to 14 in which political orientation is first introduced as a fixed component, followed by each of Models 2 to 7.

In examining Models 9 to 14 it is useful to use Models 1 and 8 as a comparison. Model 1 shows the effect of political orientation alone, while Model 8 shows the effect of all of the variables involved in the study. Models 9 to 14 illustrate that once political orientation has been taken into account, Models 2 to 7 have only limited additional effect in accounting for the receptivity measures. Of these models, Model 3 has the greatest additional influence, particularly in regard to the overall receptivity measure, and among group practitioners.

Table 5 gives the changes in the coefficients of determination, resulting from the introduction of political orientation after taking into account all other significant effects contributed by the other 37 predictors. As the table shows, the liberal-conservative dimension adds significantly to the variance explained even when all of the other significant factors are first taken into account. The influence of the political orientation measure is similarly reflected by the standardized regression coefficients for each dependent variable, taking into account all other significant predictors of that variable. In eight of the ten comparisons the standardized regression coefficient is higher for political orientation than for any of the other variables. The only exception involves the peer review index for group and nongroup practitioners. But even in these

Table 4 Coefficients of Determination[a] for Sets of Independent Predictors Relative to Measures of Receptivity (Per Cent)

		Overall Receptivity		Financing		Organized Practice		Peer Review		Physician Extenders	
		Group	Non-group	Group	Non-group	Group	Non-group	Group	Non-group	Group	Non-group
Model 1	Political orientation measures	18.9	14.4	12.3	13.7	12.7	12.2	5.5	2.5	6.2	4.7
Model 2	Social background, experience, and life style	13.1	6.6	9.0	3.7	12.2	5.3	3.7	5.7	4.4	2.4
Model 3	Community and practice structure	19.7	10.5	5.1	5.2	25.3	9.4	9.8	5.9	4.5	1.6
Model 4	Practice pressures	10.0	0.8	2.6	1.2	7.4	3.9	5.3	0.0	4.4	0.0
Model 5	Medical training and practice behavior	9.8	6.3	1.7	1.9	8.1	4.4	6.2	4.5	2.4	1.9
Model 6	Doctors' satisfactions and attitudinal orientations	5.0	5.3	2.6	3.8	3.3	4.8	1.3	2.9	1.2	1.5
Model 7	Professional affiliations	8.9	1.4	1.5	1.4	10.2	1.5	5.1	0.0	3.1	4.4
Model 8[b]	All variables free	36.5	27.0	20.1	19.3	33.9	23.3	14.1	13.6	14.3	8.5
Model 9[c]	Model 1 fixed; followed by variables in Model 2	23.8	18.5	15.6	14.0	19.6	15.0	7.7	8.0	10.5	7.2
Model 10	Model 1 fixed; followed by variables in Model 3	29.8	20.9	15.1	16.2	30.2	17.8	12.5	8.1	9.9	6.2
Model 11	Model 1 fixed; followed by variables in Model 4	23.9	15.0	13.3	14.2	16.3	15.1	9.3	2.9	9.6	4.9
Model 12	Model 1 fixed; followed by variables in Model 5	25.0	18.8	13.3	14.2	17.7	15.1	10.6	6.3	8.2	6.2

| Model 13: | Model 1 fixed; followed by variables in Model 6 | 22.4 | 17.9 | 15.4 | 16.0 | 16.0 | 15.9 | 6.4 | 4.7 | 6.7 | 5.7 |
| Model 14 | Model 1 fixed; followed by variables in Model 7 | 24.4 | 15.4 | 13.3 | 14.6 | 19.6 | 13.5 | 9.7 | 2.5 | 8.4 | 4.9 |

[a] For Models 1–8, coefficients of determination are based only on variables achieving statistical significance at the .05 level.

[b] In Model 8, all variables are free, allowing the program to select the predictors ordered by the degree to which they contribute to changes in the coefficient of determination. The coefficient of determination shown includes only those variables achieving statistical significance at the .05 level.

[c] Models 9–14—Include Model 1 fixed; followed by the introduction of the remaining variables in free form, ordered by the degree to which they contribute to the coefficient of determination. The coefficient of determination includes the total of the political orientation measures regardless of whether they achieve statistical significance. Additional variables are included only if they reach the .05 level.

Table 5 Additional Contribution of Political Orientation to the Coefficient of Determination for Receptivity Measures Following the Introduction of All Other Significant Predictors (Per Cent)

Measures of Receptivity	Additional Contribution to Coefficient of Determination by Political Orientation
1. Overall receptivity	
Group practitioners	8.3
Nongroup practitioners	8.6
2. Receptivity to federal financing	
Group practitioners	6.8
Nongroup practitioners	7.5
3. Receptivity to organized practice	
Group practitioners	4.7
Nongroup practitioners	6.6
4. Receptivity to peer review	
Group practitioners	2.0
Nongroup practitioners	1.4
5. Receptivity to physician extenders	
Group practitioners	3.8
Nongroup practitioners	3.5

cases the standardized regression coefficient is approximately as high as the other significant predictors. Almost identical results (Table 6) were obtained by using partial correlation coefficients. In examining other findings relevant to the various dependent measures, we find no other variables that are consistently important, although some are quite influential in specific cases.

Since political orientation is a crucial predictor in this study, it is interesting to review its most important correlates. As mentioned earlier, it was highly correlated with political party identification and absorbed the entire effect of party identification on receptivity to organizational change. Also, as expected on the basis of many other studies, Jewish doctors were more likely to be on the liberal side,[3,4] and Protestant doctors were more likely to be of conservative persuasion. More liberal doctors were most likely to come from larger communities and the Northeast. They were also more likely to be in group practice, particularly in larger groups and in groups on nonfee-for-service arrangements. Doctors in group practice who were more liberal also saw fewer patients, had a more limited scope of practice, had lower incomes, and were less likely to be members of their local medical societies. They were more likely to believe that physicians have responsibility to advise and care for the psychological problems of patients and that it is proper for government officials to evaluate the care patients receive. In both group and nongroup practice, physicians in internal medicine and those who had passed specialty

Table 6   Partial Correlation Coefficients and Standardized Regression Coefficients Describing the Relationships between Political Orientation and Receptivity Measures

Measures of Receptivity	Partial Correlation Coefficient[a]	Standardized Regression Coefficient	Number of Variables in Equation
1. Overall receptivity			
Group practitioners	.34	.31	8
Nongroup practitioners	.33	.30	14
2. Receptivity to federal financing			
Group practitioners	.28	.29	9
Nongroup practitioners	.29	.30	13
3. Receptivity to organized practice			
Group practitioners	.26	.23	7
Nongroup practitioners	.28	.27	16
4. Receptivity to peer review			
Group practitioners	.15	.16	7
Nongroup practitioners	.12	.12	8
5. Receptivity to physician extenders			
Group practitioners	.21	.20	5
Nongroup practitioners	.19	.19	8

[a] These data are, of course, redundant. They are provided for the reader's convenience.

boards were more liberal, while general practitioners were more conservative. Also in both types of practice, more liberal physicians agreed that the growing tendency for people to bring less serious disorders to doctors and to seek help more readily for their problems in their family lives was a good trend; these associations were modest, however.

It is clear from the analysis that the physician's political-philosophical orientation is the most consistent and most substantial predictor of our dependent measures of receptivity to organizational innovations. This orientation is more influential on the overall index, on federal financing, and on organized practice than it is on the issues involving peer review and physician extenders. In contrast, such independent variables as amount of postgraduate education, taking refresher courses, and the like had almost no predictive value at all. This suggests that the sophistication of the physician in terms of training had little to do with receptivity to organizational innovations.

Doctors in group practice, in contrast to nongroup physicians, are more favorable to all ten indicators of organizational innovation involved in this study (see Table 1). Among group practitioners the most important predictor, other than political orientation, is the number of other physicians involved in the practice. On three of the indices—overall receptivity, organized practice, and peer review—there is a substantial relationship between the number of physicians in the group and receptivity. Two other important factors among group physicians were lower income and receiving one's income in a form other than fee-for-service. Doctors with lower incomes were higher on overall receptivity, federal financing, and organized practice; and doctors on payment bases, other than fee-for-service, were more receptive to organized practice and physician extenders. These findings may reflect that doctors with lower incomes and doctors on salary perceive that they have less to lose in the implementation of organizational innovations.

Among nongroup practitioners it was more difficult to find strong and consistent predictors other than political orientation. There was, however, a limited consistency. On three of the indices—overall receptivity, peer review, and physician extenders—doctors who were more receptive tended to have a broader conception of the physician's role as measured by the types of consultations that they felt were justified. Also, on two of the indices, receptivity to peer review and physician extenders, physicians who had their specialty boards were more receptive. These results are consistent with the notion that physicians who wish to practice in a more focused way and those with specialty qualifications are less threatened by peer review and more willing to delegate tasks of little interest to them. Generally, with the exception of political orientation, the predictors of receptivity among group practitioners were quite different than among nongroup practitioners.

Thus, the findings reported here have clearly documented the hypothesis that receptivity to organizational innovations in the delivery of health care is significantly related to the political-philosophical orientation of physicians. Moreover, it is the only variable that consistently yields substantial correlations among different dimensions of receptivity and between group and non-group practitioners. This finding is not surprising or profound, but its implications are important. The debate over the future organization of health care is fundamentally a social and political discussion and not one to be determined solely on the basis of physicians' views of their work or their presumption of technical competence in this area. The future of medical-care delivery must be determined in terms of public goals and research establishing the effects of varying organizational arrangements relative to these goals.

Notes

1. Colombotos, J. (1969). "Physicians and Medicare: A Before-After Study on the Effects of Legislation on Attitudes." *American Sociological Review*, **34**:318–334.
2. Pastore, N. (1948). *The Nature-Nurture Conflict*. New York: King's Crown Press.
3. Colombotos, J. (1969). "Social Origins and Ideology of Physicians: A Study of the Effects of Early Socialization." *Journal of Health and Social Behavior*, **10**:16–29.
4. Babbie, E. (1970). *Science and Morality in Medicine*. Berkeley: University of California Press.

CHAPTER VII

Doctors in Revolt: The Crisis in the English National Health Service*

Medical activities are presently organized more for the convenience of the medical practitioner than to maximize the distribution and effectiveness of health-care delivery. As the nation comes to consider new patterns of organization and provision of services, these inevitably will be a threat to many physicians. There is growing evidence of trade union activity among physicians, and we should be prepared to anticipate that doctors will perceive social change as threatening. We, therefore, must consider how change can be brought about with minimum acrimony. It is inevitable that, if physicians should become too threatened, they will use whatever power and influence they have to thwart change or to subvert change once it occurs.

Hopefully, it is possible to learn from experience and the errors of others. In this chapter a dispute that developed between British general practitioners and the Ministry of Health is examined within the English context. The type of collective action characterizing this dispute is likely to become more prevalent, and it is important to try to minimize the destructive consequences that result from such open clashes. Whatever one's views may be on appropriate organization of medical care, it is clear that low morale among physicians is unlikely to contribute to high-quality care. While it is important to weigh physicians satisfaction against other factors, such as accessibility of care and meeting the nation's needs, any adequate system must insure that the varying roles that physicians play are reasonably rewarding and meaningful. The consequences of giving too little attention to these issues are reflected in the dispute described below.

* Adapted from a paper coauthored with Ronald G. Faich, which appeared in *Medical Care*, **8:** 442–455 (November-December, 1970).

In 1965 Britain was threatened with the withdrawal of its general practitioners from the National Health Service. Although the Health Service had been no stranger to vigorous and disruptive disputes, the 1965 conflict over remuneration and other terms of service approached revolt. As the acrimonious climate heightened, it became clear that the doctors were united as never before and that there was at least a significant segment among them that was quite prepared to bring the National Health Service to a standstill.

This chapter deals with a general issue of sociologic relevance heretofore neglected in sociologic inquiry: Under what conditions do some members of an organized professional group break ranks in situations where the profession is engaged in conflict with outside agencies concerning the conditions of service? Since such a large majority of the general practitioners in Britain were willing to submit undated resignations to their professional organization, by isolating the segment of doctors who did not, we can begin to effectively locate some of the conditions under which a professional front is broken.

Climate of the Dispute in the National Health Service

A short summary of remuneration issues and negotiations is necessary to depict the climate that characterized the situation at the time of the dispute. The continuous difficulties over remuneration that had plagued the Health Service since its inception led the Royal Commission on Doctors' and Dentists' Remuneration to recommend in 1962 that a standing body be set up for long-term and periodic income reviews.[1] Although this review body was to be independent of both the Ministry and the professional groups, it was acceptable to both. The body was expected to make recommendations on income levels to the Prime Minister every three years, thus regularizing possibilities for the adjustment of remuneration. To facilitate its deliberations, the Review Body requested that the medical profession submit a joint claim on behalf of all the National Health Service doctors (both general practitioners and consultants).* This brought to the forefront a continuing problem within the profession itself —the disagreements concerning the appropriate relative money values to be placed on the work of each of the two major medical roles. The need to present a joint claim raised bitter disputes among the doctors as to the proper differentials between GP and consultant, and seriously weakened the unity and position of the British Medical Association. When the Review Body made its first report in March 1963, it recommended an across-the-board increase of 14 percent for all doctors; it appeared unwilling to direct itself to the difficult question of differentials. On the face of it, one would have expected the doctors

---

* Consultants are doctors who practice their specialities primarily in hospitals. General practioners are, for the most part, excluded from hospital practice.

to be pleased with the award; and at first they appeared to be, but the GPs soon recognized that the manner in which they were paid would result in a net increase which was far less than the one received by consultants. Stevens[2] describes their thinking:

As the weeks went by they became progressively more uneasy, as many for the first time began to comprehend the ramifications of the global pool. There were two important factors. First, although the agreed net income of the average GP was to be increased by 14 percent (from £2,425 to £2,765), his gross income would not increase by this amount. At least one third of the ordinary GP's total income went on expenses, which were not to receive the same boost. Thus the 14 percent applied only to part of his income. The sum involved was not large, but the principle assumed enormous importance in the eyes of individuals. Second, and of greater importance, it was found that increased fee scales had already overdrawn the pool. GPs had been receiving overall a greater amount than that allowed for their average income. Thus a proportion of the 14 percent increase (£2.7 million out of a total of £7.6 million) had already been paid out. Another £0.8 million had to be left in the global pool in respect of increased earnings from other sources (e.g., hospital work). This left only £4.1 million to be distributed through raised capitation and other general medical fees: the individual GP would receive no more than a 7 or 8 percent increase in his net pay, and only 5 or 6 percent increase in relation to his gross income, including expenses. To the average GP it seemed that the consultant had received more from the Review Body than he had. General practitioners were already sensitive about their relative status, and the results of the award seemed a further blow. What made it worse [was] that this was not the fault of the Review Body or of the government, but of the pool system —and the calculations, being logical in terms of the system, had been agreed to by the GP's own nominees on the joint working party. Thus the growing resentment of GPs was frustrated by the lack of any villain but their own leaders.

The impact of the Review Body's March 1963 award was to exacerbate a feeling already existing among GPs that the British Medical Association was representing the consultants' interests against those of the general practitioner. It left the general practitioner discontented and stimulated his sense of status deprivation relative to his consultant colleagues. In October 1963, the General Practitioners' Association was formed to capture the reins of leadership from the BMA who, it maintained, was not vigorous enough in pursuing the claims of the GP. During this same period, the BMA was doing what it could to maintain its position as the representative of all doctors. After bitter disputes within the organization itself, a new memorandum was drafted to the Review Body asking them to upgrade general practice and GP income by approximately 18 million pounds a year. However, by this time, the fires of the general practitioners' discontent were well fanned, and the revolt of the more vocal GPs was on its way—a revolt not only against the National Health Service but also against the leadership of the British Medical Association. As the Review Body considered the doctors' case, the turmoil continued unabated.

Before the Review Body reported again, the Labor Party—in opposition since 1951—regained power in October 1964. Although Labor was friendly to the improvement of the Health Service, the country was operating under a strained budget. It was not clear that the Government was ready to give the Health Service highest priority for vast new appropriations over other pressing economic and social needs. However, the Labor Party had promised in its campaign to remove the two shilling prescription charge which patients were required to pay, and this promise was soon fulfilled after the Labor Government took office. This move embittered many GPs, who felt the Government's priorities were distorted; they argued that this action worsened their situation by stimulating additional patient demand. From their perspective, the Government was adding additional burdens to their already heavy work load. Although the Government took a friendly attitude toward the doctors and their problems, the elimination of prescription charges, buttressed by the suspicions of the politically conservative doctors toward a Labor Government, appeared to bring down any semblance of gentlemanly debate.

In January 1965, the Medical Practitioners' Union, coalescing elements of both the political left and right, encouraged the threat of withdrawal from the National Health Service. This idea appealed to many GPs, and already individual groups of doctors were making plans to submit their resignations if the Review Body did not produce according to demand. In early February, the Review Body rejected the contention that GP remuneration had been seriously inadequate. Although it recommended an increase of 5 1/2 million pounds, the amount fell far short of the requested adjustments costing in the vicinity of 18 to 20 million pounds. Moreover, rather than being distributed among all the doctors, the bulk of the 5 1/2 million pounds was to be used for new expense schemes.

The Review Body's report threatened even further the leadership of the British Medical Association and left it in the precarious position of losing its ability to speak for the doctors. The two more militant groups of doctors—the General Practitioners' Association and the Medical Practitioners' Union— were already encouraging their members to withdraw from the National Health Service if their demands were not met. The BMA had no course but to follow, and it began collecting undated resignations from its constituents through the British Medical Guild. Although the BMA attempted to temper its new initiative by emphasizing that it had no intention of sabotaging the National Health Service, it was clear that a significant segment of the doctors was in open revolt and that the BMA was doing its best to maintain its control. By March 17, 1965, the British Medical Guild had received 16,500 potential resignations from the nation's 22,000 general practitioners with the intention that these would be submitted by April 1.[3]

The prospects of fragmented medical leadership and the attack on the leadership of the British Medical Association were viewed with considerable concern by the Health Ministry. Since 1948, the Ministry had developed workable relationships with BMA spokesmen,[4] whom the Ministry could negotiate with in a regularized fashion and who, it knew, negotiated responsibly. Moreover, the Health Service was the creation of the Labor Government, and there is little question but that Labor felt pride in it and wished to maintain its status. The new Minister of Health, Mr. Robinson, publicly expressed his willingness to discuss ways of improving both general practice and methods of remuneration, and he disavowed responsibility for the turmoil which he attributed to warring factions of doctors in competition with one another. There was little question but that he was concerned with improving general practice and alleviating doctors' feelings of discontent, if only the doctors could agree on a politically and economically viable alternative to the structure of general practice as it existed. But the doctors were in a militant mood, and it was clear that the alternatives they were supporting were not acceptable, especially the ideas of a "fee-for-service" and disciplinary controls on patients. By March 1965, the BMA drafted a "Charter for the Family Doctor Service" which was used as a basis for discussion with the Ministry. The core of the Charter was based on the notion that doctors be paid according to their work and that their contractual obligations to the Health Service be based on a specified workweek with additional payments for assuming further responsibility. The discussions of the Charter were to serve as the basis for the new system of remuneration which was accepted by the Review Body in its report of May 1966.

If one were to solely consider the economic context of the dispute, the doctors' discontent would be difficult to understand. The contention that the differential in income between general practitioners and consultants had increased cannot be supported; indeed, there is considerable evidence that the differential had decreased.[5] Moreover, general practitioners' incomes compared favorably with the earnings of other professionals in Great Britain. The Review Committee in its report of March 1966 was unconvinced that medical earnings were substantially lower than they should be, and the generous award to doctors was made on a rather different rationale.[6] Why, then, should the general practitioner exhibit such a belligerent disposition in relation to his situation and to the National Health Service? Several factors are at once apparent.

Doctors were paid via a pool payment system, constructed on the concept of a fixed average net income.[7] Money in the pool was distributed on the basis of a complicated formula—the main component of which was a weighted capitation payment. When the Health Service originated, doctors strongly opposed the concept of a salary and supported the pool payment system. It became increasingly evident to the GP, however, that under this setup the more work he undertook, the less he earned per unit of work. In recent years, the number of general practitioners relative to the population has declined, thus resulting in a higher patient load per doctor. In 1964 and 1965, years in which much of the controversy was developing, the number of doctors in general practice decreased by 322.[8] Thus, although the average doctor was caring for a larger number of patients and devoting greater effort to his practice, the pool from which he was paid was constructed on the basis of the number of doctors rather than of the amount of work. Furthermore, the pool did not take account of changing patterns of utilization, the changing age structure of the population, and other factors that affected demand and the doctor's work load. Finally, the pool system produced a variety of inequities, depending on the viewpoint and situation of the evaluator. Thus, almost every doctor could recognize some way in which he was penalized by the pool system.

Another factor contributing to discontent was a feeling of deprivation relative to general practitioners in other English-speaking countries and to consultants within the National Health Service. As the shortage of doctors increased throughout the world, efforts were made to recruit British doctors; and medical professional journals in Britain carried numerous advertisements—especially from the United States—attempting to attract doctors by offering higher incomes, better facilities, and more responsibility than is generally available to them. During the period of dispute, the number of British doctors who had emigrated was substantial,[9] and most doctors could cite some acquaintance who was thriving in the United States, Canada, or Australia. The knowledge that more doctors were emigrating, leaving the British GP behind with more work than ever before, exacerbated the doctors' feelings of deprivation. The Review Body may have been quite right in noting that doctors were adequately rewarded in relation to other professionals in Britain, but other professionals in Britain were not the doctors' reference group.

If there was a reference group for the GPs, it was the consultants. Not only did they receive higher incomes and prestige, but also the continuing advances in medical technology sharpened the distinction between more prestigious hospital work and the uncertainty and ambiguity of the role of the general practitioner. At the same time, the consumer had become more knowledgeable about medical practice and more critical of medical services. Although there is no evidence that the average Britisher had any less respect for the general practitioner than in previous times, the professional groups in Britain view GPs with less esteem than does the working man.[10] But given the class background of the typical doctor, it is the professional man's esteem to which he is attuned. Moreover, the hostilities within the British Medical Association concerning financial differentials between the general practitioner and the consultant, stimulated by the need to present a joint claim for the whole profession which we have already reviewed, increased the salience of the entire matter and offered the general practitioners an issue on which to focus their discontent.

Finally, it is important to note that little progress had been made in defining more clearly the general practitioner's role in what is clearly a new era in scientific medicine. In October 1963, when the dispute was beginning to brew, a distinguished official committee headed by Annis Gillie reported to the Minister of Health on *The Field of Work of the Family Doctor.*[11] Abundant with high ideals and platitudes but short on facts, this report was most striking in its irrelevance to the true condition of the National Health Service. It rehashed and reintroduced many of the pet schemes which had been discussed since 1948 but which had not elicited serious interest among the doctors or their representatives. It was not at all clear how the lofty aims and aspirations of this committee could be implemented without radically changing the structure of the Health Service and opinion within the medical profession itself.

The stance encouraged by the Gillie report, as well as by many other appraisals, was that the general practitioner has a unique role in dealing with the social and psychologic problems of patients as well as in serving as a "first line of defense in times of illness, disability, and distress...." Few such advocates, however, have been able to specify how such a stance might be effectively communicated to the doctor except in the grossest generalities. Since medical education in Britain is extremely conservative and based predominantly on hospital practice, the average doctor has not assimilated such socially benevolent views. He too frequently shows the values of the medical school, which place greatest emphasis on the diagnosis and treatment of less common disorders rather than on those most frequently seen in general practice. It is difficult to see how the general practitioners' concept of their role can be changed without a prior major change in British medical education.[12]

The Research Study

On April 1, 1966, a randomly chosen sample of 1500 general practitioners in England and Wales, with unrestricted practices, was sent a long questionnaire dealing with their satisfactions and dissatisfactions, the organization of their practices, their attitudes toward medical care, their work load, and many other issues of relevance to the organization of general practice within the National Health Service. Since it was necessary to use the sampling frame from October 1, 1964, the sample of 1500 doctors yielded 1356 eligible respondents (84 percent) after excluding doctors who died, retired, left general practice, or moved from one Executive Council to another before April 1,

1966. After three communications, 60 percent of the eligible respondents returned completed questionnaires. On the fourth approach to the doctor, a shorter questionnaire was sent, and an additional 13 percent responded, yielding a total response rate of 73 percent on many key items. Basic demographic data on all doctors in the sample and the total population were provided by the Ministry of Health. This allowed for an analysis of differences between respondents and nonrespondents, and comparisons among the various waves of response allowed an analysis of doctors' views in relation to the timing of their response.

In all, the respondents constituted a good approximation of all of the doctors in the sample and in the general population. Although there is insufficient space to go into the details of our analysis here, we find that our respondents include some over-representation of young doctors, doctors in larger partnerships, and those who tend to be dissatisfied. We estimate the over-representation of such doctors at most as 10 percent in comparison with the sample and the population.

Results

The data in this paper pertain to the correlates of the doctors' reports of whether they submitted their undated resignations to the British Medical Guild in 1965 when they were requested. Of our sample, 78 percent reported that they submitted their resignation, 20 percent that they did not, and 1 percent failed to respond to the question.* The resignation rate derived for the sample is reasonably close to the 75 to 80 percent figure reported in the National Press during the period of the survey.

It should be clear that the act of submitting an undated resignation had various meanings to different doctors and that this act resulted from diverse motives. In two pretests of earlier versions of the questionnaire, among approximately 75 doctors, we asked each doctor who submitted his resignation to explain why he did so. Although a majority discussed dissatisfaction with conditions of service, professional unity and the need to support one's colleagues were frequently mentioned. Moreover, doctors appeared to differ in their perceptions of the consequences of this action. While many saw submitting undated resignations as a political move to influence the Government and strengthen the hand of the doctors' negotiators, others were quite prepared to see their resignations used in breaking away from the National Service. While some were convinced they would never be used and were quite prepared to

---

* Since continuing opportunity was available for the doctors to submit their resignation at the time the study took place, there is no reason to anticipate that doctors distorted their responses to this question in light of the need to provide a prestigious answer consistent with an event that occurred in the past, as frequently happens in postelection surveys.

withdraw them if this eventuality occurred, others perceived the resignations as a final drastic step. Several typical comments follow:

I couldn't see any prospect at all of negotiations with the government leading anywhere in dealing with the needs of the Service. By resigning we could get a new contract with the government to attract new young doctors who are now emigrating in large numbers.

General practice had come to a dead end in this country as far as advancement had gone. Government was not putting money or effort into it. Only after the negotiating committee produced a reasonable charter, I thought it reasonable to submit my resignation if consideration to the charter was not given by the government. To help to force the government's hand.

Importance of taking a definite stand or course to impress the Minister that we were serious about the problems of general practice. . . .

The future development of Health Services in this country should be decided and guided by the wishes of patients and doctors, rather than politicians and social theorists.

Importance of a united front in order to get better conditions of general practice.

I hoped (vainly, it seems) that a new Health Service would be born.

In considering the data to be presented, it is important to keep in mind that submitting one's resignation was the most common form of behavior, and that those who withheld their resignations constituted the deviant group. Since the perceived conditions of service and the climate of opinion that prevailed during this period provided strong incentive for submitting one's resignation, it seems reasonable to inquire as to what differentiated those who did not resign from the majority.

We believe that we have located several significant sources of influence in the doctors' responses to the resignation request.

First, the doctor's response is related to the stake he had in the issues at hand. Since the crisis centered around the debate concerning remuneration, the doctor's view concerning this issue most closely captures his investment in the controversy. Those doctors who report that remuneration is a problem in general practice are much more likely to submit resignations than those who do not. It is important to emphasize that investment in the money issue is not the same as economic deprivation. Although doctors with more patients earned more money within the N.H.S., they were as likely to complain about remuneration as other doctors. There were other measures of investment as well; for example, older doctors were less likely to submit resignations than younger ones. It is clear that many of the older doctors did not feel any real investment in the dispute. Several doctors anticipating retirement remarked that it was not their battle, and the dispute was less likely to draw their energy or interest.

Second, we found that the doctor's response to the resignation request was related to the *nature of the demands the conditions of service made upon him.*

Table 1 Various Aspects of the Pattern of Work among British General Practitioners in Relation to Size of Practice

Items Describing Pattern of Work	Per Cent of Doctors Reporting Pattern of Work with Patient Loads of					
	Less than 1500 (30)	1500–1999 (63)	2000–2499 (177)	2500–2999 (217)	3000–3499 (192)	3500 or more (128)
Reports that the need to work rapidly and make spot diagnoses is a very serious problem	7	16	25	32	38	45
Reports that the number of patients he must assume responsibility for is a very serious problem	7	8	9	17	27	38
Reports that having sufficient time to tend adequately to his practice is a very serious problem	17	14	19	22	38	43
Reports that the amount of time he has for each patient is a very serious problem	7	16	28	34	47	45
Reports that he is very dissatisfied with the amount of time and effort he must devote to his practice	3	5	16	23	29	26
Reports that he is very dissatisfied with the amount of time he could give to his patients	10	24	34	43	51	54

| Reports of time pressure affecting behavior—high score[a] | 30 | 27 | 42 | 49 | 51 | 46 |
| Reports of time spent on social aspects of medical practice—high score[b] | 37 | 29 | 17 | 15 | 15 | 8 |

[a] This scale is based on two items in which the doctor reports how frequently during the past month he (1) didn't have time to do an adequate examination of the patient who required it and (2) didn't have time to do what he felt was necessary for the patient. The scores are divided into two groups separated as close to the median as possible.

[b] This scale is based on three items in which the doctor reports how frequently during the past month he (1) just let the patient talk on for a half hour or more to get things off his chest (2) he began a discussion with patients about psychological factors when they came for a prescription renewal; and (3) he had to spend a half hour or more exploring the patient's social and emotional background. The scores possible are divided into two groups above and below the average of the range of scores.

Table 2   Per Cent of British General Practitioners Who Did Not Submit Resignations, by Size of Practice and Emphasis on Remuneration as a Problem

Practice Size	Reports Amount of Remuneration He Receives	N	Per Cent of Doctors Who Did Not Submit Resignations
Less than 2000 patients	Not a problem	(9)	67
	A problem, but not serious	(21)	48
	A fairly serious problem	(24)	25
	A very serious problem	(38)	24
2000 to 2499 patients	Not a problem	(19)	58
	A problem, but not serious	(38)	37
	A fairly serious problem	(63)	22
	A very serious problem	(56)	11
2500 patients or more	Not a problem	(62)	26
	A problem, but not serious	(107)	22
	A fairly serious problem	(202)	16
	A very serious problem	(165)	8

The measure that captures this dimension most effectively is the number of patients the doctor looks after. Doctors with small practices were much less likely to submit resignations than those with larger ones. Doctors respond to large practices not by continually increasing their workday, but by practicing at a different pace and style which is particularly frustrating and uncongenial. They feel deprived not only in terms of the hours they devote to their patients, but more importantly in terms of the amount of work and effort they must pack into this period of time. Such a pattern of work requires them to practice on an assembly line basis which diminishes the unique satisfactions possible in a general practice. We included several behavioral items on our questionnaire which allowed us to gauge the extent to which the doctor's pace and pattern of work were affected by the size of his practice. All of the aspects of hurried practice—spot diagnoses, inability to provide enough time for patients, failure to do an adequate examination or undertake needed action, and the like— were related to size of practice (Table 1). The size of practice variable thus encompasses not only numbers of patients, but also the manner and pace of the doctor's work, and it exerts an influence on his entire outlook. An examination of Table 2 will show the independent effects of the remuneration issue and size of practice on the resignation rate, as well as their joint influence.

On further analysis, we found that most of the items concerning general dissatisfaction and reported problems involving number of patients, time, and money substantially differentiated those groups with a higher and lower rate of resignations. For example, among doctors reporting 18 or more very or fairly serious problems in general practice only 5 percent did not submit resig-

Table 3   Relationship between Scores on Various Attitudinal Scales and Per Cent of Doctors Who Did Not Submit Resignations

Attitudinal Scales	Doctors Who Did Not Submit Resignations (%)
Endorses sacrificing attitudes	
High ($N = 315$)	25
Intermediate ($N = 291$)	17
Low ($N = 179$)	15
Agrees that Health Ministry should assume responsibility for influencing general practice	
High ($N = 159$)	41
Intermediate ($N = 311$)	19
Low ($N = 298$)	13
Rejects traditional medical role conceptions	
High ($N = 89$)	34
Moderate high ($N = 257$)	19
Moderate low ($N = 322$)	16
Low ($N = 100$)	19
Agrees that patients ought to consult for nonmedical aspects	
On 7 or more items ($N = 275$)	28
On 5 or 6 items ($N = 290$)	20
On 4 or less items ($N = 213$)	12
Assuming that the same outcome could be achieved, prefers to treat	
An illness complicated by emotional factors ($N = 151$)	28
With a clear physical cause ($N = 621$)	18

Table 4   Relationship between Various Features of Medical Practice and Per Cent of Doctors Not Submitting Resignations

Items Describing Medical Practice	Doctors Who Did Not Submit Resignations (%)
Use of diagnostic facilities	
Used 5 or less in two weeks (N = 274)	21
Used 6-9 in two weeks (N = 327)	20
Used 10 or more in two weeks (N = 124)	21
Seeks advice from other medical men concerning his practice	
Every week or so (N = 343)	19
A couple of times a month (N = 127)	20
A few times a year or less (N = 327)	21
Has ancillary help	
Yes (N = 681)	18
Wife only (N = 39)	38
No (N = 76)	28
Receives ancillary help from local health authority	
Yes—full-time (N = 49)	16
Yes—part-time (N = 143)	20
No (N = 613)	21
Undertakes paid medical work in addition to general practice	
Yes (N = 547)	20
No (N = 259)	20
Has private patients in addition to health service patients	
Yes (N = 520)	20
No (N = 288)	21
Uses an appointment system	
Yes (N = 266)	21
No (N = 535)	20

nations, while 38 percent of those reporting 5 or less such problems did not. We also found that other generalized responses such as reporting problems concerning restrictions on practice, trivial complaints, the need to issue certificates, public attitudes toward doctors, paper work, and lack of leisure time were related to rates of resignation. Since these various problem items are substantially intercorrelated and most are associated, as well, with practice size, we shall not devote any further attention to them.

There were, however, other attitudinal dimensions that showed some relationship to the rate of submission of resignations. Doctors who endorsed attitudes favorable to the idea that they should be willing to sacrifice their interests and work long and irregular hours, those who felt the Health Ministry should assume responsibility for influencing general practice in various ways, those who failed to endorse traditional medical role conceptions, those who enjoyed working with illnesses complicated by emotional factors, and those who gave greater endorsement to the idea that patients would be justified in bringing nonmedical problems to the doctor had a higher rate of failing to submit resignations than doctors who could not be categorized in this way (Table 3).

Although there were substantial relationships between submitting a resignation and particular problems of practice involving time, money, and work, problems associated with the actual conditions of medical practice were for the most part unrelated to the rate of resignation. Resignation rates did not substantially differ in relation to the use of diagnostic facilities and to seeking advice from other medical men concerning practice, using local authority ancillary help, undertaking additional paid medical work, treating private patients, and using an appointment system; nor by the extent to which the doctor reported problems in the following areas: opportunities to work in cooperation with health authority workers, having to maintain continual responsibility for patients, opportunities to have professional contacts with colleagues, limited opportunities to work within a health center arrangement, provisions for obtaining necessary ancillary help, opportunities for maintaining adequate premises, access to diagnostic services and equipment, and opportunities to improve medical skills (Table 4, 5).

Third, we found that doctors who had little social contact with other doctors were less likely to submit resignations (Table 6). We believe that the social contact variable is an indicator of the degree to which the doctor is *exposed to social pressures.* Our measures of this variable, however, are difficult to interpret since they imply several possible alternative explanations. Since the debate and resignation movement received so much attention in the medical press and general mass media, it is certain that most doctors could become aware of the issues and politics of the situation without extensive informal contacts. Moreover, all doctors were circularized in the collection of resignations by the British Medical Guild. Thus, it seems unlikely that the informational import of informal social contacts could have been significant. Rather, we feel that the social contact measure reflects the degree to which the doctor was exposed to or insulated from colleague pressure. Since the mass of doctors were submitting resignations in a militant atmosphere and advocating

Table 5 Relationship between Various Features of Medical Practice and Per Cent of Doctors Not Submitting Resignations

			Per Cent of Doctors Who Did Not Submit Resignations Among Doctors Who Described Item as					
Items Describing Medical Practice	Not a Problem (Per Cent)	N	A Problem but Not Serious (Per Cent)	N	A Fairly Serious Problem (Per Cent)	N	A Very Serious Problem (Per Cent)	N
Opportunities to work in cooperation with health authority workers	21	(431)	19	(213)	15	(97)	17	(54)
Having to maintain continual responsibility for patients	22	(245)	23	(218)	15	(151)	17	(189)
Opportunities to have professional contacts with colleagues	19	(431)	22	(205)	17	(114)	25	(52)
Limited opportunities to work within a health center arrangement	22	(407)	16	(140)	18	(94)	19	(108)
Provisions for obtaining necessary ancillary help	25	(193)	24	(173)	16	(240)	17	(202)
Opportunities for maintaining adequate premises	23	(326)	22	(177)	12	(169)	19	(135)
Access to diagnostic services and equipment	21	(494)	18	(206)	16	(77)	25	(32)
Opportunities to improve medical skills	21	(170)	25	(198)	18	(266)	16	(171)

the need for a united front, doctors who were closely allied with other doctors, but who were uncertain about their decision, must have felt considerable social pressure to participate. Since the threat of withdrawal from the Health Service conflicted with professional values, a significant number of doctors probably felt some conflict when faced with a choice. Those who were isolated from significant social contact were more insulated from social pressures of the group and probably found it less difficult to resist submitting their resignations.

If our interpretation of the meaning of social contact is correct, it is reasonable to expect that social contact would be more influential when it is more intimate than when it is more work oriented. Our data tend to support this interpretation. Such measures as frequency of discussing medical problems with other doctors or seeking advice from other doctors concerning aspects of one's practice are much weaker in influencing resignations than partnership, friendship, and social contact. Coleman and his colleagues[13] come to a some-

Table 6 Contact with Other Doctors and Per Cent of Doctors Not Resigning (Per Cent)

Measures of Social Contact	Doctors Who Did Not Submit Resignations (%)
Works by himself (N = 155)	32
Works with partners (N = 653)	17
Gets together socially with other doctors in home	
Hardly ever (N = 173)	32
A few times a year (N = 343)	20
A couple of times a month or more (N = 287)	13
No doctors among three closest friends (N = 196)	31
At least one doctor among three closest friends (N = 605)	17
Socializes with other doctors at a club or other meeting place	
Hardly ever (N = 245)	27
A few times a year (N = 297)	20
A couple of times a month or more (N = 258)	14
Belongs to informal group of practitioners	
No (N = 649)	21
Yes (N = 147)	14

Table 7   Relationship between Aspects of Professional Involvement and Rate of Resignation

Professional Involvement Items	Doctors Who Did Not Submit Resignations (%)
Reads *The Lancet*—a high quality journal	
No ($N = 691$)	17
Skims ($N = 37$)	24
Reads at least selectively ($N = 79$)	43
Intensive specialized training since medical school in social medicine, well-baby care, psychiatry, or social science	
None ($N = 686$)	20
Some ($N = 40$)	28
Publications	
None ($N = 667$)	18
One or more ($N = 139$)	29
Medical diploma	
No ($N = 675$)	18
Yes ($N = 120$)	27
Paid or honorary appointment on staff of N.H.S. hospital	
No ($N = 530$)	18
Yes ($N = 281$)	25
Member of the College of General Practitioners	
No ($N = 580$)	19
Yes ($N = 220$)	23
Member of the Royal Society of Medicine	
No ($N = 775$)	20
Yes ($N = 25$)	32

what similar conclusion in respect to the influence of the drug detail man on the time of adoption of a new drug:

> ....whether a doctor adopted gammanym immediately after its appearance or sixteen months later, it was usually the detail man who, along with direct mail advertising, reached the doctor with the first news of the new development and performed the function of informing him. Subsequently, an increasing and perhaps evaluative role was played by sources within the profession (p. 63).

Table 8 Relationship between Professional Involvement and Per Cent of Doctors Not Submitting Resignations, Simultaneously Controlling for Practice Size, Report on Remuneration, and Social Contact with Other Doctors in Home

Doctor Reports That Amount of Remuneration	Social Contact With Other Doctors Is	Doctors Who Did Not Submit Resignations (Per Cent)	N		Not Submitting Resignations When Professional Involvement Is (Per Cent)	N
Is not a problem						
Practice size is:						
Less than 2000 patients	Low	100	(6)	Low	100	(2)
				High	100[a]	(4)
	High	0[a]	(3)	Low	0[a]	(1)
				High	0[a]	(2)
2000–2499 patients	Low	53	(15)	Low	56	(9)
				High	50	(6)
	High	75[a]	(4)	Low	100[a]	(1)
				High	67	(3)
2500 patients or more	Low	29	(48)	Low	52	(21)
				High	11	(27)
	High	14	(14)	Low	0	(8)
				High	33	(6)
Is a problem but not serious						
Practice size is:						
Less than 2000 patients	Low	37	(16)	Low	45	(11)
				High	20[a]	(5)
	High	80[a]	(5)	Low	100[a]	(2)
				High	67[a]	(3)

Table 8 (Continued)

Doctor Reports That Amount of Remuneration	Social Contact With Other Doctors Is	Doctors Who Did Not Submit Resignations (Per Cent)	N	Not Submitting Resignations When Professional Involvement Is	(Per Cent)	N
2000–2499 patients	Low	42	(24)	Low	56	(9)
				High	33	(15)
	High	31	(13)	Low	33a	(3)
				High	30	(10)
2500 patients or more	Low	30	(61)	Low	30	(20)
				High	29	(41)
	High	13	(46)	Low	11	(18)
				High	14	(28)
Is a fairly serious problem Practice size is:						
Less than 2000 patients	Low	31	(13)	Low	33	(6)
				High	29	(7)
	High	18	(11)	Low	0a	(5)
				High	33	(6)
2000–2499 patients	Low	24	(38)	Low	40	(10)
				High	18	(28)
	High	21	(24)	Low	14	(7)
				High	24	(17)
2500 patients or more	Low	21	(123)	Low	29	(51)
				High	15	(72)
	High	8	(78)	Low	20	(25)
				High	2	(53)

Is a very serious problem

Practice size is:

Less than 2000 patients	Low	26	(31)	Low	31	(13)
				High	22	(18)
	High	14	(7)	Low	25ᵃ	(4)
				High	0ᵃ	(3)
2000–2499 patients	Low	11	(35)	Low	30	(10)
				High	4	(25)
	High	10	(20)	Low	17	(12)
				High	0	(8)
2500 patients or more	Low	11	(101)	Low	17	(23)
				High	9	(78)
	High	3	(62)	Low	0	(19)
				High	5	(43)

[a] Percentage is based on five or less cases.

109

In our case, the doctor had to come to some decision as to whether participating in the threatened withdrawal from the Health Service was a proper professional stance. The judgment of one's closest colleagues appeared to be most influential in this decision.

We are still left with the possibility that the results obtained are a consequence of the fact that doctors who are isolated from medical social networks are in some ways different from those who are not. We have, therefore, explored in detail the factors that differentiate doctors with varying degrees of social contact with their colleagues. These differences cannot explain the influence of social contact on the rate of resignations.

Finally, although length of hospital training and postgraduate course work were unrelated to the rate of submitting resignations, there was some evidence that doctors with considerable "professional involvement" were less likely to submit resignations. Members of the Royal Society of Medicine, those holding medical diplomas, doctors who have published papers, those who have sought special training in general practice concerns such as psychiatry, and those who read *The Lancet*, a prominent medical academic journal, were less likely to submit resignations (Table 7). We believe that men having these characteristics were more likely to hold strong professional values and, therefore, experienced greater conflict when faced with the resignation request.

The range of variation on the basis of the factors we described was substantial. For example, when we take into account the first three factors, we find that among the 62 doctors with large practices who were concerned about money and who had a lot of contact with other doctors, 97 percent submitted resignations. Among the six doctors who had the opposite characteristics, none submitted resignations. The variations within these extremes followed a consistent pattern as an examination of Table 8 will show. When we add a fourth factor—professional involvement—controlling for the other three, the number of doctors in each group becomes very small. There are 24 comparisons between doctors of high and low involvement. Seventeen of these are in the predicted direction.

In commenting on the specific situation of the doctors, we would not want to miss the more general relevance of this study. Professional groups are showing greater militancy in fighting to protect their interests, and increasingly they are using various weapons that characterize trade unionism. In situations where a professional group presents a united front in some societal conflict, it is important to understand under what conditions some portion of the group breaks ranks. On the basis of our study, we would suggest that those professionals most likely to break ranks are: (1) those who have the least investment in the issues at stake; (2) those who face the least adverse work circumstances; (3) those who are most insulated from the social pressures of the mass, and (4) those who suffer the greatest conflict between the issue at hand and professional norms.

Notes

1. Stevens, R. (1966). *Medical Practice in Modern England.* New Haven: Yale University Press, pp. 127–138, 286–300.
2. Ibid., pp. 289–290.
3. Ibid., p. 312.
4. Eckstein, H. (1960). *Pressure Group Politics: The Case of the British Medical Association.* Stanford: Stanford University Press.
5. Stevens, R., op. cit., pp. 317–318.
6. Review Body on Doctors' and Dentists' Remuneration (1966). *Seventh Report.* Cmnd. 2992, London: Her Majesty's Stationery Office.
7. For an excellent summary of the pool system, see Eckstein, H., op. cit., pp. 128–130.
8. British Ministry of Health (1965). *Annual Reports 1964.* London: Her Majesty's Stationery Office.
9. Abel-Smith, D., and K. Gales (1964). *British Doctors at Home and Abroad.* Hertfordshire: Codicote Press. Occasional Papers on Social Administration, No. 8.
10. Cartwright, A. (1967). *Patients and Their Doctors: A Study of General Practice.* London: Routledge and Kegan Paul.
11. British Ministry of Health (1963). *The Field of Work of the Family Doctor.* Report of the Subcommittee of the Standing Medical Advisory Committee. London: Her Majesty's Stationery Office.
12. See McKeown, T. (1965). *Medicine in Modern Society.* London: George Allen and Unwin.
13. Coleman, J., et al. (1966). *Medical Innovation: A Diffusion Study.* Indianapolis: Bobbs-Merrill.

PART THREE

PATIENT EXPECTATIONS AND THE ORGANIZATION OF PRACTICE SYSTEMS

CHAPTER VIII

Patient Selection and
Practitioner Networks

There are large variations in the extent to which persons identify problems, become concerned about them, and seek assistance. These differences are dependent on the manner in which problems become manifest and their severity, on the social and cultural background of the persons involved, and on family and community contexts. Once problems become manifest, a wide variety of factors influences how they are defined, the alternative solutions available for dealing with them, and sources of perceived help. Whether the person comes into care at all or where he appears in the care network is related to forces well beyond the particular character of his symptoms.

Epidemiological studies of the occurrence of illness in populations suggest that symptoms and life problems have high prevalence. Only a small segment of illness occurring in the community is brought to the attention of medical practitioners, and the presentation of complaints and the timing of such presentations are usually problematic. Although a great deal of research remains to be undertaken on perceptions and definitions of complaints and the process of seeking help, there is growing evidence that suggests that an important motivation for seeking care involves the person's larger life context, social difficulties, and psychological distress. These frequently trigger the help-seeking process, although only the medical complaint may be apparent at the outset.

In the next chapter various aspects of the presentation of bodily complaints are explored. The presentation of complaints is complex and variegated, and we have hardly begun to understand, in any systematic fashion, the many ways in which patients come to relate to medical services. In the later discussion we feature two aspects of presentation: whether the person has or lacks a psychological vocabulary to symbolize the distress experienced; and the social and cultural constraints on varying types of expression. It is suggested that many patients seeking primary medical services are motivated by life difficulties and psychosocial problems, but do not feel free to deal openly with their underlying difficulties or do not perceive the nature of their discomfort. This problem confronts the primary care physician with the sensitive and difficult task of identifying underlying life problems, but in a manner that is helpful and does not threaten or alienate the patient.

Primary medical care, of course, has many functions, and dealing with underlying life difficulties contributing to morbidity is only one facet of care. The physician must balance varying activities involved in identifying disease states, assessing their significance, deciding on appropriate treatment approaches, and managing the patient, for example. Yet, the physician must also be sensitive to patients as individuals within a family and community context, since life situations are a major source of ill health and may be a major barrier to convalescence. If he treats the presentation of the patient solely at the manifest level, his treatment may be only symptomatic, and he frequently will fail to deal with the basic underlying difficulties that brought the patient to him.

Although we tend to think of the physician's actions in individual terms, they are conditioned as much by the practice system of which he is a part and by its assumptions, as the patient's behavior is influenced by social and cultural factors. The capacity of a physician to cope with the types of complaints common in primary medical practice depends partly on his training and the constraints of practice structures. The physician in a practice setting not only manages his patients but also must manage his time to insure that he will be able to see the various patients who are waiting. He must, to some extent, balance his efforts with any patient against the allocation of his day's work and his overall responsibilities. The nature of the work and how it presses on him will affect the way he approaches the individual patient and what he is able to do.

In Chapter 10 I give data on the correlates of frustration among primary care physicians. One aspect of physician frustration is to characterize patients' problems as trivial and inappropriate. There is little evidence to suggest that such attributions have any substantial relationship to patterns of morbidity or to special characteristics of specific patient populations. Instead, I suggest that the tendency to make such attributions tells us something about physicians and the conditions of their practice.

One of our strongest findings is that the attribution of triviality to patients is related to the number of patients the doctor sees within a specified period of time. In trying to understand this relationship, we are exploring the following line of thought. Physicians are frequently faced with patients who present diffuse complaints that are difficult to deal with expeditiously. Ideally, the physician must devote a good deal of time to talk with patients—to explore the happenings in their interpersonal and psychological lives, their feelings, and reactions. Even under ideal conditions this may be difficult for the physician because of his orientations and his limited training to deal with such matters. But when he has a large number of other patients waiting to see him, the pressure of the queue puts great restraints on his behavior. If he takes too much time, he is likely to complicate his day and perhaps even anger his waiting patients. Existing pressures demand that he take only limited time to explore the patient's problem, and thus he is inclined to treat the patient symptomatically. Doctors who are less busy have greater freedom to spend more time talking with patients and exploring the sources of their distress.

Chapter 9 examines the situation of the chronically complaining patient and possible factors related to the nature of these complaints. These patients are frequently designated as hypochondriacs but this concept, as used by many doctors, is an accusatory one. It constitutes a moral condemnation of the patient and a deprecation of his plea for help. Since the physician is the accusor, however, it is usually assumed that the difficulty resides with the patient rather than with the physician's frame of reference or the nature of the interaction that occurs between physician and patient.

Within the traditional approach to medicine, the patient presents a set of complaints, and the physician through his investigation attempts to account for, explain, or find justification for it. Logically, if not empirically, the diagnostic situation involves two sets of facts: historical data and symptoms reported by the patient or other information about his condition; and further data obtained by the physician through systematic examination for abnormal signs. It is possible for physicians to hypothesize that some patients are hypochondriacs or malingerers if they notice substantial discrepancies between the patient's complaints and other findings elicited through an investigation of the complaints. Logically, there are two sources for such discrepancies: (1) the patient, for whatever reason, may exaggerate, modify, or fabricate his health status in describing his symptoms, or he may withhold or misperceive important information concerning the state of his body; and (2) the doctor's perspective affecting how he views the complaint may be limited, or his investigation of the complaint may be faulty. In short, an assessment that a patient is a hypochondriac may either be a result of the patient's presentation, the physician's approach to the patient, or both.

The interaction is more complex than the above suggests in this respect: the physician, in his independent assessment of the patient's complaint, must depend substantially on information supplied by the patient as, for example, in the medical history. Thus, even the assumed independent investigation must be filtered through the perceptions and reporting abilities of the patient, and the physician can never be sure that he has elicited all of the appropriate facts or that the information obtained is accurate. The areas in which verification of complaints can be made independently are really quite limited and constitute no adequate basis for minimizing or rejecting the patient's concern.

In view of current knowledge, there appears to be little specific treatment for patients whose complaints appear excessive in relation to their physical condition. Even under the best of conditions, it has been very difficult to meet satisfactorily the needs of such patients. Under conditions of medical practice that prevail it is becoming impossible. Modern medical practice is characterized by a growing demand on the limited manpower available and an increasing specialization of medical functions. As doctors become more specialized, they are less interested and less capable of meeting the more diffuse needs of patients suffering from psychological distress. And in accommodating to medical demand, medicine is increasingly more bureaucratized, resulting in greater frustration of such patients' needs. Bureaucratic organization of medicine is extremely useful in insuring a high level of technical care that is efficiently distributed, but it is a rather poor mode for dealing with the psychological needs of difficult patients. Some health bureaucracies recognize these difficulties, and they are attempting to develop new roles for social workers and nurses who take on some of these important responsibilities for personal care.

If the role of psychological distress in disease were limited to a handful of patients who were disordered in the way in which they oriented themselves to physical symptoms, then restructuring medicine to fit their peculiar needs would obviously not be justified. But the notion that the average patient suffering from the average disease is unaffected in any significant way by psychological or behavioral factors is clearly incorrect. Although most doctors recognize that a large proportion of patients seeking the advice and help of physicians are motivated in seeking care by psychosocial problems, it is often assumed that patients who are really "sick" are not. This incorrect assumption permeates all of medical practice and has very substantial effects on the quality of patient care. Querido and his colleagues[1] in Holland, for example, studied 1630 patients suffering from a variety of medical conditions in a general hospital in Amsterdam. They found a significant difference in the chance of recovery between patients who had to cope with problems apart from their physical illness and those who did not. The investigators found that 69 per cent of their 1630 patients had a favorable clinical prognosis on the basis of medical factors alone. But only three-fifths of these patients actually did well. The investigators found that patients who did poorly could be characterized as suffering from psychological distress. Duff and Hollingshead,[2] in an intensive study of the care received by 161 patients in a teaching hospital associated with one of the most eminent medical schools in the United States, found considerable failure on the part of doctors to appreciate psychological factors in illness, and that these failures had adverse effects on the quality of medical care. These investigators estimate, on the basis of their study, that less than half of the diagnoses on the medical service studied were accurate, and they maintain that a large proportion of the medical errors made resulted from the failure to understand the psychological and social condition of patients. The mental state of patients affected the course of their illnesses and the degree of disability following hospitalization.

The tendency for subjective factors and physical factors to be evident at the same time is characteristic of all illness, and this has considerable significance in understanding the sick. Whether, indeed, the "psychological" and the "physical" are just two different languages to describe the same events, as Graham[3] has argued, or whether they interact in some complex but poorly understood way need not deter us here. It is plain, however, that subjective factors are part of illness and its outcome.[4-6] In considering either a reaction like pain or a more elaborate syndrome like disability, we frequently find that the phenomenon of illness itself varies when different subjective states are present. As Beecher[7] and many other investigators of pain have demonstrated, there is no dependable relationship between the number of pain endings stimulated (or the extent of their stimulation) and the resultant experience of pain. Moreover, the degree of pain experienced is concomitant with changing definitions of the meaning and consequences of pain. Similarly, in illness it is apparent that the manner in which symptoms are defined and the meanings attributed to them have a pervasive effect in many instances on the condition of the patient and the physical, psychological, and social deterioration evident.

Regardless of how physicians may wish to define their work, the fact is that much of primary care activity will continue to involve patients with psychosocial and psychophysiological disorders. Problems such as alcholism, drug dependency, depression, anxiety, family problems, and stress-related symptoms are extremely prevalent; and much of the demand for medical care stems from such disorders. Although physicians may attempt to avoid primary care practice, the ones who have this role must, in some way, come to terms with the high prevalence of these conditions.

There are, of course, many physicians who have a special interest in dealing with such patients. At this point it is difficult to know clearly what distinguishes them from other physicians, although there is some evidence that they have different attitudinal orientations. They are more likely to have an interest in psychiatry and the behavioral sciences, and seem to enjoy the complexity involved in dealing with a difficult patient.

Since the structure of practice affects the way that the physician orients himself to patients, we have been continuing studies of physician orientations in different practice contexts. Our preliminary analyses suggest that forms of remuneration can affect these orientations. When physicians are extremely busy, the structure of remuneration will influence how hard they work. Our data suggest that physicians on fixed remuneration schemes, such as capitation or salary, tend to deal with a busy practice by giving each patient less time. Physicians on fee-for-service incentives are somewhat more likely to increase the hours they devote to seeing patients and are less likely to cut back on the amount of time for each patient. Prepaid group practitioners, for example, generally work on a salary basis for a specified number of hours. They deal with large numbers of patients by working more rapidly and perhaps with greater efficiency. The fee-for-service physician is more likely to feel that he owes a certain minimum of time to each patient and may deal with a large number of patients by expanding his office time.

Although our data are very limited and fragmentary, they suggest that doctors in prepaid settings are more hurried with their patients; and others who have studied prepaids have made similar observations. Salary and capitation plans limit to some extent client control over the physician, and the doctor in this context has more leeway to organize his day within the time available. He is not as dependent as the fee-for-service physician on the patient's satisfaction with the consultation. This is also reflected in patient studies where patients in prepaid settings complain of being treated impersonally and more like a "charity case."

Clearly, each particular practice form has distinct advantages and costs. The incentive in fee-for-service practice for unnecessary work is too well known to require elaboration here, but capitation and salary systems also have difficulties. Instead of becoming an advocate of one or another payment mechanism, it is more prudent to investigate the advantages and costs of each, and search for combinations of incentives that achieve whatever aims we wish most to promote. If, indeed, it is true that the nature of patient demand and payment incentives in prepaid group practice lead the physician to behave more impersonally and to give less attention to patients' life situations, and if we think these are important qualities, then we must develop the conditions within prepaid practice that bring about the desired goals. There is a variety of possibilities that are available: new forms of paraprofessional personnel to assist the physician, patient education programs, greater client input in practice policy making, and checks against hurried and impersonal physician behavior, for instance. Rather than glorify one or another practice model, it is imperative that we learn more about the less desirable consequences of each and that we develop measures that alleviate or eliminate them.

If we consider the discussion in the larger context of this book, then it raises important questions of public policy. It has been maintained that significant motivation for access to medical care stems from underlying psychosocial difficulties in the population. These problems will require time and empathy from physicians and other health workers. But as government responds to the demand for greater access on behalf of the population, it wishes to achieve it within limited economic expenditures. It thus increasingly emphasizes efficiency and management; it attempts to create conditions where physicians and clinics can see more patients as expeditiously as possible. But as the pressures for efficiency and productivity increase, it will give physicians less rather than more time to deal with patients' human problems.

As we consider the political issue of insured access to medical care, we tend to be unfocused in respect to the question of what kind of care. Extended access, which is solely a product of increased efficiency and improved management, will not involve the necessary resources to adequately provide sensitive and responsive primary care. For patients presently without adequate access, entrance into the system is of first priority. But we had better be careful not to neglect just what we wish to provide, once access is insured, and to build the necessary structures to see that it is properly delivered.

It is clear that there is a great deal more that we need to know about how to manage health problems that reflect life difficulties. We need to consider the relevance of varying health structures and new health workers in providing care that is responsive. Although the need is evident, the solutions are unclear. But if we fail to raise the appropriate issues, we are unlikely to develop relevant answers.

Notes

1. Querido, A. (1959). "An Investigation into the Clinical, Social, and Mental Factors Determining the Results of Hospital Treatment." *British Journal of Preventive and Social Medicine*, **13**:33–49.

2. Duff, R. S., and A. Hollingshead (1968). *Sickness and Society*. New York: Harper.

3. Graham, D. (1967). "Health, Disease, and the Mind-Body Problem: Linguistic Parallelism." *Psychosomatic Medicne*, **29**: 52–71.

4. Hinkle, L. (1973). "The Effect of Exposure to Culture Change, Social Change, and Changes in Interpersonal Relationships, Upon Health." Paper presented at the Conference on Stressful Life Events, The City University of New York, June 1973.

5. Rahe, R.H. (1972). "Subjects' Recent Life Changes and Their Near-Future Illness Reports." *Annals of Clinical Research*, 4:250–265.

6. Wolff, H. (1968). *Stress and Disease*. 2nd ed. Springfield, Ill.: Thomas.

7. Beecher, H. (1959). *Measurement of Subjective Responses*. New York: Oxford University Press.

CHAPTER IX

Social Psychologic Factors Affecting the Presentation of Bodily Complaints*

Patients often recognize symptoms for which they seek medical assistance, but, on the basis of a history and physical and laboratory examination, the physician cannot obtain evidence to account for or justify the patients' complaints.[1] Such patients conform in part to Gillespie's concept of hypochondria, which he viewed as "a persistent preoccupation with the bodily health, out of proportion to any existing justification and with a conviction of disease."[2] There is considerable disagreement, however, on the appropriate formal definition of hypochondria,[3] and it may be incorrect to apply the same designation to profound and persistent hypochondrical syndromes associated with psychiatric illness and the type of hypochondriasis usually seen in general practice.

Perceptions of Symptoms

Estimates derived from British and American morbidity surveys indicate that three of four persons have symptoms in any given month for which they take some definable action such as use of medication, bed rest, consulting a physician and limiting activity.[4] In addition, persons experience many other symptoms, which they regard as trivial and which they ignore. Investigators believe that it is pointless to attempt to measure symptoms that do not receive some type of treatment or special attention since they occur commonly and have too little impact to be reported accurately in household surveys.[5,6] Yet

* Adapted from a paper appearing in the *New England Journal of Medicine,* **286**:1132–1139 (May, 1972).

such symptoms overlap appreciably with typical presenting complaints among patients seeking medical care.[7]

The major task of this chapter is to suggest how normal attribution processes develop in the definition of symptoms. As an initial formulation, it appears that persons tend to notice bodily sensations when they depart from more ordinary feelings. Each person tends to appraise new bodily perceptions against prior experience and his anticipations based on the experiences of others and on general knowledge. Many symptoms occur so commonly throughout life that they become part of ordinary expectations and are experienced as normal variations. Other experiences, such as a young girl's first menstruation, might be extremely frightening if prior social learning has not occurred, but would ordinarily be accepted as normal if it had. In analyzing responses to more unusual symptoms it is instructive to examine situations in which normal attribution processes become disrupted as a consequence of special kinds of learning, and in this regard hypochondriasis among medical students is an interesting example.

The Case of the Medical Student

It has frequently been observed that medical students experience symptom complexes that they ascribe to some pathologic process. This syndrome appears to have high prevalence—approximately 70 percent.[8,9] Factors contributing to the development of this syndrome usually include social stress and anxiety, bodily symptoms and detailed but incomplete information on a disease involving symptoms similar to the bodily indications perceived by the student. Hunter, Lohrenz, and Schwartzman describe the process as follows.

The following constellation of factors occur regularly. The student is under internal or external stress, such as guilt, fear of examinations and the like. He notices in himself some innocuous physiological or psychological dysfunction, e.g., extrasystoles, forgetfulness. He attaches to this an undeserved importance of a fearful kind usually modeled after some patient he has seen, clinical anecdote he has heard, or a member of his family who has been ill.[9]

It is not clear from such descriptions to what extent each of the components— stress, bodily symptoms and external cues—is necessary to the process and what specific role each plays. Since both stress and bodily symptoms are extremely common among students in general—and the phenomenon in question does not appear to occur so dramatically or with equal prevalence among them—it seems reasonable to suspect that the medical student's access to more detailed medical information contributes greatly to the attribution process.

An experiment by Schachter and Singer[10] helps to explain how information affects emotional response. Subjects were told that the experimenters were interested in the effects of a vitamin compound called Suproxin (a nonexistent substance) on their vision, and these subjects were given an injection. Each subject was then asked to wait, while the drug took effect, in a room with another student who appeared to be a subject who had received the same injection, but who was really a confederate of the experimenter.

The injection received was epinephrine bitartrate (adrenaline), whereas subjects in control groups received a saline solution (the placebo). Some of the subjects who received epinephrine were told to anticipate heart pounding, hand tremor and a warm and flushed face; this group was correctly informed. A second group receiving epinephrine was given no information about what to expect; this group was called the ignorant group. A third group receiving epinephrine was incorrectly informed that their feet would feel numb, that they would have itching sensations, and that they would get a slight headache; this group was called the misinformed group. While the subject was waiting for the "experiment" to begin, the confederate of the experimenter went into a scheduled act in which he slowly worked himself into a "euphoric" state playing imaginary basketball, flying paper airplanes, hula-hooping, and so on. During this period the subject was observed behind a one-way window, and his behavior was rated in terms of relevant categories. Later, he was asked to report as well his subjective feelings. Three additional groups were studied in a variation of the same situation: another epinephrine informed group; an epinephrine ignorant group; and a placebo group. In this second situation the confederate simulated anger instead of euphoria. Thus, it is possible to assess the influences of epinephrine, the various expectations subjects are given for their bodily experiences, and the different environmental cues (i.e., an angry or euphoric confederate).

Subjects who received an injection of epinephrine and who had no correct or appropriate explanation of the side effects that they experienced (particularly the epinephrine misinformed group) were most affected in their behavior and feeling states by the cues provided by the student confederate. The nature of the emotion—whether anger or euphoria—was influenced by the behavior of the confederate. Schachter and Singer believe that emotion involves a two-stage process requiring physiologic arousal and a definition of it. They maintain that the same internal state can be labeled in a variety of ways, resulting in different emotional reactions. External influences on definitions of internal states are particularly important when persons lack an appropriate explanation of what they are experiencing.

With the use of the Schachter-Singer formulation, "medical students' disease" can be characterized as follows. Medical school exposes students to continuing stress resulting from the rapid pace, examinations, anxieties in dealing with new clinical experiences and the like. Students, thus, are emotionally aroused with some frequency, and like others in the population, they experience a high prevalence of transient symptoms. The exposure to specific knowledge about disease provides the student with a new framework for identifying and giving meaning to previously neglected bodily feelings. Diffuse and ambiguous symptoms regarded as normal in the past may be reconceptualized within the context of newly acquired knowledge of disease. Existing social stress may heighten bodily sensations through autonomic activation, making the student more aware of his bodily state, and motivating him to account for what he is experiencing. The new information that the student may have about possible disease and the similarity between the symptoms of a particular condition and his own symptoms establish a link that he would have more difficulty making if he were less informed. Moreover, the student—in the process of acquiring new medical information—may begin to pay greater attention to his own bodily experiences and may also attempt to imagine how certain symptoms feel. This tendency to give attention to bodily feelings may assist the development of the syndrome.

Woods, Natterson and Silverman[8] found that, contrary to usual belief, "medical students' disease" was not an isolated experience linked to a particular aspect of medical training, but occurred with relatively equal frequency throughout the four years of medical school. Thus, the syndrome's occurrence may depend on the coincidental existence of student arousal, the presence of particular bodily feelings, and cues acquired from new information about disease that seems relevant to existing symptoms.

Hunter, Lohrenz, and Schwartzman,[9] on the basis of their study, conclude that symptom choice is influenced by "a variety of accidental, historical and learning factors, in which the mechanism of identification plays a major role." Yet there appears to be a variety of factors that may increase the probability of the occurrence of the syndrome, and it is important to inquire under what conditions concern about illness in contrast to alternative definitions will become manifest. The normal person may have a variety of symptoms without experiencing a fear of illness. Many investigators of hypochondriacal patients note that reported symptoms tend to be diffuse and may change from one occasion to another. Such patients often report numerous complaints referring to a variety of organ systems, or they report nonlocalized symptoms: insomnia, itching, dizziness, weakness, lack of energy, pain all over, and nausea, for example.[11-13] Kenyon,[14] in reviewing 512 patient case records at the Bethlem Royal and Maudsley hospitals, found that the head and neck, abdomen and chest were the regions of the body most frequently affected, and that the most typical complaints were headache and gastrointestinal and musculoskeletal symptoms. Striking features of almost all descriptions of hypochondriacal patients, particularly in early stages, are the lack of specificity of complaint and similarity to frequently occurring symptoms in normal populations. Moreover, many of the complaints tend to be of symptoms that commonly occur under stress and that epidemiologic studies show to have very high prevalence in ordinary community populations.[15,16] The common occurrence of such symptoms and their diffuseness establish conditions under which widely varying attributions may reasonably occur. Incorrect attributions may occur as well in existing organic disease because of the diffuseness of symptoms, referred pain, particular characteristics of the patient or some combination of these factors.

It is noteworthy that "medical students' disease" terminates readily and within a relatively short time. Woods and his colleagues report that the syndrome sometimes disappears spontaneously, but more often through further study of the illness or by direct or covert consultation with an instructor or physician. They suggest that it is "reassurance" that limits the condition, but the term is exceedingly vague and has a variety of meanings. Most reports in the literature concerning more persistent hypochondria suggest that such patients are not easily reassured, and thus it would be useful to have more specific understanding of the mechanism by which "medical students' disease" is short-circuited.

One way in which the medical student discovers errors in attribution is through a further understanding of diagnostics. As he learns more about the disease, he may discover that the attribution he made does not really fit or that a great variety of symptoms that commonly occur may be characteristic of the clinical picture. Another possibility is that the stress in the student's life that is fluctuating subsides with some relief in his anxiety, and his awareness of his symptoms may decline. How the incorrect attribution comes to be corrected has never been studied, but possibly the student's growing knowledge of symptomatology sharpens his judgment about his own complaints. If clear knowledge is indeed necessary to disconfirm the attribution adequately, the syndrome should be more persistent when knowledge is disputed and uncertain. In this light, it is of interest that "medical students' disease" of a psychiatric character appears to be less transient and more chronic than such syndromes that develop around fears of physical illness.[8] In the psychiatric area it is more difficult to separate the attribution from the entity to which the attribution is made.

Another issue concerns the origins of the initial attribution of illness. The conclusion reached by Hunter, Lohrenz, and Schwartzman[9] that identification plays a major part has already been noted, and this appears to be the most generally accepted psychiatric point of view. The concept of identification as used by the authors in this respect is more descriptive than explanatory, and it encompasses the observation often made that the patient will frequently focus on a disease that affected a loved one. An examination of cases described in the literature suggests that the localization and definition of the complaint may depend on idiosyncrasies or may be fortuitous. Ladee[3] reports the observation of Orbán concerning a veterinary surgeon who felt a pain in the right lower part of his abdomen. Apparently, he feared an incipient bowel obstruction rather than appendicitis, and Ladee explains that appendicitis is rare among cattle whereas ileus is frequent. Felix Brown,[17] in a thoughtful review of 41 cases of hypochondria, notes the important influence of topical suggestions. Many commentators have also observed how frequently symptoms of a particular kind follow publicity given to the illness or death of a well known personality or a dramatic mass-media demonstration concerning some disease.

It appears that the concept of identification may be too diffuse and imprecise in encompassing such varied phenomena as the association between mother and child, audience and public figure, and the occurrence of a stomach pain and seeing a movie concerning a person with stomach cancer. An alternative perspective from which to analyze such influences would involve consideration of factors affecting the perception of personal vulnerability.

Perceptions of Personal Vulnerability

Although persons may vary widely in their sense of invulnerability—which appears to be linked with their levels of self-esteem—psychologic survival generally depends on the ability of people to protect themselves from anxieties and fears involving low-risk occurrences to which all persons are exposed or dangers that they are powerless to prevent.[18,19] Feelings of invulnerability are threatened under circumstances of greatly increased risk such as combat and new and difficult experiences, but even under these conditions, persons generally manage to maintain a relatively strong sense of invulnerability through various psychologic defense processes and coping actions. However, a "near-miss" can dramatically undermine one's sense of invulnerability and may lead to extreme anxiety and fear reactions. The death of a close friend or coworker in combat,[20] being involved in an automobile accident in which others are killed or suffer bodily injury, and learning that someone who is defined as having comparable ability to oneself has failed an important examination that one is intending to take[21] serve to threaten the sense of security.

Basic to the undermining of a sense of invulnerability are social comparison processes. It is much less difficult to explain injury to people of unlike characteristics without threat to oneself in that one can attribute the injury to aspects of the person that are different from one's own. When such persons are more like oneself—in terms of age, sex, life style or routine—it is much more difficult not to perceive oneself at risk, and personal intimacy or physical proximity similarly increases feelings of vulnerability.

Various studies suggest that self-esteem is an intervening variable between situation and response. Although the role of self-esteem is not fully clear, one possibility is that persons with high self-esteem see themselves as more capable of dealing with threatening situations and, thus, are less vulnerable.[22] The awareness that one is able to cope and that one has had success in the past in dealing with adversity insulates the person from anxiety.[23] This concept of the self-esteem effect appears most reasonable in cases in which coping ability can affect the situation and realistically reduce threat; it is not so obvious that self-esteem reduces a sense of threat of impending illness, although many writers on hypochondria note specifically that low self-esteem is associated with this syndrome. A sense of confidence may generalize to situations even when it is not particularly realistic, or may lead persons to focus less on bodily indications. This is clearly an area for more focused inquiry.

Some symptoms present in a fashion that makes them difficult to ignore, and many symptoms are sufficiently impressive in their occurrence or sufficiently disruptive of normal functioning so that variation in response is relatively limited. Moreover, many symptoms occur so as not to allow alternative attributions readily. Hypochondria developing around a fear that one has a fractured leg or an extremely high fever is not found ordinarily; indeed, the response to such symptoms is not mediated in any influential way by social and cultural variables. But when symptoms are more diffuse, variation in response is more likely to occur.

In sum, it has been maintained that most ordinarily occurring symptoms are considered normal or explained in conventional frameworks, as when muscle aches are attributed to unaccustomed physical activity or indigestion to overeating. When such ordinary symptoms occur concomitantly with emotional arousal, and when they are not easily explained within conventional and commonly available understandings, external cues become important in defining the character and importance of such bodily feelings. Such cues may be fortuitous, or they may be the consequence of prior experience, cultural learning or personal need for secondary gain. The manner in which sociocultural and psychologic contexts condition attributional responses requires further examination.

Social and Cultural Influences on Response to Symptoms

From very young ages, children more or less learn to respond to various symptoms and feelings in terms of reactions of others to their behavior and social expectations in general. As children begin to mature, clear age and sex patterns become apparent, and the children become clearly differentiated in the manner in which they respond to pain, their risk-taking activities, and their readiness to express their apprehensions and hurts.[24] Learning influences the tendency of males as compared with females to take more risks, to seek medical care less readily, and to be less expressive about illness and appear more stoical.

The role of cultural differences in identification and response to illness has been described nicely by Zborowski[25] and has been amplified in a variety of other studies.[26] Zborowski, in studying reactions to pain in a New York City hospital among various ethnic groups, noted that whereas Jewish and Italian patients responded to pain in an emotional fashion, "Old Americans" were more stoical and "objective," and Irish more frequently denied pain. He also noted a difference in the attitude underlying Italian and Jewish concern about pain; although the Italian patients primarily sought relief from pain and were relatively satisfied when such relief was obtained, the Jewish patients appeared to be concerned mainly with the meaning of their pain and the consequences of pain for their future health and welfare. Thus, different attributional processes appeared to form the basis of these manifest similarities. Zborowski reported that Italian patients seemed relieved when they were given medication for pain, and their complaining ceased. In contrast, Jewish patients were reluctant to accept medication and appeared to have greater concern with the implications of their pain experience for their future health.

Other studies have similarly found that ethnic groups differentially report symptoms and seek medical assistance for them, and vary in the extent to which they are willing to accept psychologic interpretations of their complaints.[27,28] It is unclear whether the ethnic differences, noted in the literature, are a result of the fact that children with particular prior experiences and upbringing come to have more objective symptoms, interpret the same symptoms differently, express their concerns and seek help with greater willingness, or use a different vocabulary for expressing distress. Such distinctions are important.

Responses to Perceived Illness and Vocabularies of Distress

It is apparent that social learning will affect the vocabularies persons use to define their complaints and their orientations to seeking various kinds of care. It is reasonable to expect that persons from origins where the expression of symptoms and seeking help is permissible and encouraged will be more likely to do so, particularly under stressful circumstances. In contrast, in cultural contexts where complaining is discouraged, persons experiencing distress may seek a variety of alternative means for dealing with their difficulties. Zborowski, in describing the "Old American" family, stressed the tendency of the mother to teach the child to take pain "like a man," not to be a sissy and not to cry. Such training, according to Zborowski, does not discourage use of the doctor, but it implies that such use will be based on physical needs rather than on emotional concerns. One might, therefore, anticipate that persons with such backgrounds might be reluctant to express psychologic distress directly, but might express such distress through the presentation of physical complaints. Kerckhoff and Back,[29] in a study of the diffusion of a hysterical illness among female employees of a Southern mill alleged to be caused by an unknown insect, found that the prevalence of the condition was high among women under strain who could not admit they had a problem and who did not know how to cope with it.

Pauline Bart,[30] in comparing women who entered a neurology service, but who were discharged with psychiatric diagnoses, with women entering a psychiatric service of the same hospital, found them to be less educated, more rural, of lower socioeconomic status, and less likely to be Jewish than those who came directly to a psychiatric service. Bart suggests that these two groups of women were differentiated by their vocabularies of discomfort, which affected the manner in which they presented themselves. She also observed that 52 percent of the psychiatric patients on the neurology service had had a hysterectomy as compared with only 21 percent on the psychiatric service. The findings suggest that such patients may be expressing psychologic distress through physical attributions and, thus, expose themselves to a variety of unnecessary medical procedures.

Most of the understanding of the patient's complaint comes from observation of that part of the process that brings the patient into contact with the physician. It should be clear that this tends to focus on only a segment of the entire sample and excludes patients with comparable problems who do not seek assistance. Various analysts of the medical consultation, such as Balint,[31] note that the symptoms that the patient presents are frequently of no special consequence, but serve to establish a legitimate relation between patient and doctor. He maintains that the presentation of somatic complaints often masks an underlying emotional problem that is frequently the major reason the patient has sought help. Certainly, a complaint of illness may be one way of seeking reassurance and support through a recognized and socially acceptable relation when it is difficult for the patient to present the underlying problem in an undisguised form without displaying weaknesses and vulnerabilities contrary to expected and learned behavior patterns. The emphasis that Balint places on the symptom as a front for underlying emotional distress, although characteristic of some patients, neglects the fact that many patients who are more receptive to psychologic vocabularies may also be viewed as hypochondriacal.

The response to bodily indications may also depend on the social acceptability of certain types of complaints, and even the nature and site of the complaint, according to Balint, is a matter frequently negotiated between patient and physician. Harold Wolff[32] has also noted that minor pains from certain parts of the body may be more frequent because they are culturally more acceptable and because they bring greater sympathetic response. Hes,[33] in a study of hypochondriac patients referred to a psychiatric outpatient clinic, noted the inhibition of emotional expression as a result of culturally determined taboos on complaining about one's fate and a culturally determined excessive use of bodily language. He found these conditions particularly characteristic of Oriental Jewish women, who made up a major proportion of his patients with hypochondria.

Mechanic and Volkart[34] examined the influence of stress and inclination to use medical facilities among 600 male students at a major university. Stress (as measured by indexes of loneliness and nervousness) and inclination to use medical facilities (as measured by anticipated behavior given hypothetical illness situations) were clearly related to the use of a college health service during a one-year period. Among students with high stress and a high inclination to use medical facilities 73 percent were frequent users of medical facilities (three or more times during the year), but among the low-inclination-low-stress group, only 30 percent were frequent users of such services. Among those of high inclination, "stress" was an important influence in bringing people to the physician. Seventy-three percent of persons experiencing high stress used facilities frequently, although only 46 percent did so among those with low stress.[35] A similar trend was observed among those who were less inclined to seek advice from a doctor, but the relation between stress and actually seeking advice was substantially smaller and not statistically significant. These data support the interpretation that stress leads to an attempt to cope; those who are receptive to the patient role tend to adopt this particular mode of coping more frequently than those who are not so receptive. The previous discussion also suggests that when stress helps initiate a medical contact, the contact may be presented through a vocabulary of physical symptoms that frequently impress the physician as trivial or unimportant. A very similar study was carried out with comparable results among British women using two general-practice panels within the English National Health Service.[36]

The impression emerging from these studies is that there are at least two major patterns of behavior that physicians tend to regard as hypochondriacal. The first consists of patients who have a high inclination to use medical facilities and a willingness to use a vocabulary of psychologic distress, openly complaining of unhappiness, frustration and dissatisfaction.[37] The more common and difficult patient to deal with is one who has a high receptivity to medical care but who lacks a vocabulary of psychologic distress. Such patients tend to present the doctor with a variety of diffuse physical complaints for which he can find no clear-cut explanation, but he cannot be sure that they do not indeed suffer from some physical disorder that he has failed to diagnose.

Patients who express psychologic distress through a physical language tend to be uneducated or to come from cultural groups where the expression of emotional distress is inhibited. Such patients frequently face serious life diffi-culties and social stress, but the subculture within which they function does not allow legitimate expression of their suffering nor are others attentive to their pleas for support when they are made. Because of their experiences these patients frequently feel, sometimes consciously but more frequently on a level of less than full awareness, that expression of their difficulties is a sign of weakness and will be deprecated. They thus dwell on bodily complaints, some that are ever present, and others that are concomitant with their experience of emotional distress. These patients are often elderly, lonely and insecure, and they may be inactive enough to have time to dwell on their difficulties. When such patients seek out physicians they may use their physical symptoms and complaints as a plea for help.

Effects of Emotional Distress on Symptoms

It has been suggested at various points that emotional arousal appears to heighten the experience of symptoms, and in this regard the literature on reac-tions to pain is noteworthy. Beecher[38] has reported the failure of 15 different research groups to establish any dependable effects of even large doses of morphine on pain of experimental origin in man. He has found it necessary to distinguish between pain as an original sensation and pain as a psychic reac-tion. As Beecher notes, one of the difficulties with most forms of laboratory pain is that they minimize the psychic reaction, which has an essential role in pain associated with illness. For example, in a comparative study he found that civilian patients undergoing surgery reported strikingly more frequent and severe pain than wounded soldiers with greater tissue trauma. He observed that such variations resulted from varying subjective definitions, and concluded that there is no simple, direct relation between the wound per se and the pain experienced.

A variety of reports both of an anthropologic nature and in the experimen-tal literature indicate how a person's definition of a painful experience condi-tions how much pain he is willing to tolerate and what he will endure without protest. In experimental situations persons can be given instructions and incentives to endure severe pain stimulation.[39-41] Here it is difficult to separate what people may feel from their willingness to control expression patterns, but many such reports suggest that when there is strong positive motivation, peo-ple will undergo extraordinary pain without complaint. Also, if intensely involved in some pattern of behavior, they may not become immediately aware of severe body trauma.[42]

The reactive component in illness has long been recognized as an important aspect not only in defining the condition but also in the patient's response to treatment and in the course of the illness. Imboden and his colleagues have studied prolonged convalescence in chronic brucellosis and influenza, in which they argue that emotional stress concomitant with the course of the illness may become intermingled with symptoms of the illness in such a way that the end point of the illness becomes confused with continuing emotional distress.[43,44] They note that symptoms of emotional distress may be attributed to the physical illness well beyond the normal course of the infection, which may serve to maintain the patient's self-concept.

The studies on prolonged convalescence suggest some of the conditions under which misattribution may occur. For example, the course of influenza and brucellosis is likely to leave the patient fatigued, with a lack of energy and interest, weakness and a variety of other somatic symptoms. These symptoms may also accompany depression and other emotional distress. The similarity in the symptoms makes it reasonable for the patient to attribute these symptoms after the illness to the persistence of the illness. The similarity that makes the errors of attribution more likely also makes it difficult for the physician to determine when the symptoms are a product of an emotional problem and when they are complications of the physical illness. Thus, the physician may unwittingly reinforce the patient's confusion.

The manner in which physicians may come to reinforce particular patient tendencies is suggested by a variety of reports.[45,46] Zola,[45] for example, on the basis of a study of patients for whom no medical disease was found, suggests that the patient's cultural background influenced how he presented his symptoms and, thus, how the doctor evaluated them. Although the ethnic groups studied did not differ in the extent of their life difficulties, Italians, who are more emotional in the presentation of symptoms and give more attention and expression to pain and distress, were more likely to be evaluated as suffering from a psychogenic condition.

Treating the Chronic Complainer—Correcting Errors in Attribution

In a classic paper, Felix Brown[17] defined bodily complaints in five ways: partly on a physiologic or somatic level, associated with anxiety; symbolic of something else; consistent with mood disturbance, usually depression; by substitution or conversion of an affect, usually anxiety, with more or less elimination of the affect; and with more or less conscious purpose for the patient—purposive hypochondriasis.

The first three groups are most typical of the chronic complainer seen in ordinary medical practice. Ordinarily, it is believed that doctors must provide general reassurance, which relieves the patient's level of distress, but if the implications of some of the theoretical statements made earlier are followed, it should become clear why reassurance alone may not be the most effective approach. Frequently, the interpretation that the patient has made of his symptoms is a provisional and vague definition, and, as Balint indicates, this attribution is readily changed by the physician's suggestions. The physician may be able to alleviate the patient's distress to the extent that he can provide the patient with benign interpretations of his distress that are credible and to the extent to which he can reassure him and bolster his esteem and sense of mastery. To provide general reassurance alone may have no effect on the patient's perspective relevant to the meaning of his symptoms, although it may contribute to the alleviation of anxiety. Providing alternative attributions is difficult because they not only must relieve anxiety but must be culturally and psychologically acceptable to the patient as well. For example, if the patient has learned that a psychologic expression of distress is unacceptable, such an interpretation by the physician may be of little use to the patient, may exacerbate his anxiety, and may disrupt the relation between doctor and patient.

The suggestion that the attribution the doctor provides must be credible means that it must be consistent with what the patient is experiencing and likely to experience in the future. If not, it may serve to arouse the patient's anxiety further and will not be taken seriously. Some evidence on this matter comes from a study by Rickels and his colleagues[47,48] on the effects of placebos. Suggestibility is an important factor in the medical situation, and placebos have been found to alleviate distress in a wide range of medical disorders.[26] Rickels and his colleagues, however, found that patients with prolonged experience with anxiety and the use of tranquilizing drugs do poorly when treated by placebos, and many suffer a worsening of their anxiety state. Patients who are attuned to their inner feelings and have had experiences with psychoactive drugs do not experience placebos as credible. The impact of the suggestion effect is hardly equal to the patients' past experiences of true relief of their symptoms with tranquilizers, and the failure of the placebo to reduce their anxieties to the level they expect may alarm them and make them think that they are more upset than usual.

Such an interpretation is offered by Storms and Nisbett[49] in a study of insomniac subjects. These subjects were given placebos to take before going to bed; some were told that the pill would increase their arousal, and others that it would decrease it. The former reported that they got to sleep more quickly than previously, whereas the latter reported that they took longer to get to sleep than before. Storms and Nisbett believe that the subjects who thought that their arousal was due to the pill felt less upset and could fall asleep more easily, but those who continued to feel arousal despite the fact that the pill was to reduce their arousal defined themselves as particularly upset. Although caution is required in generalizing to clinical situations, such studies illustrate how the efficacy of the doctor's interpretations of his patient's problems will depend on the extent to which they are credible in terms of the patient's experiences and the extent to which he anticipates the patient's reactions to symptoms and treatment.

The adequacy of the doctor's management of the patient is also likely to depend on the kinds of expectations and instructions he provides the patient in preparation for what lies ahead. Whether doctors say anything or not, patients will anticipate and acquire expectations of the course of their condition, how they expect to feel, what is likely to happen and the like. To the extent that the patient is not instructed, his expectations may be highly contrary to what is likely to occur, and this discrepancy may alarm the patient and disrupt his management. Various experimental studies suggest that very modest instruction and information have an important effect on patient outcomes,[50,51] and on facilitating preventive health actions.[22]

Egbert and his colleagues,[50] for example, selected a random group of patients undergoing surgery and gave them simple information, encouragement and instruction concerning the impending operation and means of alleviating postoperative pain. The researchers, however, were not involved in the medical care of the patients studied, and they did not participate in decisions concerning them. An independent evaluation of the postoperative period and the length of stay of patients in the experimental and control groups showed that communication and instruction had an important beneficial effect.

In a similar experimental study by Skipper and Leonard,[51] children admitted to a hospital for tonsillectomy were randomized into experimental and control groups. In the experimental group patients and their mothers were admitted to the hospital by a specially trained nurse, who attempted to create an atmosphere that would facilitate the communication of information to the mother and increase her freedom to verbalize her anxieties. Mothers were told what routine events to expect and when they were likely to occur, including the actual time schedule for the operation. The investigators found that the emotional support reduced the mothers' stress and changed their definition of the hospital situation, which in turn had a beneficial effect on their children. Children in the experimental group experienced smaller changes in blood pressure, temperature and other physiologic measures; they were less likely to suffer from postoperative emesis and made a better adaptation to the hospital, and they made a more rapid recovery after hospitalization, displaying fewer fears, less crying, and less disturbed sleep than children in the control group.

In sum, credible instructions provided in a sympathetic and supportive way that help people avoid attributional errors and that avoid new reasons for anxiety might be more helpful to the complaining patient than blanket reassurances that provide no alternative framework for understanding his symptoms. Reassurance that does not take into account the patient's assessment of the threat that he faces might serve only to mystify him and to undermine his confidence in his physician. The literature contains frequent reports not only of patients with hypochondria who went from one doctor to another but also of repeated cases in which the patient appeared to get gratification in disconfirming the doctor's appraisal. Therapeutic approaches that facilitate the patient's coping efforts may be particularly useful with these difficult patients.

Notes

1. Gardner, E. A. (1970). "Emotional Disorders in Medical Practice." *Annals of Internal Medicine,* **73:**651–653.

2. Gillespie, R. D. (1928). "Hypochondria: Its Definition, Nosology, and Psychology." *Guy's Hospital Reports,* **8:**408–460.

3. Ladee, G. A. (1966). *Hypochondriacal Syndromes.* Amsterdam: Elsevier.

4. White, K. L., et al. (1961). "The Ecology of Medical Care." *New England Journal of Medicine,* **265:**885–892.

5. National Center for Health Statistics (1964). *Health Survey Procedure: Concepts, Questionaire Development, and Definitions in the Health Interview Survey.* PHS Publication No. 1000, Series 1, No. 2. Washington D.C.: U.S. Government Printing Office.

6. Mooney, H. W. (1963). *Methodology in Two California Health Surveys, San Jose (1952) and Statewide (1954–55).* PHS Monograph No. 70. Washington D.C.: U.S. Government Printing Office.

7. Mechanic, D., and M. Newton (1965). "Some Problems in the Analysis of Morbidity Data." *Journal of Chronic Diseases,* **18:**569–580.

8. Woods, S. M., et al. (1966). "Medical Students' Disease: Hypochondriasis in Medical Education." *Journal of Medical Education,* **41:**785–790.

9. Hunter, R., et al. (1964). "Nosophobia and Hypochondriasis in Medical Students." *Journal of Nervous and Mental Diseases,* **139:**147–152.

10. Schachter, S., and J. E. Singer (1962). "Cognitive, Social, and Physiological Determinants of Emotional State." *Psychological Review,* **69:**379–399.

11. Katzenalbogen, S. (1942). "Hypochondriacal Complaints with Special References to Personality and Environment." *American Journal of Psychiatry,* **98:**815–822.

12. Greenberg, H. P. (1960). "Hypochondriasis." *Medical Journal of Australia,* **1**(18): 673–677.

13. Robins, E., et al. (1952). "'Hysteria' in Men: A Study of 38 Patients so Diagnosed and 194 Control Subjects." *New England Journal of Medicine,* **246:**677–685.

14. Kenyon, F. E. (1964). "Hypochondriasis: A Clinical Study." *British Journal of Psychiatry,* **110:**478–488.

15. Srole, L., et al. (1962). *Mental Health in the Metropolis: The Midtown Manhattan Study.* New York: McGraw-Hill.

16. Leighton, D. C., et al. (1963). *The Character of Danger: Psychiatric Symptoms in Selected Communities.* New York: Basic Books.

17. Brown, F. (1936). "The Bodily Complaint: A Study of Hypochondriasis." *Journal of Mental Science,* **82:**295–359.

18. Janis, I. L. (1951). *Air War and Emotional Stress: Psychological Studies of Bombing and Civilian Defense.* New York: McGraw-Hill.

19. Wolfenstein, M. (1957). *Disaster: A Psychological Essay.* New York: Free Press.

20. Grinker, R. R., and J. P. Spiegel (1945). *Men Under Stress.* Philadelphia: Blakiston.

21. Mechanic, D. (1962). *Students Under Stress: A Study in the Social Psychology of Adaptation.* New York: Free Press.

22. Leventhal, H. (1970). "Findings and Theory in the Study of Fear Communications." In L. Berkowitz (ed.), *Advances in Experimental Social Psychology,* Vol. 5, New York: Academic Press pp. 119–186.

23. Lazarus, R. S. (1966). *Psychological Stress and the Coping Process.* New York: McGraw-Hill.

24. Mechanic, D. (1964). "The Influence of Mothers on Their Children's Health Attitudes and Behavior." *Pediatrics,* **33:**444–453.

25. Zborowski, M. (1952). "Cultural Components in Responses to Pain." *Journal of Social Issues,* **8**(4):16–30.

26. Mechanic, D. (1968). *Medical Sociology: A Selective View.* New York: Free Press.

27. Mechanic, D. (1963). "Religion, Religiosity, and Illness Behavior: The Special Case of the Jews." *Human Organization,* **22:**202–208.

28. Fink, R., et al. (1969) "The 'Filter-Down' Process to Psychotherapy in a Group Practice Medical Care Program." *American Journal of Public Health and the Nation's Health,* **59:** 245–260.

29. Kerckhoff, A. C., and K. W. Back (1968). *The June Bug: A Study of Hysterical Contagion.* New York: Appleton-Century-Crofts.

30. Bart, P. B. (1968). "Social Structure and Vocabularies of Discomfort: What Happened to Female Hysteria?" *Journal of Health and Social Behavior,***9:**188–193.

31. Balint, M. (1957). *The Doctor, His Patient, and the Illness.* New York: International Universities Press.

32. Wolff, H. G. (1963). *Headache and Other Head Pain.* Second Edition. New York: Oxford University Press.

33. Hes, J. P. (1968). "Hypochondriacal Complaints in Jewish Psychiatric Patients." *Israel Annals of Psychiatry and Related Discipliness,* **6:**134–142.

34. Mechanic, D., and E. H. Volkart (1961). "Stress, Illness Behavior, and the Sick Role." *American Sociological Review,* **25:**51–58.

35. Mechanic, D. (1963). "Some Implications of Illness Behavior for Medical Sampling." *New England Journal of Medicine,* **269:**244–247.

36. Mechanic, D., and D. Jackson (1968). "Stress, Illness Behavior, and the Use of General Practitioner Services: A Study of British Women." Mimeo, Department of Sociology, University of Wisconsin.

37. Kadushin, C. (1958). "Individual Decisions to Undertake Psychotherapy." *Administrative Science Quarterly,* **3:**379–411.

38. Beecher, H. K. (1959). *Measurement of Subjective Responses: Quantitative Effects of Drugs*. New York: Oxford University Press.

39. Lambert, W. E., et al. (1960). "The Effect of Increased Salience of a Membership Group on Pain Tolerance." *Journal of Personality,* **28:**350–357.

40. Ross, L., et al. (1969). "Toward an Attribution Therapy: The Reduction of Fear Through Induced Cognitive-Emotional Misattribution." *Journal of Personality and Social Psychology,* **12:**279–288.

41. Blitz, B., and A. J. Dinnerstein (1971). "Role of Attentional Focus in Pain Perception: Manipulation of Response to Noxious Stimulation by Instructions." *Journal of Abnormal Psychology,* **77:**42–45.

42. Walters, A. (1961). "Psychogenic Regional Pain Alias Hysterical Pain." *Brain,* **84:**1–18.

43. Imboden, J. B., et al. (1959). "Brucellosis. III. Psychologic Aspects of Delayed Convalescence." *Archives of Internal Medicine,* **103:**406–414.

44. Imboden, J. B., et al. (1961). "Symptomatic Recovery from Medical Disorders: Influence of Psychological Factors." *Journal of the American Medical Association,* **178:**1182–1184.

45. Zola, I. K. (1963). "Problems of Communication, Diagnosis, and Patient Care: The Interplay of Patient, Physician and Clinic Organization." *Journal of Medical Education.* **38:** 829–838.

46. Brodman, K., et al. (1947). "The Relation of Personality Disturbances to Duration of Convalescence from Acute Respiratory Infections." *Psychosomatic Medicine,* **9:**37–44.

47. Rickels, K., and R. W. Downing (1967). "Drug- and Placebo-Treated Neurotic Outpatients: Pretreatment Levels of Manifest Anxiety, Clinical Improvement, and Side Reactions." *Archives of General Psychiatry,* **16:**369–372.

48. Rickels, K., et al. (1966). "Previous Medication, Duration of Illness and Placebo Response." *Journal of Nervous and Mental Diseases,* **142:**548–554.

49. Storms, M. D., and R. E. Nisbett (1970). "Insomnia and the Attribution Process." *Journal of Personality and Social Psychology,* **16:**319–328.

50. Egbert, L. D., et al. (1964). "Reduction of Postoperative Pain by Encouragement and Instruction of Patients: A Study of Doctor-Patient Rapport." *New England Journal of Medicine,* **270:**825–827.

51. Skipper, J. K. Jr., and R. C. Leonard (1968). "Children, Stress, and Hospitalization: A Field Experiment." *Journal of Health and Social Behavior,* **9:**275–287.

CHAPTER X

Correlates of Frustration among British General Practitioners*

There is growing evidence of discontent and frustration among general medical practitioners throughout the world. This is reflected in an unwillingness of doctors to accept roles as general practitioners, in increasing threats of strikes and boycotts among doctors, and in an outpouring of angry rhetoric. With the growth of medical technology, the increasing development of hospital medical care, and growing specialization, those doctors who continue to perform a wide variety of roles within the community appear to have not only many of the same obligations as in previous times, but additional ones as well. At the same time, these doctors have suffered a loss of status relative to more specialized practitioners, and they experience greater uncertainty than ever before as to how they might best function. Explanations of the frustrations among general practitioners give more or less emphasis to such factors as the structural conditions under which doctors practice, their attitudes toward general practice, the nature of their medical education, and the character of the demands made upon them.[1] The purpose of this chapter is to examine–within one medical context–the influence of various factors on the degree of frustration experienced by doctors continuing to perform such generalized roles.

The context of this article is the National Health Service of England and Wales. The data reported here come from a random national sample of general practitioners who were surveyed in 1966 during the peak of an angry confrontation between general practitioners and the government. One need do no more than peruse the letters to the *British Medical Journal* during 1965 and 1966 to appreciate the high level of emotion and frustration that characterized the dispute.

The analysis in this chapter is based on 772 respondents. To facilitate the analysis, 41 doctors were excluded from the sample because they failed to respond to 10 percent or more of the questions. In the remaining cases, where

* Adapted from a paper appearing in the *Journal of Health and Social Behavior,* **11:**87–104 (June, 1970).

data on a particular question were missing, the respondents were assigned to the mean response of those replying to that question. The demographic profile of the sample used in the analysis was almost identical to the profile of all respondents, and the sample profile was remarkably similar to that of all general practitioners in England and Wales with unrestricted practices. A detailed description of the sample in relation to the total population of general practitioners is provided elsewhere.[2]

The major issue to be examined here is whether the inevitable frustrations of general practice are alleviated through modern forms of medical organization and by particular orientations of general practitioners that make them more receptive to a broad spectrum of problems they are likely to encounter frequently.[3] We shall view frustration in terms of three different indicators. The first indicator is one we shall refer to as *trivial consultations*; it comes from a previous study by Ann Cartwright[4] and asks the doctor to estimate the proportion of his office consultations that he feels to be trivial, unnecessary, or inappropriate.* We make the assumption that reports indicating a high proportion of trivial cases tell us more about the practitioner than about his patients. In her study Cartwright followed up on two-fifths of the doctors in her sample and asked them to make a record of one day's consultations, indicating whether or not they felt each consultation was or was not warranted. One-fifth of the consultations reported were regarded as unwarranted, and doctors tended to record as trivial a smaller proportion of cases than they estimated in the earlier questionnaire. Cartwright's belief[5] that doctors who report a large proportion of their cases as trivial, unnecessary, and inappropriate "were exaggerating their irritation or being illogical" appears reasonable. She has also shown that this estimate is an excellent predictor of a variety of aspects of the doctor and his practice.

Similar assumptions are made in the case of our other two indicators. For the second indicator, which will be referred to as *harassment reported*, fourteen types of patients that doctors regard as difficult, annoying, and unreason-

Table 1   Intercorrelations among Indicators of Frustration

	Harassment Reported[a]	Practice Realistic
Trivial consultations	−.37	.25
Harassment reported	−	−.19

[a] Negative correlations between harassment and the other two indicators result from the manner in which the variables have been scored.

* References to trivial consultations in this chapter indicate all cases that the doctor reports to be trivial, unnecessary, or inappropriate.

able are described. In each case the doctor is asked to report how often he sees the type of patient described (frequently, sometimes, seldom, or never).* Although doctors obviously see such patients from time to time, it seems highly unlikely that doctors would see such patients frequently. Moreover, we do not believe that such patients are very differently distributed among practices, and some data relevant to this point will be reported later. We thus developed a score on these items by simply summing the number of individual types of patients that the doctor reports that he sees frequently. We assume that such reports reflect the doctor's feelings of harassment rather than any objective situation.

The third indicator, referred to as *practice realistic*, requires the doctor to estimate how realistic various general practice functions are under present conditions of practice organization and with an average-size practice. Fifteen functions are described, varying from such general ones as adequately screening out patients with physical disorders to such specific ones as undertaking routine screening through cervical smears.† In each case the doctor is asked to

* The following types of patients were included: (1) a patient who insisted that you visit him in his home even though you felt reasonably certain that the visit was not really necessary; (2) a patient who complained that you kept him waiting too long; (3) a patient who insisted on referral to a consultant although you did not regard the referral as necessary; (4) a patient who insisted that you authorize a particular test although you felt the test unnecessary; (5) a patient who insisted that you prescribe a particular medication which you felt was inappropriate; (6) a patient who insisted on a medical certificate which in your opinion was unnecessary; (7) a patient who has threatened to write to the local executive committee to complain about you; (8) a patient who threatened to leave your practice; (9) a patient who visits your surgery frequently but pays little attention to your prescribed regimen; (10) a patient who lacks gratitude although you have conscientiously taken care of him; (11) a patient who does not accord you the respect and courtesy you deserve; (12) a patient who asked you to make dishonest statements in filling out a medical certificate; (13) a bereaved patient who blames you for the death of a relative; and (14) a neurotic patient who persistently complains although you are doing all you can to help him.

Forty-four percent of the sample report that none of these events occurs frequently; 36 percent report that one or two of these events occurs frequently; 10 percent report that three or four of these events occur frequently; and 9 percent report that five or more of such events occur frequently.

† The items included in this indicator are as follows: (1) to provide a high standard of medical care; (2) to provide a high-quality doctor-patient relationship; (3) to adequately screen out patients with serious physical disorders; (4) to know the histories of most of your patients; (5) to maintain a proper record system; (6) to provide care for the varied psychosocial problems you encounter in your practice; (7) to be able to treat not only the patient, but the consequences of his illness for his family; (8) to follow psychiatric patients outside the hospital; (9) to allow patients the opportunity to talk out their problems; (10) to provide continuity of care; (11) to advise on and care for psychological problems of patients; (12) to keep abreast of new developments in medicine; (13) to provide good preventive care; (14) to visit your patients in the hospital; and (15) to undertake routine screening through cervical smears.

Of our sample, 8 percent felt that none of these functions was either quite or somewhat realistic; 23 percent felt that 1–4 were realistic; 31 percent felt that 5–8 of these functions were realistic; 23 percent felt that 9–12 of these functions were realistic; and 15 percent felt that 13 or more of these functions were realistic.

Table 2 Some Correlates of the Dependent Variables (Per Cent)

	Trivial Consultations[a]			Practice Realistic			Harassment Reported		
	High	Low		No	Yes		High	Low	
	Reports 25% or More as Trivial ($N = 455$)	Reports Less than 25% as Trivial ($N = 317$)	r^b	Scores of 0–6 ($N = 336$)	Scores of 7 or More ($N = 436$)	r^b	One or More Occurs Frequently ($N = 432$)	None Occurs Frequently ($N = 340$)	r^b
1. Agrees that bringing less serious disorders to doctors is a good trend ($N = 286$)	30	48	−.31	27	45	−.19	34	41	.20
2. Strongly agrees that the NHS does not protect doctors from unreasonable demands by patients ($N = 556$)	79	62	.16	79	67	.12	81	61	−.16
3. Strongly agrees patients are too demanding ($N = 354$)	62	23	.44	54	39	.17	61	27	−.33

4. Reports that in the past month a patient became hostile to him ($N = 353$)	50	40	.13	51	42	.09	51	39	−.20
5. Reports that quite a few times or more patients in the past month were hypochondriacs ($N = 292$)	48	23	.29	43	34	.17	49	24	−.33
6. Reports that he found himself dealing with family disputes and marital discord quite a few times in the past month ($N = 246$)	35	27	.10	35	30	.04[c]	39	23	−.22
7. Reports that many times in the past month he had to spend a large proportion of his day doing things that require no real skill or experience ($N = 275$)	45	23	.31	46	28	.20	47	21	−.30
8. Low inducement in general practice scale—Highest Score ($N = 235$)	33	26	−.18	40	23	−.24	38	21	.24

[a] The categorization used here is desirable in light of Cartwright's finding in her study of consultations that, on the average, 20 per cent were regarded as trivial, unnecessary, or inappropriate.

[b] Product-moment correlation. In each case these correlations are based on all the available data. The percentages in this table and those that follow are meant to give a better picture of some of the differences. The groupings in the tables, however, are extremely crude and do not use much of the detail available in the data.

[c] r does not achieve statistical significance at the .05 level. Since the variables used in this paper differ in the extent to which they are skewed, and since some are dichotomous, the significance level is not a particularly reliable index. It has some heuristic value, however.

indicate whether the function is quite realistic, somewhat realistic, somewhat unrealistic, or very unrealistic under present conditions. This question was scored by summing the number of items to which the doctor responds either quite or somewhat realistic.

The use of this estimate of what is realistic as an indicator of frustration is not as justifiable on its face as the use of the other two indicators. The extent to which doctors regard various functions as realistic will depend on their abilities to organize their practice, to work rapidly, and to cope with large numbers of patients in a relatively thorough fashion. It is reasonable, however, to assume that doctors who believe that many elements of good medical practice are unrealistic are doctors who are frustrated in their work.

Table 1 shows the product-moment correlations among the three indicators of frustration. The average correlation among the three indicators is .27, the highest correlation (−.37) is between trivial consultations and harassment reported, and the lowest correlation (−.19) is between realistic practice and harassment reported.

To some extent it is possible to evaluate our assumption that the three questions are indicators of frustration by examining the correlations between these indicators and various questions we believe depict in some fashion the doctor's frustration. Table 2 provides data on each of the indicators and on various other items: the doctor's attitude toward the trend for patients to bring less serious problems to doctors; the doctor's belief that the National Health Service does not protect doctors from unreasonable demands from patients; the doctor's response that patients are too demanding; his report that in the past month patients became hostile to him; his response that many of his patients have been hypochondriacs; his report that he found himself frequently dealing with family disputes and marital discord; his response that he spent a large proportion of his days doing things requiring no real skill and experience; and his view that there was low inducement for good medical practice. Of the 24 correlations between these items and our three indicators, only one did not reach statistical significance. The average correlations between these items and trivial consultations, practice realistic, and harassment reported were .24, .16, and .25, respectively.

Implicit in the discussion of our indicators has been an assumption that although the proportion of problem patients may vary somewhat from practice to practice, it is unlikely that the large variations in response to our indicators could be explained by the fact that different doctors have varying kinds of patients. Although we have limited data to test this assumption, we can in part assess its validity by seeing to what extent responses to these indicators vary from one region to another. We also asked doctors to estimate the social class background of their patients, and we can consider to what extent these indicators vary by the reported social class characteristics of the doctors' patients. Tables 3 and 4 provide the relevant data.

Table 3 Regional Variations and Indicators of Frustration (Per Cent)

Regional Variation	Trivial Consultations		Practice Realistic		Harrassment Reported	
	High — Reports 25% or More as Trivial (N = 455)	Low — Reports Less Than 25% as Trivial (N = 317)	No — Scores of 0-6 (N = 336)	Yes — Scores of 7 or More (N = 436)	High — One or More Occurs Frequently (N = 432)	Low — None Occurs Frequently (N = 340)
Northern region	08	06	09	06	08	06
East and West Riding region	09	09	09	10	11	08
North Midland region	08	07	06	09	08	07
Eastern region	10	14	10	13	10	13
London and Southeastern region	18	18	20	17	18	19
Southern region	05	12	07	08	06	10
Southwestern region	09	09	09	09	07	11
Midland region	11	12	11	12	12	11
Northwestern region	14	10	13	11	14	10
Welsh region	07	03	07	05	06	05

Table 4   Indicators of Frustration and Doctors' Reports of the Social Class Status of Their Patients (Per Cent)

| | Doctors' Reports that Their Patients Are Mainly: | | | |
| | Upper Middle Class and Above | Lower Middle Class | Working Class | |
Indicators of Frustration				Total
Trivial Consultations				
Reports 50 per cent or more trivial ($N = 187$)	13	33	54	100
Reports as trivial 25 per cent but less than 50 per cent ($N = 268$)	09	47	44	100
Reports as trivial 10 per cent but less than 25 per cent ($N = 224$)	12	55	33	100
Reports less than 10 per cent trivial ($N = 93$)	11	53	37	101
			$r = -.09$	
Practice Realistic				
Low (Score of 2 or less) ($N = 156$)	08	44	48	100
(Score of 3–6) ($N = 180$)	11	46	44	101
(Score of 7–10) ($N = 231$)	13	46	40	99
High (Score of 11 or more) ($N = 205$)	11	50	39	100
			$r = -.06$[a]	
Harassment Reported (Number of Frequent Responses)				
None ($N = 340$)	12	51	37	100
One ($N = 175$)	12	47	41	100
Two ($N = 108$)	07	50	43	100
Three or more ($N = 149$)	10	33	57	100
			$r = .15$	

[a] does not achieve statistical significance at the .05 level.

An examination of Table 3 shows that when one considers doctors who are high or low on the various indicators of frustration, very large differences do not appear from region to region—certainly not enough to explain the large differences among doctors on these indicators. There is some tendency, however, for doctors who practice in the Southern Region to be less frustrated and those in the Welsh and Northwestern Regions to be more frustrated. Table 4 shows some relationship between the class characteristics of patients and their responses to various indicators of frustration. In general, doctors who report the highest proportion of trivial consultations and those who report the highest levels of harassment are more likely to report that their patients are primarily working class. A similar trend obtains in respect to the practice-realistic indicator, although the difference is more modest. Overall, these variations are not sufficiently large to influence other findings; in the strongest case patients' social class explains slightly more than 2 percent of the total variance. It would be interesting to consider whether the differences observed result from varying types of complaints among patients from varying class backgrounds, or whether they reflect something about the communication between doctors and working-class patients. Unfortunately, our data are not sufficient to carry this issue further.

An Examination of Correlates of Frustration among General Practitioners

The independent variables used in this analysis are summarized in Table 5. Because of the amount of information available, we can discuss only some of these variables. Emphasis will be given to those factors of greatest significance in explaining frustration. Our independent variables are divided into three groups: (1) characteristics of the doctor and factors describing him, such as his educational background; (2) characteristics of the doctor's practice and professional behavior and affiliations; and (3) doctor's attitudinal orientations. The third category, which contains expressions of general inclinations, includes items that are "least objective" and most difficult to interpret, since responses to some of these items may also be manifestations of the doctor's frustration.

Table 6 shows the relationship between our three indicators of frustration and doctor's age, sex, parental background, and three indices of the doctor's educational background. In most instances these relationships are very small and do not reach statistical significance. There are some exceptions, but they are not consistent across the three frustration indicators, and thus we cannot place high reliance on them. Older doctors are more likely to feel that certain standards of practice are realistic. Postgraduate course work appears to insu-

Table 5 Independent Variables Used in the Analysis of Frustration Indicators

Doctor's Personal Characteristics and Educational Background	Practice Organization and Professional Behavior	Doctor's Attitudinal Orientations
1. Age	7. Daily patient office load	25. Doctor's social orientation to medicine
2. Sex	8. Has a medically trained assistant	26. Attitude toward G.P.'s responsibility for psychiatric patients
3. Father's occupational level	9. Number of partners	27. Attitude toward management of psychiatric patients
4. Amount of hospital training	10. Has an appointment system	28. Attitude toward the Ministry of Health
5. Postgraduate course work	11. Number of private patients	29. Attitude toward sacrificing one's own interests
6. Education in social medicine, psychiatry, and the behavioral sciences	12. List size	30. Reported uncertainty in decision making
	13. Access to hospital beds	31. Reports he would practice differently outside the NHS
	14. Has a hospital appointment	32. Overall satisfaction with general practice
	15. Town size of practice location	33. Estimate of a reasonable patient load
	16. Use of diagnostic facilities	34. Strongly agrees that even a very busy doctor has an obligation to know his patients personally
	17. Professional consultations	35. Doctor's patient load relative to number of patients he reports he can reasonably handle
	18. Receives help from a local authority attachment	
	19. Total practice time spent during previous day	
	20. Member of the College of General Practitioners	
	21. Member of British Medical Association	
	22. Does some regular psychotherapy	
	23. Reports that he seeks out patients' problems and provides supportive care	
	24. Number of professional journals read	

Table 6 Personal Characteristics and Frustration (Per Cent)

Personal Characteristics	Trivial Consultations			Practice Realistic			Harassment Reported		
	High — Reports 25% or More as Trivial (N = 455)	Low — Reports Less than 25% as Trivial (N = 317)	r	No — Scores of 0-6 (N = 336)	Yes — Scores of 7 or More (N = 436)	r	High — One or More Occurs Frequently (N = 432)	Low — None Occurs Frequently (N = 340)	r
1. Age (51 years of age or older) (N = 219)	26	32	.06[a]	24	32	.15	26	31	−.04[a]
2. Sex—male (N = 717)	94	92	.04[a]	95	92	.04[a]	94	92	−.04[a]
3. Father's occupational level—professional and intermediate (N = 629)	80	84	−.07[a]	78	84	−.03[a]	79	84	.09
4. Training—above median category in hospital training—3½ years or more (N = 224)	31	27	−.02[a]	31	28	.02[a]	28	30	−.03[a]
5. Course work—none in past five years (N = 265)	37	31	.08	39	31	.11	36	32	−.04[a]
6. Education in psychiatry, social medicine, and the behavioral sciences (N = 189)	23	26	.04[a]	22	26	.04[a]	24	26	−.02[a]

[a] r does not reach statistical significance at the .05 level.

151

Table 7 Factors Describing Practice Organization and Professional Behavior and Frustration (Per Cent)

Pratice Organization and Professional Behavior	Trivial Consultations			Practice Realistic			Harassment Reported		
	High Reports 25% or More as Trivial (N = 455)	Low Reports Less than 25% as Trivial (N = 317)	r	No Scores of 0–6 (N = 336)	Yes Scores of 7 or More (N = 436)	r	High One or More Occurs Frequently (N = 432)	Low None Occurs Frequently (N = 340)	r
7. Daily patient load—sees 50 or more patients a day during busy period (N = 421)	61	46	−.28	57	52	−.11	60	48	.22
8. Has an M.D. assistant (N = 76)	07	14	.10	09	11	.03[a]	07	14	−.11
9. Number of partners: four or more (N = 79)	10	10	.03[a]	07	13	.05[a]	11	10	.01[a]
10. Has an appointment system (N = 261)	31	39	−.14	30	37	−.06[a]	31	37	.08
11. No private patients (N = 272)	39	29	.15	37	34	.06[a]	39	30	−.08
12. List size—3000 patients or more (N = 308)	42	37	−.11	35	44	.11	41	38	.06[a]
13. Bed access—yes (N = 420)	51	60	−.11	50	58	−.04[a]	51	58	07
14. Hospital appointment—yes (N = 269)	33	37	−.06[a]	34	36	.02[a]	32	38	.07

15. Town size—100,000 or more (N = 263)	39	27	-.13	35	35	34	-.05[a]	37	30	.07
16. Use of diagnostic facilities—above median category in number of procedures used (N = 283)	35	39	.10	35	38	38	.06[a]	35	38	-.07[a]
17. Professional contacts—above median category (N = 333)	42	44	.07[a]	41	45	45	.07[a]	42	45	-.08
18. Help from local authorities—none (N = 582)	77	73	-.10	76	75	75	.04[a]	75	76	.00[a]
19. Total practice time spent during previous day—above median category (N = 332)	44	41	-.08	46	41	41	-.04[a]	45	40	.07[a]
20. Member of the College of General Practitioners (N = 216)	24	34	-.13	23	32	32	-.12	25	31	.11
21. Member of the British Medical Association (N = 655)	83	87	-.07[a]	82	87	87	-.11	83	88	.10
22. Does some regular psychotherapy (N = 172)	21	24	-.01[a]	22	23	23	-.01[a]	22	23	-.01[a]
23. Reports that he seeks out patients' problems and provides supportive care (N = 465)	59	62	.08	54	65	65	.16	57	64	-.06[a]
24. Reads three or more professional journals (N = 229)	26	34	.05[a]	29	30	30	.02[a]	29	30	-.04[a]

[a] r does not reach statistical significance at the .05 level.

Table 8 Doctors' Attitudinal Orientations and Indicators of Frustration (Per Cent)

Attitudinal Orientations	Trivial Consultations			Practice Realistic			Harassment Reported		
	High	Low		No	Yes		High	Low	
	Reports 25% or More as Trivial (*N* = 455)	Reports Less than 25% as Trivial (*N* = 317)	*r*	Scores of 0–6 (*N* = 336)	Scores of 7 or More (*N* = 436)	*r*	One or More Occurs Frequently (*N* = 432)	None Occurs Frequently (*N* = 340)	*r*
25. Social orientation to medicine—Above median category (N = 348)	36	58	−.34	39	50	−.20	42	49	.16
26. Attitude toward G.P.'s responsibility for psychiatric patients—believes in almost all cases such care is G.P.'s responsibility (N = 264)	29	41	−.23	30	38	−.17	32	37	.09
27. Attitude toward management of psychiatric patients—believes G.P. should manage difficult psychiatric patients by himself (*N* = 239)	29	34	−.10	29	33	−.09	31	31	.08

28. Attitude toward the Ministry of Health—above median category in acceptance ($N = 248$)	29	37	.17	26	37	.13	30	35	−.04[a]
29. Attitude toward sacrificing one's own interests—above median category ($N = 307$)	37	44	.12	33	45	.20	35	45	−.14
30. Low reported uncertainty in decision making—below median category ($N = 304$)	36	44	−.17	32	45	−.15	35	45	.22
31. Reports would practice differently outside NHS ($N = 451$)	64	50	−.20	69	50	−.22	65	50	.18
32. Overall high satisfaction with general practice—above median category ($N = 362$)	36	62	−.35	33	59	−.33	39	57	.25
33. Under present arrangements feels he can look after 2500 patients or more ($N = 244$)	28	37	.08	12	47	.40	29	35	−.09
34. Strongly agrees that even a very busy doctor has obligation to know patients on a personal basis ($N = 288$)	34	43	−.13	30	43	−.14	33	43	.15
35. Reports that he looks after more patients than he reasonably can handle ($N = 487$)	67	57	.15	72	56	.17	67	59	−.10

[a] r does not reach statistical significance at the .05 level.

155

late doctors from frustration on two of the indicators, but to a modest degree. Doctors who report the highest proportion of trivial cases, and those who believe practice standards are unrealistic, are least likely to have had postgraduate course work. On the whole, however, we must conclude that personal characteristics of doctors and their educational background have little influence on the frustration they experience.

Table 7 presents data describing the relationships between the frustration indicators and variables characterizing the doctor's practice organization and professional behavior. The most striking fact concerning this table is that, for the most part, practice organization and professional behavior have no great impact on the indicators of frustration. The one variable that stands out among the eighteen described in the table is the number of patients the doctor sees in his office during a typical busy day. Doctors who see more patients tend to regard a higher proportion of their patient load as trivial and report greater harassment. Although this variable is less influential in relation to the practice-realistic indicator, its influence is statistically significant. Another factor consistent across all three indicators is membership in the College of General Practitioners, although its overall influence is more modest than that of the previously mentioned variable. What is perhaps most important in this table is that such factors as number of partners, whether the doctor has a hospital appointment, whether he does regular psychotherapy, his reading of professional journals, his use of diagnostic facilities, professional consultations, and the like have relatively little influence on the degree of frustration experienced by the doctor.

The number of patients a doctor sees on a particular day appears to be an important indicator of how he must work. Doctors who process patients in large numbers and who must work rapidly tend to have a very different style of work than doctors with smaller patient loads, and the former may often find patients with psychological and social complications a nuisance within the context of their practice. The influence of patient load can be seen by considering that while doctors with larger practices tend to agree more than those with smaller practices that high quality practice is possible, yet those who process many patients on a given day are higher than other doctors on this frustration indicator. Moreover, it should be clear that the number of patients the doctor sees during a single day is a better predictor of frustration than list size. Apparently it is not the number of patients one cares for or how long one works that is most important, but rather the pressure patient load places on the mode of the doctor's practice.

Table 8 presents data on the relationship of eleven attitudinal variables and the three indicators of frustration. Here a radically different picture emerges. We find that the doctors' attitudinal predispositions are substantially and consistently related to the degree of frustration reported. Doctors who are more frustrated have a lesser social orientation to medical care, report considerably greater uncertainty in making decisions, are less likely to believe that psychiatric patients are their responsibility or that they should manage psychiatric patients by themselves, report that they would practice differently outside the National Health Service, are less likely to feel a personal obligation to patients, feel they have too many patients, and the like. Although Table 8 provides data on only one indicator of general dissatisfaction, we tend to find a rather substantial relationship between almost every indicator of dissatisfaction and the three indicators of frustration. ﹀

As noted earlier, these data must be viewed with some caution since such attitudinal measures might be regarded as occupying part of the same general domain as the dependent variables. Those who report many exasperating experiences tend to be the same people who report uncertainty, negativism, and dissatisfaction. Both types of reports may stem from the same general response tendencies. After examining hundreds of relationships among the various indicators available, we obtained the strong impression that a certain amount of the frustration and dissatisfaction is embodied in the personalities and orientations of the doctors themselves. Events in 1965–66 might have brought out their most negativistic orientations, and the data appear to reflect an interaction between historical events and modal personality characteristics. One might speculate that many of the personalities drawn to medical practice were increasingly ill-fitted for dealing with growing patient lists and changing conditions of practice, which helped undermine the general practitioner's status and sense of self-confidence. Those with positive attitudinal orientations and a sense of medicine as a social endeavor appear to have adapted more readily to some of the less favorable changes in the general practitioner's conditions of work.

The Cumulative Effect of Various Independent Variables

Although our variables differ in their degree of skewness, and some are dichotomous, the use of a multiple regression analysis will provide some idea of their cumulative influence. Obviously, many of our independent variables are intercorrelated among themselves, and thus our presentation of zero-order relationships include considerable redundancies. Although it is not realistic to attempt a causal model with the data at hand, it is instructive to consider the combined effects of the most influential variables in the analysis.

If we consider the six variables relevant to the doctors' background and educational experiences, it is clear that they explain from 1.4 to 4 percent of the total variance of the three indicators of frustration. This confirms our earlier observation that this group of variables has minimum influence on the dependent variables. If we consider the eighteen variables describing the doctors' practice organization and professional behavior, the degree of variance explained among the frustration indicators varies from 8 to 13 percent. In the case of each dependent variable, a small number of independent variables explains most of the influence. The number of patients the doctor sees during a busy day is the most important predictor of trivial consultations and harassment reported and one of the most influential factors affecting realistic practice.

The number of patients seen on a busy day accounts for more than half of the total variance of harassment reported that can be explained by the group of eighteen predictors. In the case of the practice-realistic variable, five of the eighteen predictors account for four-fifths of the total variance: (1) doctors' reports that they seek out patients' problems and provide supportive care; (2) smaller list size; (3) smaller number of patients seen on a busy day; (4) membership in the College of General Practitioners; and (5) membership in the British Medical Association. Finally, in the case of trivial consultations, the number of patients seen by the doctor on a busy day explains almost two-thirds of the total variance accounted for by the eighteen variables. Most of the remaining variance that can be explained is accounted for by five other variables: (1) is not a member of the College of General Practice; (2) has fewer private patients; (3) has no appointment system; (4) has no medically trained assistant; and (5) has no bed access.

A somewhat different picture emerges in respect to the group of attitudinal variables. These eleven independent variables account for 12 percent of the variance of harassment reported, 23 percent of the variance of trivial consultations, and 28 percent of the variance of practice realistic. Once again, in each case a small number of variables accounts for most of the variance explained by the entire group of variables. In the case of harassment reported, overall satisfaction with general practice and uncertainty in making decisions account for almost four-fifths of the variance explained. In the case of practice-realistic the doctor's estimate of a good number of patients, his overall satisfaction, and his attitude toward sacrificing his own interests account for approximately 85 percent of the total variance explained. Finally, in the case of trivial consultations, overall satisfaction, social orientation to medicine, and the doctor's attitude toward the management of psychiatric patients account for approximately 85 percent of the explained variance. Since there is a considerable degree of overlap among the various attitudinal orientations—and with the exception of overall satisfaction different variables are most influential for each of the dependent variables—it is impossible to specify precisely which aspects of these attitudinal orientations are most important.

The Relationship between Frustration and Performance

There still remains the question central to our entire analysis, a difficult one to answer definitively: Is there any relationship between the quality of a doctor's performance and the degree to which he feels frustrated? If no such relationship exists, then the previous analysis, however interesting, has no great importance. Data in Table 7 show very little relationship between most patterns of practice believed by medical care experts to be desirable and our indicators of frustration. Less frustrated doctors tend to use more diagnostic procedures, but such relationships are very modest and reach statistical significance in only one of three instances. Few of our practice measures deal with patient-care performance, however.

Four other items of information from the doctors in our sample are pertinent to this question, however. Each doctor was asked to indicate how often in the past month he did not have time to do an adequate examination of a patient, and how often he did not have time to do what was necessary for the patient. These questions do not establish standards and are, thus, open to different interpretations, but they may give us some indications of the doctors' perceptions of the quality of their performance. We also asked doctors how frequently in the past month they had issued prescriptions (excluding repeat prescriptions) without seeing the patient. Most experts would agree that such behavior constitutes low-quality medical care. Finally, we asked doctors to report how frequently in the previous month they gave patients certificates although they were not really convinced that the patient was too sick for work. Although this last item is more difficult to interpret, it seems reasonable to argue that doctors who engage in such behavior are either insecure, insufficiently motivated, or amenable to considerable client control. None of these traits would be viewed as assets on the part of the doctor. Table 9 presents data showing the relationship between these four items and the three indicators of frustration.

As an examination of the table shows, all four performance items are significantly related to all three indicators, in some cases to a substantial degree. Although these data cannot be viewed as definitive, they strongly suggest that frustrated doctors tend to be poorer doctors and are more willing to take undesirable short cuts.

Discussion and Conclusion

One of the more impressive findings of this study has been the failure to account for differences in frustration by objective factors characterizing the doctor, his educational experiences, the structure of his practice, and profes-

Table 9 Reports on Performance and Dependent Variables (Per Cent)

Performance Reports	Trivial Consultations			Practice Realistic			Harassment Reported		
	High	Low		No	Yes		High	Low	
	Reports 25% or More as Trivial (N = 455)	Reports Less than 25% as Trivial (N = 317)	r	Scores of 0–6 (N = 336)	Scores of 7 or More (N = 436)	r	One or More Occurs Frequently (N = 432)	None Occurs Frequently (N = 340)	r
1. Reports that he didn't have time to do an adequate examination quite a few times or more during past month (N = 216)	34	20	.20	39	20	.25	36	15	−.28
2. Reports that he didn't have time to do what he felt was necessary for the patient quite a few times or more during past month (N = 232)	36	21	.16	41	22	.25	38	20	−.20
3. Reports that he issued prescriptions (excluding repeat prescriptions) without seeing the patient quite a few times or more during past month (N = 109)	17	10	.11	17	12	.12	19	09	−.20
4. Reports he gave patients certificates although he wasn't really convinced that patient was too sick for work quite a few times or more during past month (N = 202)	35	14	.28	34	20	.16	39	09	−.41

sional orientations. With the exception of the number of patients that doctors deal with on a busy day, no other variable of an objective kind has a large effect on the degree of frustration experienced by doctors. Our data strongly suggest that doctors who must cope with a very large daily patient load must adapt their practice to these demands and function somewhat differently from those who have smaller patient loads. This requires doctors to take various short cuts, some of which violate professional standards and which they find upsetting.

These findings have considerable practical significance, but they must be viewed with great caution. On the face of it, they tend to contradict the hope on the part of many medical care experts that doctors' frustrations can be significantly alleviated through the stimulation of group practice, the use of ancillary help, more organization of practice, more intensive educational and professional experience, and the like. Our findings suggest that there is little difference among doctors who vary on these factors. Nevertheless, our sample may not have offered enough variety of organizational forms and practice variations to make a fair assessment of the question. Although many of the doctors in our sample practiced in groups, few practiced in well-organized groups with effective use of ancillary personnel. Although there were large variations in educational background among the doctors in the sample, for the most part the education was all of the same character—it emphasized the hospital practice of medicine in contrast to social and preventive aspects of medicine. Although many of the doctors had bed access and hospital appointments, it was clear that they did not all feel welcome as equal participants in hospital contexts. Thus, although the findings here are disconcerting, they are hardly a definitive answer to the issues posed by medical care experts the world over.

We did find a reasonably large influence of attitudinal orientations on the degree of frustration experienced by doctors. After reviewing these data in many different ways, we obtained the impression that there are complex attitudinal predispositions among doctors that significantly influence their responses, irrespective of the organization of their practices or the conditions of service. This is supported by the fact that attitudinal variables explain a considerable amount of variance even after all of the background and practice variables are introduced. It is also very possible that these are deep-rooted personality tendencies that are not easily modified by educational programs or changes in the organization of medical care.

General practice as an activity is radically changing under modern conditions of medical care. The general practitioner, if he is to be successful, must have a social and preventive orientation as well as a technical one, and he must be able to obtain gratification from situations where he deals with people in circumstances of great uncertainty and where basic knowledge is frequently absent. Yet many of the students selected by medical schools in both England

162   CORRELATES OF FRUSTRATION AMONG GENERAL PRACTITIONERS

and the United States do not have particularly strong personal motives to engage in such practice, nor does their training reinforce such motives if they are present. Many medical students have entrepreneurial orientations and strong scientific-technical perspectives. Moreover, there are strong biases among medical school admissions committees toward selecting students with background in the "hard" rather than the behavioral sciences, and there is a large overrepresentation of students from higher socioeconomic groups. In England, for example, less than 2 percent of our entire sample came from families whose fathers had partly skilled or unskilled occupations. This situation exists despite the availability in recent years of government grants to able students accepted by the medical schools. This fact is interesting in light of the earlier observation that doctors who seem to be most frustrated are overrepresented among those with working-class practices.

Notes

1. Mechanic, D. (1968). *Medical Sociology: A Selected View*. New York: Free Press.
2. Faich, R. (1969). "Social and Structural Factors Affecting Work Satisfaction: A Case Study of General Practitioners in the English Health Service." Unpublished Ph.D. thesis, University of Wisconsin.
3. For such arguments, see: Great Britain, Ministry of Health (1965). *The Field Work of the Family Doctor*. London: Her Majesty's Stationery Office; College of General Practitioners (1965). *Report of a Symposium on the Art and the Science of General Practice*; or, *The Problems of General Practice*. Torquay: Devonshire Press; Great Britain, Royal Commission on Medical Education (1968). *1965–68 Report*, Cmnd. 3569. London: Her Majesty's Stationery Office.
4. Cartwright, A. (1967). *Patients and Their Doctors: A Study of General Practice*. London: Routledge & Kegan Paul.
5. *Ibid.*, p. 45.

PART FOUR

STRESS, SOCIAL ADAPTATION, AND THE PROVISION OF MENTAL HEALTH SERVICES

CHAPTER XI

Social Structure and Personal Adaptation: Some Neglected Dimensions

The study of social adaptation is usually pursued without seriously considering the pervasive influence of social structural variables on personal and social adaptation. Traditional approaches to adaptation have developed from psychodynamic studies and ego psychology, and there has been a continuing tendency to view mastery of the environment in terms of intrapsychic mechanisms that allow individuals to psychologically control environmental stimuli impinging on them and to maintain a state of personal comfort. Recently, with growing emphasis on environmental mastery and effective performance, some investigators have broadened their scope of study to include such concerns as the learning and use of skills and the direct manipulation of the environment, but this new development has not been very systematically developed. Almost all investigators, regardless of their orientations, fail to consider the relationship between social structure and mastery.

From a social psychological point of view, it has become apparent to investigators of stress that adaptation must be considered in terms of the relationship between external physical and social demands on the person and his resources to deal with these demands.[1] It has become commonplace to consider the potentialities for adaptation in terms of the fit between person and environment, and even therapeutic approaches are frequently based on achieving a more congruent fit. Since the approach to adaptation has been primarily a psychological one, the person-environment fit, usually considered, is an attitudinal fit or one based on how the person perceives himself in relation to the environment. Only recently has there been greater emphasis on the issue of whether the person's actual skills are capable of dealing with true external demands.

Successful personal adaptation has at least three components at the individual level.

1. The person must have the capabilities and skills to deal with the social and environmental demands to which he is exposed. For the sake of simplicity, I shall designate these skills as coping capabilities. These capacities involve not only the ability to react to environmental demands but also the capabilities to influence and control the demands to which one will be exposed and at what pace.

2. Individuals must be motivated to meet the demands that become evident in their environment. Individuals can escape anxiety and discomfort by lowering their motivation and aspirations, but (as we shall see later) there are many social constraints against this mode of reducing stress. As motivation increases, the consequences of failing to achieve mastery also increase, and the level of motivation is frequently an important prerequisite for experiencing psychological discomfort.

3. Individuals must have the capabilities to maintain a state of psychological equilibrium so that they can direct their energies and skills to meet external in contrast to internal needs. Much of the psychological literature on adaptation concerns itself with this third dimension—one that I call "defense." Although psychologists who have studied stress have viewed defense as an end in itself, it is reasonable to consider defense as a set of mechanisms that facilitates continuing performance and mastery. Defenses that may be very successful in diminishing pain and discomfort may be catastrophic for personal adaptation if they retard the enactment of behavior directed toward real threats in the environment. To state the matter bluntly: such a defense as denial—a persistant and powerful psychological response—will do a drowning man no good!

There is still another kind of person-environment fit that is rarely discussed in the literature on stress and adaptation, but it is probably the most important of all. This fit between the social structure and environmental demands is probably the major determinant of successful social adaptation. Man's abilities to cope with the environment depend on the efficacy of the solutions that his culture provides, and the skills he develops are dependent on the adequacy of the preparatory institutions to which he has been exposed. To the extent that schools and informal types of preparation are inadequate to the tasks men face, social disruption and personal failure will be inevitable, no matter how effective the individual's psychological capacities are. Similarly, the kinds of motivation that people have and the directions in which these motivations will be channeled will depend on the incentive systems in a society—the patterns of behavior and performance that are valued and the patterns that are condemned. Finally, the ability of persons to maintain psychological comfort will depend not only on their intrapsychic resources but also—and perhaps more importantly—on the social supports available or absent in the environment. Men depend on others for justification and admiration, and few men can survive without support from some segment of their fellows.[2]

Certainly, the foregoing is obvious. As every beginning student of sociology learns in the first few weeks, solutions to life tasks become institutionalized and tend to be cumulative through the generations. Men learn through the experience of others, and solutions to environmental demands and challenges are taught from one generation to another. The ability of men and societies to adapt to the conditions of their lives depends largely on the adequacy of such institutionalized solutions.

The influence of social structure is, of course, more complicated than this discussion suggests. The community not only defines solutions to environmental challenges but also imposes new challenges through the social values it perpetuates. On the most primitive levels, the community defines territoriality, mobility, the pattern of fertility, food acquisition and use, mating, and social responsibility. But complex social structures also involve a large and varied set of demands that impinges on almost every aspect of life from survival to the most trivial of interrelationships.

Institutionalized solutions to environmental problems must change as the problems themselves change. To the extent that preparatory and evaluative institutions in a society are fitted to the types of problems people in the society must face, then most persons are likely to acquire the skills and capacities to meet life demands and challenges. But with rapid technological and social change, institutionalized solutions to new problems are likely to lag behind, and the probability increases that a larger proportion of the population will have difficulties in accommodating to life problems. Generally, the literature on stress and coping has aided the myth that adaptation is dependent on the ability of individuals to develop personal mastery over their environment. Indeed, most psychological studies of adaptation are studies of individuals and not of groups. But even a superficial thrust into the anthropological literature indicates how interdependent men are, even in the most simple of societies, and how dependent they are on group solutions in dealing with environmental problems. It becomes clearer and clearer that major stresses on modern man are not amenable to individual solutions, but depend on highly organized cooperative efforts that transcend the efforts of any individual man, no matter how well developed his personal resources are.

The Influence of Social Networks on Adaptive Behavior

Although the literature on stress often refers to group influences on adaptation to stress, these references are frequently vague. Men relate to groups in a great many ways, and they may relate to the same group in different ways. Many groups define values and goals, and serve as a reference point from which individuals can evaluate themselves. Or they may serve to encourage persons and help to allay anxiety. But the most important consideration, from the perspective of this chapter, is that group organization and cooperation allow for the development of mastery through specialization of function, pooling of resources and information, developing reciprocal help-giving relationships, and the like. It is an important truism that men are highly interdependent, and only through complex organization are the more complicated jobs of the community fulfilled. The effectiveness of individuals in many spheres of action is dependent almost exclusively on the maintenance of viable forms of organization and cooperation that allow important tasks to be mastered.

Much of the confusion in the stress literature results from viewing stress as a short-term single stimulus instead of a complex set of changing conditions that have a history and a future. Man must respond to these conditions through time and must adapt his behavior to the changing character of the stimuli. Thus, mastery of stress is not a simple repertoire; it is an active process over time in relationship to demands that are themselves changing, and that are often symbolically created by the groups within which man lives and new technologies which such groups develop. Adaptation itself creates new demands on man that require still further adaptations in a continuing spiral.[3]

Moreover, many demands are ambiguous and intangible; they are created out of the social fabric and social climate that exist at any time. Challenges, therefore, are a product of the transaction between man and his environment, and many of the demands to which man must adapt are demands that he himself has created. People, to some extent, can affect the particular demands to which they will be exposed and the pace of exposure. They can select from alternative environments and reference groups in testing themselves against their environments. They not only respond but require other persons and groups to respond to them. This complex interplay between men involves adaptive techniques that are infrequently referred to in the study of short-term single stressors. Men pace themselves; they selectively seek information in relation to their needs for developing solutions, on the one hand, and protecting their "selves" on the other; they anticipate future situations and plan solutions that they test; they frequently select the grounds on which their adaptive struggles will take place and carefully choose appropriate spheres of action. In short, they are more than seeds carried by the winds, or at least they can act as if they are.

One of the most impressive tests of the limits and potentialities of man's adaptive capacities occurs in situations where men must live in controlled environments that are contrary to their values and goals, and situations where men are victims of arbitrary power such as in concentration camps and prisons. We know from these situations that men often lose hope and become apathetic, accepting their fate without a fight. But we also know that, even under the most desperate and unencouraging circumstances, men succeed in developing competing forms of social organization that allow them to resist their oppressors and may allow them to survive. Eugene Kogon,[4] a longterm resident of Buchenwald, describes the underground organization of inmates under the most hellish of conditions.

There were a number of effective means by which the prisoners could assert their interests. They were all based on two essential prerequisites: power inside the camp, and a well organized intelligence service. . . . Functional cohesion was insured by the prisoner intelligence service. Such a service was built up in every camp from the very outset. Reliable key members of the ruling group—or the group seeking power—were systematically wormed into all important posts, sometimes only after bitter and complex maneuvering. There they were able to observe everything that happened in the ranks of the SS and the prisoners, to obtain information on every personnel shift and policy trend, to overhear every conversation....Every detail had its official "runners" ostensibly appointed in order to maintain liaison with the numerous scattered SS offices. Actually three fourths of their time was taken up by work on behalf of the prisoners (pp. 254–255).

Kogon describes in detail how the underground organization was successful in controlling work assignments and reassignment of inmates to other camps and outside work details, and how they were successful in hiding and protecting valuable members of the underground from the SS. Kogon concedes that the prisoners were not strong enough to forestall general SS directives involving mass liquidations and similar actions, but they had vast influence on matters involving "the ordinary minutiae of camp life."

The type of organization that Kogan dramatically describes has been similarly observed in prisons,[5,6] mental hospitals,[7] military organizations,[8] and many other organizational contexts. To the extent that participants in organizations do not share the goals and values of its managers and authorities, an informal organization emerges that often impedes directives and programs that threaten the welfare of organizational participants. I have described the principles underlying the power of such subordinate personnel elsewhere;[9] I simply mention here that much of organizational power stems from small decisions made on daily tasks, or what Kogon calls "ordinary minutiae." Since higher-status organizational participants wish to be relieved of such burdensome "dirty work" or are dependent on others to perform it for other reasons, the dependency relationship and access to the performance of daily work give the subordinate considerable opportunity for effective vetoes on organizational policies.

As solutions to important problems become more complex, these problems are less likely to be resolved by individual initiative and action. Instead, they are likely to depend on the ability of men to work out organized solutions involving group actions. Within this context, we must note that individuals who may be effective persons from a psychological perspective may be unfitted because of their values and individual orientations for the kinds of group cooperation that are necessary in developing solutions to particular kinds of community problems. Thus, many effective copers may become impotent in influencing their environment because of their resistance or inability to submerge themselves into cooperative organized relationships with others.

There are many examples in modern life where men's disdain for organized participation interferes with effective performance. In the sphere of medicine, for example, the development of technology and associated growing costs of medical care require new forms of medical practice better fitted to the needs of the population than the highly individualized practice of medicine. Even in the absence of economic disincentives, doctors who are highly individualistic in their orientations tend to be reluctant to work within more organized practice settings.[10] Similarly in science, team research is becoming more of a necessity because of the costs and expansion of technology and specialized knowledge. Yet, there are strong resistances to working cooperatively among many scientists who are highly individualistic and competitive in their orientations.[11] Or, to consider another example, it is clear that organization of various aspects of the work force into groups that can bargain collectively is more effective than each man bargaining for himself. Although collective action is developing among a variety of professionals, there are very strong values in the higher professions that mitigate against collective action. To move more directly into the political realm, the futility of individual action in contesting such actions as the Vietnam war or the ABM in contrast to collective opposition is evident. Group action is not necessarily effective, but it may provide at least a fighting chance.

In considering the conditions under which men will confront their environment, the symbolic aspects of threat and adaptation are extremely important. It is rarely the most oppressed who rise up to the challenges of their fate, but usually the people who have had a taste of the possibilities of improving their condition.[12] Revolutions feed on faith and rarely occur when men see no way out. The unwillingness of many concentration camp victims to oppose their murderers may have resulted partly from the uncertainty of their individual fates but, more likely, such efforts seemed futile and hopeless. In contrast, when men have hopes of success they are often willing to take on the most powerful of adversaries. All of this is, of course, very speculative. It would be better for students of coping and adaptation to invest greater attention to the question of how men see their environment and their own potency in meeting that environment.

I must comment on a serious misconception that runs throughout the stress literature: the notion that successful adaptation requires an accurate perception of reality. There is perhaps no thought so stifling as to see ourselves in proper perspective. We all maintain our sense of self-respect and energy for action through perceptions that enhance our self-importance and self-esteem, and we maintain our sanity by suppressing the tremendous vulnerability we all experience in relation to the risks of the real world.[13] It is the beauty of symbolic environments that they allow men to enhance their sense of self-importance and the community to persist at the same time. Most men tend to rate themselves and their qualities somewhat higher than their fellows would rate them, and the social contract among men allows each to control the definition of the situation, to some extent, on matters most close to his own self-interest. When the contract breaks down, one can usually locate groups that help sustain one's own self-definition, and social life is organized so loosely that most men can manage to sustain comforting self-perceptions.

The appropriate criterion for evaluating various defensive processes is the extent to which such defenses facilitate coping and mastery. Obviously, if defensive processes reach too far beyond what is acceptable to one's fellows, they create difficulty and interfere with successful adaptation. But many misperceptions of reality aid coping and mastery, energize involvement and participation in life endeavors, and alleviate pain and discomfort that would distract the person from successful efforts at mastery. Reality, of course, is a social construction and, to the extent that perspectives are shared and socially reinforced, they may facilitate adaptation, irrespective of their objective truth. As W. I. Thomas noted many years ago, if men define situations as real, they are real in their consequences.

There are other concepts that have been emphasized by psychologists who study stress that are probably more important to their own self-conceptions than they are for most people. A variable like "accessibility to self" may have some importance for introspective psychologists, but there is no good evidence that relates such variables to successful adaptation. In fact, there is reason to believe that in many life endeavors too much self-awareness or introspection retards successful coping efforts. Many "successful" copers tend to be rather insensitive to their own intrapsychic experience and tend to orient themselves more to their outer environment than to their inner world.[14] Some very successful performers are truly public personalities in that they orient themselves outwardly and tend to have no very elaborate inner life. In contrast, there are persons who, by their abilities to see complexities in every issue, find it difficult to mobilize to attack any issue.

Some Problems in the Theory and Methodology of Stress Studies

If we take the position that adaptation is anticipatory as well as reactive, and that men frequently approach their environment with plans, the study of such processes requires a different approach. Within this view, man attempts to take on tasks he feels he can handle, he actively seeks information and feedback, he plans and anticipates problems, he insulates himself against defeat in a variety of ways, he keeps his options open, he distributes his commitments, he sets the stage for new efforts by practice and rehearsal, and he tries various solutions. One cannot study these activities effectively within an experimental mode that subjects man to specific stimuli and only measures limited reactions to these stimuli. But methodological models to successfully study such active processes of coping are very much undeveloped, and the lack of richness in the experimental stress literature reflects the unavailability of a successful experimental technology for studying adaptive attempts over time.

No matter how much we may lament the fact, the development of fields of study follows the development of research technologies more than theoretical problems. In the stress field, we have been the victim of many technologies that were useful and interesting in their own way, but that diverted researchers from basic issues. Perhaps most prominent have been the clinical-interview and psychological-assessment techniques, popular among ego psychologists. The clinical interview depended too fully on retrospective reports, and the structure of such data in the absence of controls allowed each investigator to promote his favorite set of conceptions. Similarly, the use of personality-assessment tools frequently allowed the investigator to explain but not illuminate performance differences. Thus we learned that men achieved because they had a need for achievement, that they were prejudiced because they were authoritarian, and that they did not participate in organizations because they were alienated. This form of absorption-by-naming took on the character of a popular sport and, although each of these conceptions involved an underlying theory of personality, the theory itself was either discredited or forgotten while the technologists continued to use the various measures that they could correlate with a host of other information. Because the study of stress has been somewhat limited by the fashionable methodologies of the past few decades, the picture of adaptation that emerges from the literature is one that depicts man as reactive and individualistic and his mode of coping as largely intrapsychic.

The major exception to this generalization has been the study of disasters and other life stresses under natural conditions. Approaches to natural stresses can follow a quasi-experimental design and, under some conditions, can utilize appropriate comparison groups. These studies, for the most part, present a much richer picture of the complexity of social adaptation and related factors.

But in view of the complexity of such situations, it is often difficult to ferret out precisely the variables that are most influential in modes of adaptation. The literature on social adaptation would benefit substantially from a richer interaction between field studies, more precise laboratory experiments, and more experimentation that utilizes simulations of real situations. There are obvious ethical barriers in simulating stressful life circumstances, but there are many real circumstances that are amenable to study by using experimental methodologies. Also, we must develop more complex experimental models that do not restrict so closely the subject's opportunity to exercise his adaptive repertoire in dealing with laboratory situations. We must provide richer opportunities for subjects than the option of pushing one lever or another. Investigations that involve a particularly impressive use of quasi-experimental models under natural circumstances are the study by Epstein[15] of paratrooper exercises and Skipper and Leonard's study[16] of response to the stress of hospitalization and tonsillectomy.

It is likely that in the near future we have most to learn from field studies of adaptation to particular stress events over time. This kind of involvement requires greater emphasis on prospective and processual studies. Since this need has been expressed many times before, let me emphasize more specific considerations instead of the more general points.

Clearly, we must go beyond people's subjective reports of how they feel and how they have responded to particular stressful circumstances. These reports are particularly dubious when they cover events retrospectively, since we know that part of the process of adaptation involves the subtle restructuring of the individual's attitudinal set toward events that have taken place.[17,18] Successful adaptation requires changes in attitudes and perspectives that are sufficiently subtle so that the person hardly recognizes the changes himself. Large and sudden modifications of attitudes and perspectives are likely to produce new stresses and, indeed, when such large changes occur, this is in itself evidence of difficulties and disruptions in successful adaptation. We, thus, must be suspicious of reconstructions of the past as true representations of what really took place.

But even reports of events involving continuing activities and use of short recall periods may have dubious reliability. If we are not to throw the baby out with the bathwater, we have to devote considerable effort to defining what kinds of reports are generally trustworthy and what kind are not. We can anticipate that persons will more reliably report their sex, age, family composition, and similar matters than they will their mental status and marital happiness, for instance. Even when dealing with "harder" variables, persons frequently distort their responses: women, for example, have a tendency to underestimate their age; very old people tend to overestimate their age; and many others tend to report their age in round numbers. In contrast, reports on such variables as loneliness have very low test-retest reliability.[19] To some extent, this is characteristic of all mood responses, which may widely vary from one day to another. Investigators, however, must be reasonably clear about the degree of reliability of measures that their studies require and the general range of reliability of varying measures that they might utilize.

Consider, for example, data dealing with people's reports of their use of medical services. These data may or may not be worthy of collection, depending on the interests of the investigator and the research question he is asking. If the investigator wants to know whether a person has been to a dentist, a doctor, or has been hospitalized during the preceding year, respondent reports will provide a reasonably reliable approximation. If, for some reason, small differences in the utilization of medical services are important to the study, then it is reasonably clear that respondent reports will be too biased to be of any use.[20] Similarly, if an investigator wishes to note no more than crude differences between social categories on some measure of utilization, respondent reports will serve his purpose more than if he wishes to assign specific reliable scores to individual persons. Even in the case of more crude analyses of such data, respondent reports are likely to be unacceptable if there is reason to believe that there are systematic biases in reporting among different social groups.

Reports on matters such as having a heart condition, obtaining surgery, being hospitalized, and going to a doctor are reasonably "hard" because these situations will have required specific actions on the part of the respondent, which are not routine. But most studies of stress involve questions about very ordinary things that involve routine behavior and common attitudes, and such data are particularly suspect. For example, in family studies when identical questions are asked of husband and wife concerning routine activities in the family, husband-wife correlations are small.[21] Similarly, we know, for example, that what mothers tell you about themselves and what they tell you about the behavior of their children tend to be more highly correlated than data obtained independently from mother and child.[22] Too frequently, investigators end up studying the subject's tendencies to respond and little else.

It is extraordinary that there are so few efforts to obtain independent data on behavior, since it is often accessible to research investigators with some effort. It is possible, for example, to obtain medical and other records that allow some assessment of the value of what people tell you. These records, of course, have their own sources of unreliability, but investigators are on much firmer ground if they have both respondent and record data available to them. We need, in general, further development of behavior ratings that are likely to depict more satisfactorily the variables we are really interested in rather than the measures more ordinarily used. This is not a simple task, but it is one we will have to assume at some point. Persons who deceive themselves that in the future we will develop a simple paper-and-pencil test to measure coping or adaptive potentialities are bound to be disillusioned. The concern we face is so complex and multifaceted that when we do develop some adequate measures, they are likely to be very complex ones. I think that these measures will have to be in the form of behavioral tests, and that the ordinary pencil-and-paper tests are incapable of the task.

At the theoretical level, one of the largest tasks that stress researchers face is the development of models that specify, in a predictive sense, under what conditions one set of adaptations will develop in contrast to another set. If the study of adaptation is to develop as a theoretical area, then we must do more than describe the array of behaviors characteristic of persons' adaptive attempts; we must begin to specify the relative probabilities that, under given circumstances, one coping attempt will follow rather than another. This theoretical approach will depend on rich field studies that depict the scope of alternatives, followed by more controlled laboratory studies that attempt to determine the conditions under which one or another form of behavior follows. In short, theoretical needs require a range of methods and, if investigators do not choose to be eclectic themselves, at least some dialogue among approaches must be maintained.

A more sophisticated theoretical approach is beginning to emerge from this kind of interaction. It is promising, for example, that experimentalists who previously took the view that people avoided "discomforting information" are now more appreciative that sometimes they do and sometimes they don't, and the entire matter is more complicated than earlier views suggested.[23] It may be too early to suggest convergences, but it may be that persons seek out information contrary to their views and perspectives when such information is important to their future coping efforts; discomforting information may primarily be avoided when it is believed to be of little utility. Or, to consider another example, early studies were concerned with the simplistic question of whether high interactors were more or less successful at various tasks. There is a growing appreciation of the fact that there are different kinds of interaction (which I previously referred to as interaction for instrumental purposes and interaction for the purposes of support), and also that interaction may not only facilitate activity and support people but also arouse competition and anxiety and lead to interference with effective performance.[24, 25] Variables such as the rate of interaction are too crude to be informative theoretically in understanding adaptation.

It is encouraging that social psychologists in general are moving away from using their concepts to absorb existing data and are giving increasing efforts toward developing an understanding of the contingencies affecting behavior. For example, when dissonance theory[26] first became fashionable it was frequently used to explain the results of a variety of studies by citing a dissonance explanation. Recently, however, there have been more serious attempts to specify, on the basis of various contingencies, the likely route of dissonance reduction. Similar efforts are taking place in the study of social comparison processes. It has been very common for social scientists to explain data after the fact by arguing that a person's behavior was a result of choosing particular reference groups. The more interesting issue—and one that is now receiving more attention—concerns the conditions under which identification with varying possible reference groups occurs. Ego psychology has similarly been handicapped by the failure to specify, in any rigorous way, the conditions under which one set of defenses will occur in opposition to another mode of adaptation, and under what conditions particular defenses will be selected. The literature abounds with discussions of particular defenses in isolation from others. Thus, we find discussions dealing with compensation (i.e., the tendency to do particularly well in some areas to overcome inadequacies in others) without awareness of a literature on status congruency (the psychological tendency to maintain one's various statuses at approximately the same level), which appears in opposition to it. The theory of compensation argues that people strive toward maintaining unequal levels of performance, whereas the theory of status congruency maintains that people strive toward maintaining equal levels of rank. These contradictions lead to theoretical contributions because they suggest that important intervening variables have been neglected. In the example cited it is likely that people tend to compensate when a particular dimension of their status or performance is blocked or unalterable. However, when there is opportunity to perform in any of several spheres, it may be that the need for congruency is dominant. I know of no specific data that clearly resolve the contradiction, but the recognition of a contradiction raises new issues.

In conclusion, I think that it would be advisable to pursue studies of adaptation with two particular models in mind. (1) On the one hand, we need more emphasis on field studies of adaptive struggles over time. Further attention must be given to collecting data at various points in time in contrast to using retrospective reports. Moreover, such studies should give greater emphasis to the development of behavioral measures. (2) At the same time, we should be pursuing a variety of cross-sectional studies that link particular adaptive strategies and coping devices to effective behavior on a variety of life tasks. Although there are many cross-sectional type studies in the stress area, few are concerned with the relationship of what people do in respect to how effective they are. In the past, more than a reasonable proportion of the total research effort has gone into attempts to link personality traits with effectiveness and, in many ways, this has been a disappointing effort. My guess is that greater emphasis on coping strategies themselves will provide a greater payoff. Finally, I believe that a field progresses when there is constant interplay between studies in natural settings and more precise experimental investigation. We should do all we can to nurture the bridges that make such collaboration possible and fruitful.

Notes

1. McGrath, J. (ed.) (1970). *Social and Psychological Factors in Stress*, New York: Holt, Rinehart and Winston.

2. For an elaboration of the views stated above, see D. Mechanic (1970). "Some Problems in Developing a Social Psychology of Adaptation to Stress." In J. McGrath (ed.), *ibid.*

3. See Dubos, R. (1965). *Man Adapting*, New Haven: Yale University Press.

4. Kogon, E. (1958). *The Theory and Practice of Hell*, New York: Berkely Medallion Books.

5. Sykes, G. (1958). *The Society of Captives*. Princeton, N.J.: Princeton University Press.

6. Sykes, G., and S. Messinger (1960). "The Inmate Social System." In R. Cloward et al., *Theoretical Studies in Social Organization of the Prison*. New York: Social Science Research Council, pp. 5–19.

7. Goffman, E. (1961). "The Underlife of a Public Institution: A Study of Ways of Making Out in a Mental Hospital." In E. Goffman, *Asylums: Essays on the Social Situation of Mental Patients and Other Inmates*. New York: Doubleday, pp. 173–320.

8. Cohen, A. (1966). *Deviance and Control*. Englewood Cliffs, N.J.: Prentice-Hall, pp. 78–80.

9. Mechanic, D. (1962). "Sources of Power of Lower Participants in Complex Organizations." *Administrative Science Quarterly*, 7:349–364.

10. See, for example, D. Mechanic (1968). "General Medical Practice in England and Wales." *New England Journal of Medicine*, 279:680–689.

11. Hagstrom, W. (1965). *The Scientific Community*. New York: Basic Books.

12. Runciman, W.G. (1966). *Relative Deprivation and Social Justice*. Berkeley: University of California Press.

13. Wolfenstein, M. (1957). *Disaster: A Psychological Essay*. New York: Free Press.

14. See, for example, studies of the psychological characteristics of astronauts, that is, S. Korchin and G. Ruff (1964). "Personality Characteristics of the Mercury Astronauts." In H. Wechsler and M. Greenblatt (eds.), *The Threat of Impending Disaster*. Cambridge: M.I.T. Press.

15. Epstein, S. (1962). "The Measurement of Drive and Conflict in Humans." In M.R. Jones (ed.), *Nebraska Symposium on Motivation*. Lincoln, Nebraska: University of Nebraska Press, pp. 127–209.

16. Skipper, J. K. Jr., and R. C. Leonard (1968). "Children, Stress and Hospitalization: A Field Experiment." *Journal of Health and Social Behavior*, 9:275–287.

17. Davis, F. (1963). *Passage Through Crisis: Polio Victims and Their Families*. Indianapolis: Bobbs-Merrill.

18. Robins, L. (1970). "Follow-up Studies of Behavior Disorders in Children." In E. H. Hare and J. K. Wing (eds.), *Psychiatric Epidemiology*. London: Oxford University Press.

19. Nefzger, N., and A. Lilienfeld (1959). "Item Reliability and Related Factors in a Community Survey of Emotionality." *Sociometry*, 22:236–246.

20. Mechanic, D., and M. Newton (1965). "Some Problems in the Analysis of Morbidity Data." *Journal of Chronic Disease*, 18:569–580.

21. Brown, G., and M. Rutter (1966). "The Measurement of Family Activities and Relationships." *Human Relations*, **19**:241–263.

22. Mechanic, D. (1964). "The Influence of Mothers on Their Children's Health Attitudes and Behavior." *Pediatrics,* **33**:444–453.

23. Freedman, J., and D. Sears (1965). "Selective Exposure." In L. Berkowitz (ed.), *Advances in Experimental Social Psychology*, Vol. 2, New York: Academic Press, pp. 57–97.

24. Mechanic, D. (1962). *Students Under Stress: A Study in the Social Psychology of Adaptation.* New York: Free Press.

25. Hall, D. (1969). "The Impact of Peer Interaction During an Academic Role Transition." *Sociology of Education*, **42**:118–140.

26. Festinger, L. (1957). *A Theory of Cognitive Dissonance.* Evanston, Ill.: Row Peterson.

CHAPTER XII

Sociology of Mental Health

In the past two decades, sociologists have carried out a variety of studies examining factors related to the occurrence and course of psychiatric and behavior disorders, reactions to illness and deviance in the population, the help-seeking and help-giving process, the organization and functioning of psychiatric facilities, community processes affecting the provision and character of mental health services, and the larger moral and institutional influences affecting definitions of mental health, mental illness, and the social uses of psychiatry. This chapter examines the developments and trends in the field from a critical perspective and suggests some more promising areas of inquiry for the coming years.

The Concepts of Mental Health and Mental Illness

The strengths and weaknesses of the sociological contribution are partly dependent on the ambiguities of psychiatric thinking and psychiatric practice and, more specifically, the existing confusions concerning concepts of psychiatric disorder, variabilities in diagnostic practices, and problems in reliability of assessment.[1-4] Basic to this confusion are continuing disagreements as to the nature and scope of the concepts of mental health and mental illness. Of course, all concepts of health and illness are arbitrary constructions that arise from social and cultural processes. In the health area in general, certain adaptations are defined as disease when they cause distress, failures in social functioning or death, or when they lead to behavioral reactions that are disturbing to the community. In modern society there is a continual dialogue between the attributions of "sickness" and "badness" to various reactions and behaviors, and it is the social process that defines which distinctions will be made and under what circumstances.

One also confronts a dialogue between philosophical concepts of disease and more pragmatic concepts. At one extreme we find such concepts as the one propounded by the World Health Organization, which defines health as a state of "complete physical, mental and social well-being and not merely the absence of disease and infirmity." At the other extreme we find rather limited disease concepts characteristic of the approach to psychiatric practice in many European countries and associated with an organic perspective. Basic to the debate is whether mental health and illness (indeed, all health and illness) should be viewed as adaptive responses to the physical and social environment, or whether focus should be given to inborn defects of the organism and specific noxious agents in the environment. Whatever the particular approach, there is growing appreciation in all areas of medicine that disease and infirmity are a product of a complex interaction between organisms, the environments in which they develop and live, and various specific agents in the environment. Most of the chronic diseases require a more complex approach than was characteristic of the germ theory.

The more specific approaches to mental illness reflect, in various ways, the philosophical debate described above. In general terms, the varying approaches can be characterized in one of three ways: (1) medical models, (2) development models, and (3) reactive models. To understand much of the research on mental disorder, we must be clear on the larger perspective within which it is undertaken.

The Medical Model

In the mental health area, it has been extremely fashionable to be critical of the medical model, but there is continuing confusion about the nature of the model and its advantages and defects.[5] Stated briefly, the medical approach is the attempt to identify clusters of signs and symptoms that are causally related and that may be indicative of some underlying disorder. The identification of such clusters, referred to as diagnosis, makes use of basic scientific knowledge and clinical research to obtain information on the etiology of the cluster, its likely course, and appropriate treatment. In areas where medical science is developed, the correct identification of clusters of symptoms and signs—the diagnosis—then suggests a variety of information useful to the clinician in the management of his patients. Once he has identified the patient's problem, he immediately can take advantage of the established knowledge concerning disease. In short, the medical model is a heuristic model that is neither good nor bad, right or wrong. The appropriate issue concerns the usefulness of the model under varying circumstances, and whether the informational gains from adopting it are greater than the stigmatic consequences of the definition of the problem.[6]

I think that it is unproductive to debate the appropriateness of the medical model to psychiatric phenomena. In some areas, a precise diagnostic appraisal may be useful in establishing how the condition is to be managed; too frequently the diagnostic process is ritualistic, and the course of treatment does not follow in any direct way from the diagnostic assessment. This partly may result from the fact that many American psychiatrists do not view diagnosis seriously, since they are most commonly psychodynamic and developmental in their perspectives. I believe that focused research on the psychiatric diagnostic process and its relationship to treatment would be more useful than continuing polemics over whether the medical model is appropriate for psychiatry.

Relevant to the use of any model of care is the consideration of its value and its adverse effects. Too frequently, the value of psychiatric approaches and interventions have been emphasized without sufficient exploration of the adverse consequences. In a valuable historical study of Worchester State Hospital, Grob[7] found that the emphasis on an organic perspective, in which illness was viewed as inherent to organisms, contributed toward neglect of environmental measures that could alleviate the course of mental conditions. Focused research on the consequences of therapeutic interventions should give more attention to negative and positive consequences. What, for example, are the costs of community psychiatric programs for family distress,[8] impact on the development and self-esteem of children of the mentally ill,[9] or on the fertility of schizophrenic women?[10] What effect does drug-dependence have on self-esteem, a sense of mastery, and performance generally? How do varying psychiatric labels or treatments affect the life chances of patients so labeled? Too much intervention research defines the problems of rehabilitation too narrowly and tends to exclude important social factors that are relevant to the quality of life and social functioning.

Developmental Models

Most of American psychiatric, psychological, and social work practice is based on a historical or developmental model of human behavior. Emotional or behavioral disturbances are seen as adaptations to the complex factors impinging on the organism. Certain adaptations come to be defined as problems because they cause personal distress or social disruption in the family or community.

Although the developmental model is a general perspective, it encompasses points of view and methods of approach that differ in fundamental ways. For example, although both operant conditioning and psychodynamic approaches are developmental in their conceptions of etiology, operant conditioning implies approaches to treatment that can be imposed on patients as passive participants, whereas psychodynamic approaches usually require active participation of the patient with an assumption that insight or catharsis is vital to behavior change. In short, some developmental views are behavioristic while others treat the phenomenology of the patient as central.

Considerable attention has been given to the influence processes underlying behavior change in therapeutic situations and in seeking commonalities that explain patient improvement in response to therapeutic approaches varying widely in assumptions and modes of operation.[11] Recently, learning theories have been given prominence; approaches based on learning theories are extremely promising, but their utility in a wide range of situations is yet to be fully demonstrated.

Varying models of treatment involve different assumptions concerning the types of participation and roles that patients must be able to assume for effective treatment. We have learned that such assumptions may result in the exclusion of certain patients from treatment, as was common in psychodynamic therapies that put great emphasis on the ability of the patient to verbalize and that tended to exclude patients from underprivileged backgrounds.[12,13] On inpatient services, there has been growing emphasis on a variety of milieu therapies that require certain types of orientations and participation.[14] We have little knowledge of the impact of such therapies on varying populations of patients with different backgrounds, types of disorder, age, and sex. We know little about the consequences of varying population compositions or the manner in which ward social structures are manipulated to maintain social control, although attempts to describe ward atmospheres and their correlates are proceeding.[15,16] These are basic issues for study, since operational procedures have been extremely faddish and have not been based on establishing the efficacy of one or another approach.

Reactive Models

Considerable attention, in recent years, has been devoted to the impact of varying societal reactions on disturbed behavior and, particularly, to coercive and involuntary treatment. The reactive approach, building on sociological theories of deviance, is concerned less with the initial causes of disturbance and more with the reactions to it and resulting consequences.[17,18] Reactive models are based on the assumption that disturbance stems from a variety of biological, psychological, and social factors, but that the course of such behavior is importantly influenced by the manner in which the community responds to it. Erving Goffman's observations at Saint Elizabeth's hospital[19] gave great impetus to such study, and Lemert's[20] theory of the societal reaction provided a strong theoretical base for a variety of inquiries. In brief, the theory maintained that the reactions to certain types of disapproved behavior affected the opportunities for conventional adjustment, increased the forces toward continued deviance, and had major effects on the defined person's self-conceptions and future behavior. Observations made in a variety of contexts, such as among the Hutterites,[21] suggested that when the community responded to disturbed behavior in an accepting and nurturant fashion, the aggressive manifestations of mental illness seen in more coercive contexts were absent. Through such observations and studies, the ideology of moral treatment was rediscovered, which argued that coercive and degrading treatment of the mentally ill compounded their disorders and aggravated their most disturbing manifestations. With the assistance of the newly introduced psychoactive drugs in the late 1950's, administrators, mental health personnel, and patients' families were able to develop sufficient confidence to respond less coercively to the mentally ill.[22]

Associated with the growing realization of the impact of coercive and involuntary treatment was a variety of studies demonstrating the extent to which the rights of mental patients were violated in civil commitment[23] and in other legal procedures such as incompetency to stand trial.[24] The studies demonstrated that these measures were largely used to control lower class and powerless members of the society who had few resources to protect themselves against arbitrary action. Communities had come to depend on such processes to rid themselves of bizarre and annoying members. These procedures were frequently in violation of statutory requirements and due process of law, and communities rarely invested the necessary resources to provide decent treatment and care to such unfortunates. The writings of Thomas Szasz[25,26] and others brought public attention to this problem and a strong movement for the legal rights of the mentally ill was initiated, which has resulted in some landmark court rulings concerning the right to treatment, due process, and other legal protections. Some of these rulings are discussed in Chapter 14.

Associated with the reactive approach was a variety of studies dealing with the manner in which mental illness was defined in the community and how persons with varying symptoms and difficulties were selected into treatment. Clausen and his colleagues,[27,28] for example, illustrated in detail the strong tendency to normalize disturbing behavior until it became so disruptive that the family could no longer cope with it. Many other studies on rehospitalization of the mentally ill showed that while families were frequently willing to maintain persons who performed poorly, they had difficulty in coping with bizarre and frightening symptomatology, and such behavior frequently led to rehospitalization.[29-32]

At the same time, various studies were undertaken of how persons come to define themselves as having a psychological problem and the factors affecting the tendency to seek psychiatric care.[33,34] Systematic differences were observed in the propensity to seek care by sex, social class, region, and ethnic background. Although some populations could define problems in psychological terms and seek help, others primarily would express these problems through the presentation of organic complaints. Such differences could be traced to educational and cultural background as well as to a variety of psychosocial factors.[35] In general, patients tend to seek out practitioners who share their world view and social orientations,[36] and some studies have also suggested that practitioners tend to make similar types of selections.[37] In epidemiological studies of help-seeking, it has become evident that there is large overlap in psychological state between treated and untreated populations. In the case of more mild disorders, social and cultural factors are frequently more important in seeking treatment than the nature of the disorder. In conditions of greater severity, the social selection is less marked. Thus, one finds very strong selection in who comes into treatment for neurotic symptoms, but much less selection in disorders such as schizophrenia.[38]

The reactive approach has been extremely useful in understanding the community context of care. At times, the importance of social labeling and the societal reaction has been exaggerated, but it is reasonably clear that reactive processes influence who considers themselves as sick, who seeks care and of what kind, and the course of the disorder. The classic study of Hollingshead and Redlich on social class and mental illness, for example, demonstrated in a dramatic fashion how assumptions about patients, and the types of care provided to various groups, had a profound effect on the prevalence of psychiatric disorders in the various social strata.

As mental health services are more community oriented, and more concerned with identifying disorders at early stages, they are more likely than ever to deal with patients who are selected into treatment on the basis of social and social-psychological factors. Under such conditions, it is more important than ever to understand the differences between disorder and illness behavior. Various investigators have suggested the possible dangers of treating, in profound ways, transitory symptoms that may come into care not because of the severity of the disorder but because of the propensities of families to seek treatment for one of its members, or difficulties in coping with more mild problems because of other factors affecting the patient or his family.[39] A better understanding of these problems will contribute to more sophisticated approaches to treatment in community-care situations.

The Epidemiology of Mental Disorders

The existing confusion about the character of psychiatric disorders creates profound problems of case-finding for epidemiologists in psychiatry. Epidemiological approaches in psychiatry have come to depend on varying concepts of disease, disorder, and disability, and it has been difficult to achieve comparability across studies and among nations having varying diagnostic approaches. Existing epidemiological studies are frequently based on treated incidence and prevalence, incorporating profound selection biases, and they use a variety of dependent variables that are in no sense comparable. These variables include such diverse indicators as happiness, psychophysiological complaints, psychotic symptomatology, behavior problems, and social functioning. Despite the difficulties of these investigations, they have clearly provided evidence of the importance of such variables as social class, age and sex roles, residence, social mobility, ethnic and cultural differences, and community networks, although the precise role of each of these factors in various disorders remains an issue that requires continued research. Although awareness of such factors presently informs the psychiatrist's perspectives and practice, future efforts must be organized around more precise conceptions of psychiatric phenomena and more adequate and sophisticated case-finding.

In considering the definition of disorder, one is constantly confronted with the basic controversies among psychiatrists who adopt disease in contrast to developmental and reactive conceptions. Although the use of treated rates may serve as the basis for the study of limited and particularly profound disorders, it is pointless to pursue the study of the epidemiology of less severe disorders by using treated cases. Thus, the emphasis in recent years, has been placed on community surveys of psychiatric disorder;[40-43] these studies have been extremely expensive and face difficult methodological problems. The most frequent indicators used are psychophysiological symptoms that have proved useful in differentiating treated and untreated populations. Such indicators, however, are only a small part of the universe of psychiatric symptomatology and are not necessarily representative of psychiatric disorder in general. Moreover, many of the indicators used are characteristic of both physical and psychiatric disorders and may have a different meaning in varying populations.[44] For example, the report of such symptoms in a young, healthy population may be more likely to indicate psychological disorder, but in an older population, where there is more physical illness, such reports may be indicative of other health problems. Therefore, the comparability of these indicators among varying population groups is not assured.

At a more general level, some studies have concentrated on measures of happiness as indicators of general well-being.[45] Happiness appears to be a product of two types of factors that are relatively independent of one another: the absence of psychophysiological types of distress, and the number of positive events. These studies draw attention to the fact that well-being must be viewed not only in terms of the absence of symptoms but also in terms of the presence of supporting experiences. Studies have shown, for example, that community leaders may have more psychophysiological distress than the public at large, but they also experience more events supportive of their status and self esteem.[46] Psychophysiological indicators are highly susceptible to environmental fluctuations and may be fundamentally different from other indicators measuring symptoms that are less responsive to changes in the social environment such as the psychotic-type symptoms (hallucinations and delusions, for instance).

Most epidemiological studies have neglected the behavior disorders and social functioning that constitute a major part of psychiatric practice. Although some attention has been given to alcoholism, drug use, and other forms of troublesome behavior, these problems are so highly prevalent that they deserve greater research effort. Similarly, the emphasis on symptoms has resulted in neglecting social adjustment in work, family life, and the community. Each of these dimensions involves difficult problems of measurement but, if we are to take advantage of the possible fruits of epidemiological study, we must give greater attention to more adequate classification and to improved measurement of important categories of behavior.

Let us review briefly some of the methodological difficulties that require careful research.

1. Symptoms vary in their responsivity to fluctuations in the environment and we need better understanding of the nature of such fluctuations.

2. Different symptoms have varying implications for successful social functioning; indeed, there is evidence that some neurotic symptoms may contribute to effective motivation and performance, while others are profoundly handicapping.[47]

3. Varying symptoms differ in their social epidemiology and, unless we have greater specificity of dependent variables, we will tend to confuse important issues. For example, neurotic diagnoses are made more commonly in women, and personality disorders are defined more commonly in men. By selecting some disorders and excluding others, one will produce different epidemiological pictures of the distribution of disorder.

4. Varying symptom patterns may be more or less genetically based and, to treat them as the same, may confuse important issues.

5. There are profound measurement problems in differentiating symptoms of physical and psychiatric disorders in varying populations, in dealing with varying conceptions of the social undesirability of symptoms in different populations, in tapping a representative sample of aberrant symptoms in epidemiological surveys, and in dealing with differential response biases in interview studies.

All of these methodological issues deserve concentrated study if we are to obtain maximum advantage from efforts in psychiatric epidemiology.

The value of comparable measures of psychiatric disorders is illustrated by the NIMH collaborative study of schizophrenia in England and the United States. By using a standardized instrument, similarly administered in the two countries, this study demonstrated that the reported varying prevalence of schizophrenia in the two countries was a product of variabilities in diagnostic criteria.[48] When the same criterion was applied in the two countries, the proportion of schizophrenics was similar. Without arguing the issue of which definition of schizophrenia is the more correct one, it is apparent that there is value in standardizing definitions so that communication is facilitated among researchers and practitioners.[49]

Major Sociological Perspectives Concerning Psychiatric Disorders

Generally, sociological views of psychiatric disorders fall within three general perspectives. These perspectives are not unrelated to varying concepts of mental disorder, but they involve somewhat different distinctions than those made earlier in the discussion of models of disease. These sociological approaches are not mutually exclusive, and it is common to hold eclectic conceptions based on all three.

The Social Stratification Perspective

The social stratification perspective is a major one, directing much sociological effort in a variety of areas. Considerable impetus for this perspective came from the theoretical discussion by Robert Merton[50,51] in his theory of anomie in which he saw deviant adaptations (including mental illness) as a response to aspirations blocked by inadequate means to achieve them. Merton maintained that while the social structure induced common aspirations it differentially provided the means to achieve them in varying social groups. Thus, rates of deviance in varying social strata could be viewed in terms of the effects of social structure. Many other sociologists emphasized a stratification perspective with no elaborate theory except that the conditions in varying social contexts, associated with social differentiation, resulted in varying rates of disorders. Some sociologists view the social class structure as a variable sufficient in itself, while those of a more social-psychological persuasion attempt to understand how socialization in varying social strata results in different values, skills, and concepts of self, for example.[52,53] Although the influence of social class on psychiatric disturbance and treatment has been appreciated for decades, the Hollingshead-Redlich study in New Haven focused widespread interest on class differences, and for the first time social class became a variable of real concern to psychiatrists.

One of the most persistent themes over several decades concerns the observed relationship between social stratification and mental illness, and particularly the association between social class and schizophrenia.[54-57] The observation of a disproportionate number of schizophrenics in the lowest social strata, noted in studies undertaken throughout the world, has generated a variety of conceptions concerning the role of social structure in the occurrence and course of mental illness. Although the evidence is not fully consistent and is much debated, I think the data show that the disproportionate occurrence of schizophrenia in the lowest social strata is a consequence of genetic selection and either downward social mobility or failure to move upward with one's age cohort as a result of the debilitating consequences of the disorder.[58] Some interpret the evidence as suggesting that this class difference is partly a product of social causation related to the class structure.[59] Further research to clarify the existing situation is required. Less debatable is the fact that social class has effects on the course of schizophrenia and other disorders by exposing lower-class patients to treatment and community conditions that tend to exacerbate the more debilitating effects of their disorders.[60] There has been some work that attempts to better understand the hospital and community conditions that are most conducive to limiting disability associated with chronic schizophrenia and other disabling psychiatric disorders,[61,62] but much more work along these lines is necessary.

Some social epidemiological investigations, in recent years, have described the course of specific symptoms and syndromes.[63] Although studies designed to follow the natural course of psychiatric disorders are expensive and difficult to conduct, they are of very high priority because they help to distinguish the more transitory conditions from conditions that are more persistent and that are likely to result in continuing disability. Furthermore, they help to specify needed interventions and a more effective use of treatment resources. Finally, they clearly point to symptoms that tend to be transitory and that do not necessarily require treatment or conceivably may be prolonged by inappropriate treatment. An important and provocative finding, established on the basis of two followup studies in Saint Louis, is that antisocial behavior in childhood persists into adulthood with compounding difficulties while the natural history of neurotic type symptoms is less noxious.[64,65] The process through which such outcomes occur has not been established, but it would be productive to give greater attention to prospective studies by using various populations and methodologies. Since the antisocial syndrome is more common in the lower social strata and among blacks, these studies provide further reason to explore social stratification hypotheses.

Societal Reaction and Labeling Theory

A major aspect of the sociological effort in the study of psychiatric disorders deals with the social processes through which patients are identified and treated and the consequences for the patient's self-identity and future social performance. Sociological work on labeling[66,67] and stigma[68] has sensitized practitioners and administrators to the importance of the environment and regimen on self-conception, self-confidence, self-reliance, and patients' potentialities for future performance. We have learned that social expectations in treatment can have important effects in encouraging inactivity and dependency or activity and attempts to cope more effectively.[69] In particular, the debilitating effects of long periods of inactivity and dependence have been shown to have substantial adverse effects on motivation and future social adaptation.

Much of the work in this tradition goes beyond a more narrow concept of mental illness and seeks to understand the social psychological antecedents for self-concepts and personal efficacy.[70-76] It has been maintained, with some empirical support, that official processing by mental health and correctional agencies can have adverse effects on the self-images of those processed and that social stigma associated with labeling may restrict occupational and interpersonal opportunities. In its more audacious forms, labeling theory has maintained that official processing of mental patients results in more organized and chronic conditions,[77] but empirical support has been inconsistent with this more extreme formulation.[78]

Models Dealing with Social Resources, Stress, and Coping

As the concept of mental health has broadened, greater attention has been devoted to studying social stress, coping effectiveness, and the social resources available to support vulnerable persons during periods of difficulty. Recently, greater attention has been given to considering multidimensional models that see failures in functioning and personal distress as resulting from complex circumstances in which social stress taxes coping efficacy and available supporting resources.[79,80] Concepts of stress differ; some emphasize life changes, regardless of how they are defined by the person concerned;[81-83] others emphasize the importance of anticipation and the definition of the situation.[84]

At the levels of institutions and communities, sociologists have studied how a person's capacities, skills, and defenses have been conditioned by the social networks to which they belong, by societal incentives, and by the quality of social and cultural preparation for the life problems they must face.[85-87] Inadequacies stem not only from personal incapacities but also from the failure of social organizations to adapt to changing technology and cultural and social change. Complex organizations are instruments to achieve various goals and must be examined from this perspective.[88,89]

The failures of large custodial hospitals and penal institutions in rehabilitating clients have been well documented and, beginning with Goffman's descriptions and analyses, the effects of total institutions on patients have been explored in many ways. These studies have demonstrated that inactivity, dependency, and hopelessness contribute toward personal deterioration. Less attention, however, has been given to a more balanced consideration of the gains and liabilities of hospital and community care under varying circumstances. Not all hospitals are necessarily bad for all patients, and the organization of community care and ambulatory services requires carefully planned systems of resources that provide the necessary assistance to meet patient needs and to minimize social costs for the family and community.

In the case of schizophrenia, the most disabling major chronic disorder, the importance of drug intervention has been effectively illustrated in a controlled community experiment carried out by Pasamanick and his colleagues.[91] A follow-up study of these patients suggests the difficulty of maintaining a reasonable level of functioning without aggresive community care.[92] Similarly, in hospitals, it is difficult to achieve effective performance among schizophrenic patients over extended periods of time. There seem to be limitations on resources, time, and patience, and patients frequently cannot sustain progress over long periods of time. We still know very little about how to sustain long-term patients with serious psychiatric disorders, and much more research is necessary to attack this problem in a more focused way.

Overall Directions for Future Sociological Research on Psychiatric Disorders

I have already argued the importance of focusing more specifically on particular disorders and on improved classification. Here I explore the general issues relevant to sociological efforts in a variety of fields but particularly germane to work on mental disorders.

1. Confusion Concerning the Strength of Association. Too frequently, investigators are content to demonstrate the importance of one or another variable without giving consideration to the magnitude of the observed relationship or its practical significance. Too many studies produce theories based on small effects in large samples, which reach statistical significance but which have only limited importance. We should move beyond the point of demonstrating effects without considering the degree of association and its import within the total picture.

2. Failure to Specify Intervening Processes. Much of the work on mental disorders is atheoretical and is based on very simple global hypotheses about effects without specifying the intervening processes contributing to these effects. For example, too many studies posit a relationship between social class or social stress and mental illness without attempting to examine the processes through which the antecedent variables affect the dependent variable. We are beyond the point of demonstrating such effects, and more sophisticated models are necessary to achieve fruitful results.

At the other extreme, one finds enormously complex models that cannot be effectively captured in empirical work. Thus the field tends to be characterized by very simple research on a limited number of variables or very complex models supported by anecdote. More attention must be given to examining multifactor models of greater complexity in rigorous designs.

3. *The Need to Develop Sociological Models that Take Account of Evidence in Genetics and Related Fields of Inquiry.* Many of the issues of concern in the study of mental disorders have important biological, genetic, and psychological components.[93,94] In developing more elaborate conceptions consistent with the complexity of the phenomenon it is crucial to take into account the effects of important variables from other fields. Increasingly, we may have to move toward developing interactive models that take into account genetic vulnerabilities, psychological factors, and social influences. It is conceivable, for example, that social stress is important in schizophrenia only among persons who are genetically vulnerable and who are exposed to specific environmental contexts. These problems will require greater collaboration between psychiatrists, sociologists, and geneticists.

4. *Importance of Distinguishing between Etiological Factors and Those Affecting the Course of Disease.* Although the distinction between incidence and prevalence is an important one in epidemiology, the difficulty of obtaining incidence data has resulted in many investigators using prevalence rates to study etiology. Therefore, there has been a continuing confusion in the literature between factors central to the occurrence of mental disorders and those primarily important in affecting its course. These factors may be the same or similar, but they need not be. Also the literature on mental disorders demonstrates persistent confusion between the factors resulting in the initiation of help-seeking and those resulting in the disorder diagnosed.

From a practical standpoint, it is difficult and frequently impossible to separate illness from illness behavior or disease from disability. But these distinctions must be kept constantly in mind if we are to avoid compounding errors.

Neglected Areas for Sociological Inquiry on Psychiatric Disorders

Throughout this chapter, I have suggested various areas in which I believe efforts have been productive and where further work is warranted. Here I explore areas for further research that are of vital importance.

1. Psychiatric Illness in General Medical Practice. The vast proportion of psychiatric morbidity in the population is treated within the context of general medical practice. Although it is difficult to precisely estimate the proportion of patients who have psychosocial and psychiatric difficulties, it is widely agreed that such patients constitute a significant proportion of all primary medical care.[95] Although some of these patients present psychiatric and family difficulties in psychological terms, many more present vague physical symptomatology including headaches, lack of appetite, insomnia, nervous stomach, aches and pains, and listlessness. It is believed that many of these patients suffer from depression, anxiety states, and a variety of psychosocial difficulties. Although general practice is the main route into care for psychiatric conditions, it has been badly neglected as an area of study and we know relatively little about the natural history of these conditions, the preparedness of physicians to recognize and deal with them, types of drug therapy and treatment provided, and referral into speciality care, for example.[96-98]

In studying psychiatric illness and services, investigators have generally failed to view help-seeking for psychiatric conditions within a larger epidemiological framework. Frequently persons in distress present common physical symptoms to physicians, but the initiation of the medical consultation was basically motivated by the underlying distress and not the symptoms presented. We need much more work on the identification of symptoms in the population, the attributions persons make in attempting to understand them, and how they come into help networks.[99] We also need more practical efforts oriented toward improving the capacity of general physicians, internists and pediatricians to deal with these problems, and behavior disorders in general.[100] We need more basic work on the manner in which patients construe symptoms, the vocabularies they use to describe them, their modes of presentation in seeking help, and the conditions under which they conform with medical advice.[101,102]

Greater attention is also required in considering the social and psychiatric care available to patients on general medical units. There is evidence that these patients frequently face difficult social and psychological problems that require management of their life situations and emotional state.[103] Efforts to develop better cooperation between medical and psychiatric efforts in hospitals are also necessary.

2. Greater Study is Required of the Psychological and Social Problems of Aging. There are more old persons in the population than ever before, and a disproportionate number of them are women. The existing mortality trends suggest that there will be very large numbers of aged widows in the future who survive their husbands by many years. In view of the social mobility and values characteristic of American life, these persons often lead lives of great isolation and suffer from despair and unhappiness. Although the

NEGLECTED AREAS FOR SOCIOLOGICAL INQUIRY

general situation has been well documented, considerable research is necessary on social and mental health services that can contribute to enhancing the lives of many of these elderly people. Similarly elderly men, especially those with more narrow interests, suffer from considerable discontinuity between their work lives and retirement. Their bases for self-esteem are often undermined, and they lapse into inactivity resulting in personal deterioration and unhappiness.

3. The Social Functioning of Mental Patients in Community Contexts. Following the middle 1950's, and the introduction of psychoactive drugs and new administrative policies in mental health, the emphasis in care moved from the hospital to the community and intermediate facilities such as halfway houses and day hospitals. The resident population in mental hospitals substantially decreased, the number of admissions to hospitals increased, and the average length of stay was substantially diminished. This trend, buttressed by the new technology of drugs, new therapeutic attitudes, research demonstrating the damaging influences of the custodial hospital and economic motives based on a desire to control hospital costs for the mentally ill, has resulted in the present situation.

Despite changing practices, there has been very little research on the effectiveness of new treatment institutions (particularly community mental health centers) and on the quality of life of mental patients living with their families or by themselves. Limited studies suggest very low levels of social functioning, particularly among chronic schizophrenic patients, and significant costs for those who deal with them. Very little sociological study has been devoted to the networks of services allegedly providing effective community care, or how they can best be organized to deal with problems of living, housing, work, and interpersonal relationships.

As emphasis has shifted to the community, the earlier trend of studies of mental hospitalization has declined.[104-106] We have relatively few studies of hospitals following the changes in the late 1950's, and almost no attention has been given to studying the adequacy of newly emerging psychiatric units in general hospitals. There has been some study of halfway houses and day hospitals, but the move away from studying total institutions is probably too sharp a shift in sociological interests.

4. Study of the Relationships between Psychiatry and other Social Institutions. Stating with the classic paper by Davis[107] on the mental hygiene movement, sociologists have continued to focus on psychiatric practice as an ideological and social movement. Psychodynamic practice, which began as a small subculture concentrated in major urban areas and of particular attractiveness to specific social and ethnic groups, has diffused throughout the population so that both practitioners and patients are more like the general population in social characteristics than two or three decades ago. Psychiatric concepts have permeated intellectual and social thought, and psychiatric interpretations are more readily used than in the past.

As psychiatry has come to concern itself with a wide range of social phenomena, many societal dilemmas and difficulties have been shifted to the psychiatric realm, and psychiatrists play an increasing role in the legal and criminal justice system, organizational life, and in social decisions within the community. Psychiatry is used by both clients of psychiatrists and by social organizations to handle problems that would be difficult to cope with within more usual forms of conflict resolution. Although Szasz's contention that psychiatry is a modern form of witchcraft,[108] and performs the same social functions for society, is overstated, it is clear that psychiatrists perform a variety of roles, and that the uses of psychiatry require continued scrutiny and analysis.

As the society in general becomes more conscious of individual rights and due process of law, institutional psychiatry will require greater attention. Instead of guessing at such matters as future dangerousness which has great importance for the fate of individuals, we will need far better measures of what kinds of behavior are dangerous to others and require involuntary care. Clearly, coercion is used in psychiatry too frequently, and the implications of this for patient and society not only require analysis on a social and legal basis but also, in terms of its consequences, for effective treatment and rehabilitation.

Hollingshead and Redlich first demonstrated how varied psychiatrists performing different social roles were in their values and life orientations, and it is well appreciated that certain types of psychiatrists come to be selected for particular roles. In the *Fifth Profession*,[109] Henry and his colleagues also demonstrated the similarities in orientations among psychotherapists from varying fields of endeavor: psychiatry, psychology, and social work. We need more study of the characteristics of psychiatrists and the activities they choose to pursue, since it is likely that psychiatrists will play important roles in decision processes that relate to social issues and philosophy of life.[110] Similarly, as psychiatric interventions increase, some raise important ethical issues that must be considered in light of the orientations of the persons that perform them. Indeed, as psychiatry moves more boldly into behavioral conditioning, and perhaps even revives psychosurgery in new forms, it will be important for the public to participate in the ethical debate.

5. Developing the Basic Science Necessary to a Preventive Social Psychiatry. Although there has been much emphasis on crisis intervention and on prevention in recent years, basic knowledge necessary to promote such work is generally lacking. We have a very limited conception of the natural history of various psychiatric disturbances that become manifest in childhood, and we are not clear on the conditions conducive to psychiatric illness in the population at large.[111] Although poverty and lack of positive reinforcement contribute to unhappiness and other indicators of distress, poverty's precise relationship to behavior disorders and the psychoses is poorly understood. There is an obvious need for longitudinal and ecological studies over time, which investigate the complex interactions between ethnicity and culture, and poverty and deprivation. These studies must focus not only on symptoms but also on the constructive forces that result in normal psychological and social development in deprived and impoverished circumstances.

6. Studies of the Newly Emerging Mental Health Professions. In recent decades, there has been considerable elaboration of the mental health professions and greater team efforts in dealing with psychiatric disturbance. Innovative programs using lay therapists and new mental health workers have been encouraged, and new types of services including mental health advocacy have been initiated. Few of these programs have been systematically studied in terms of their efficacy or the types of roles and participation they develop relative to more traditional psychiatric practices. To keep from moving from one fad to another, these new types of services and work require careful evaluation.

7. Study of Alcoholism and its Consequences. Although the study of the sociological aspects of alcoholism was highly developed in the 1950's, [112,113] attention to this area seemed to diminish in the 1960's. Yet alcoholism has become a major cause of family and social difficulties, a main cause of physical illness, and a significant contributor to morbidity and mortality resulting from motor vehicle accidents.[114,115]

One of the difficulties in the sociological study of alcoholism has been the lack of fruitful hypotheses to pursue relative to etiology and treatment and rehabilitation. Similarly, although social and cultural understanding of alcohol use in various societies is fairly well developed, few new hypotheses are available.

One of the most interesting conceptions of alcohol use in sociology was developed by Bales,[116] and further work along the lines of viewing alcohol as adaptive behavior within culturally permissive conditions should be done. Furthermore, exploration of the relationships between eating and drinking patterns within various cultural groups might merit further study. Most important, perhaps, alcoholism must be examined and explored within its larger social context, taking into account cultural attitudes toward the use of alcohol, changing social relationships and forms of social organization, social change and social stress, and drinking as a form of coping behavior. From a treatment perspective, industrial programs to deal with alcoholism deserve careful study, and particularly the use of incentives to encourage treatment and rehabilitation.

8. Studies of the Social Organization of Work and Alienation. With changing values and behavior, and higher levels of education in the population, work alienation is likely to become a more profound problem resulting in a variety of difficulties. Very little attention has been given to work settings in relation to mental health, and such studies are likely to yield valuable knowledge to deal with newly emerging social problems.[117,118]

9. Studies of Changing Social Roles and Family Organization. The technology of birth control, women's liberation, changing sexual patterns, and newly emerging social consciousness are having profound effects on personal aspirations, male and female roles, and family organization. Change is occurring rapidly enough in this area to create considerable intergenerational conflict and personal ambivalence. These phenomena deserve careful sociological study.

10. The Study of New Psychological and Social Movements. Intense psychological experience in groups has become a national pasttime and an important commercial venture. A large number of new psychological and mystical cults are developing among the young, which are indicative of attempts to seek meaning amidst the confusions of modern living. Kurt Back,[119] in studying sensitivity training developments, has suggested that these must be understood as attempts to find meaning and fulfillment in a society where life is more segmented and less intimate. To some extent, these movements may be attracting a disproportionate number of confused and distressed persons, and their recruitment and effects are worthy of considerable attention. Are they helpful or do they compound personal difficulties?

11. Study of Influence Processes and Behavior Change. Many of the major public health problems our society faces are direct results of the social structure and social patterns of behavior: obesity, alcoholism, drug addiction, violence, smoking, poor preventive health practices, and poor nutrition. Many of these problems are not easily amenable to personal intervention, but the processes by which personal behavior can be effectively changed deserve careful study. The studies should focus not only on therapist-client influence processes but also must emphasize the organizational auspices and supports that are facilitative of influence and change.

Summary

Although this chapter focused on practical issues directly relevant to the treatment of the mentally ill, attention was given to more general problems that are basic to an effective attack on mental health problems. In emphasizing today's pressing problems, it is too easy to neglect the more general issues that are basic to future progress in dealing with mental disorders. We must remain aware of how little we really know and give support to fundamental efforts that will direct our attempts at intervention in the future. Greater attention must be given to improved concepts and measures of psychiatric conditions and disabilities, to specifying more clearly the factors intervening between social and environmental conditions and individual distress and pathology, and to separating and understanding more clearly the factors causing distress and illness, the process of help-seeking, and factors affecting the course and outcome of illness and disability. We have reached the point where greater cooperation is necessary among the relevant behavioral disciplines and where parochial efforts from the viewpoint of one or another discipline will be of less value. Although the importance of longitudinal and prospective studies has been emphasized from the viewpoint of a variety of disciplines, there are many difficulties and complexities in successfully executing such investigations. Psychiatry no longer can remain a parochial discipline relying on anecdote and clinical experience. It must build on its basic biological and social disciplines, and must develop as an investigatory and analytic field.[120] In the long run, the practice of psychiatry and its utility as a helping profession will depend on the scope and integrity of its basic sciences.

Notes

1. Dohrenwend, Bruce, and Barbara Dohrenwend (1969). *Social Status and Psychological Disorder*. New York: Wiley.
2. Mechanic, D. (1970). "Problems and Prospects in Psychiatric Epidemiology." In E. H. Hare and J. Wing (eds.), *Psychiatric Epidemiology*. London: Oxford University Press.
3. Jahoda, M. (1958). *Current Concepts of Positive Mental Health*. New York: Basic Books.
4. Sells, S. B. (ed.) (1968). *The Definition and Measurement of Mental Health*. National Center for Health Statistics, United States Department of Health, Education, and Welfare.
5. Lewis, A. (1953). "Health as a Social Concept." *British Journal of Sociology*, 4:109–124.
6. Mechanic, D. (1968). *Medical Sociology: A Selective View*. New York: Free Press.
7. Grob, G. (1966). *The State and the Mentally Ill*. Chapel Hill, N. C.: University of North Carolina Press.
8. Brown, G., et al.(1966). *Schizophrenia and Social Care*. London: Oxford University Press.
9. Rutter, M. (1966). *Children of Sick Parents: An Environmental and Psychiatric Study*. New York: Oxford University Press.
10. Shearer, M., et al. (1968). "Unexpected Effects of an 'Open Door' Policy on Birth Rates of Women in State Hospitals." *American Journal of Orthopsychiatry*, 38:413–417.
11. Frank, J. (1961). *Persusasion and Healing: A Comparative Study of Psychotherapy*. Baltimore: Johns Hopkins Press.
12. Hollingshead, A., and F. Redlich (1958). *Social Class and Mental Illness*. New York: Wiley.
13. Myers, J., and L. Schaffer (1954). "Social Stratification and Psychiatric Practice: A Study of an Out-Patient Clinic." *American Sociological Review*, 19:307–310.
14. Cumming, J., and E. Cumming (1962). *Ego and Milieu*. New York: Atherton.

15. Moos, R.H., and P. S. Houts (1968). "Assessment of the Social Atmospheres of Psychiatric Wards." *Journal of Abnormal Psychology,* **73:**595–604.

16. Moos, R.H. (1968). "Differential Effects of Ward Settings on Psychiatric Patients." *Journal of Nervous and Mental Diseases,* **147:**386–393.

17. Lemert, E. (1951). *Social Pathology: A Systematic Approach to the Theory of Sociopathic Behavior.* New York: McGraw-Hill.

18. Schur, E. (1971). *Labeling Deviant Behavior: Its Sociological Implications.* New York: Harper and Row.

19. Goffman, E. (1961). *Asylums: Essays on the Social Situation of Mental Patients and Other Inmates.* New York: Doubleday-Anchor.

20. Lemert, E., (1951) op. cit.

21. Eaton, J., and R. Weil (1955). *Culture and Mental Disorder.* New York: Free Press.

22. Mechanic, D. (1969). *Mental Health and Social Policy.* Englewood Cliffs, N.J.: Prentice-Hall.

23. Scheff, T. (1966). *Being Mentally Ill: A Sociological Theory.* Chicago: Aldine.

24. Hess, J. H., and T.E. Thomas (1963). "Incompetency to Stand Trial: Procedures, Results, and Problems." *American Journal of Psychiatry,* **119:**713–720.

25. Szassz, T. (1963). *Law, Liberty and Psychiatry.* New York: MacMillan; and Szasz, T. (1970). *Ideology and Insanity: Essays on the Psychiatric Dehumanization of Man.* New York: Doubleday-Anchor.

26. Summary of Activities of the National Council on the Rights of the Mentally Impaired, July, 1972.

27. Clausen, J., and M.R. Yarrow (eds.) (1955). *The Impact of Mental Illness on the Family. Journal of Social Issues,* No. 11, entire issue.

28. Schwartz, C. (1957). "Perspectives on Deviance—Wives' Definitions of their Husbands' Mental Illness." *Psychiatry,* **20:**275–291.

29. Freeman, H., and O. Simmons (1963). *The Mental Patient Comes Home.* New York: Wiley.

30. Angrist, S., et al. (1961). "Tolerance of Deviant Behaviour, Post-hospital Performance Levels, and Rehospitalization." *Proceedings of the Third World Congress of Psychiatry.* Montreal, pp.237–241.

31. Angrist, S., et al. (1968): *Women After Treatment: A Study of Former Mental Patients and their Normal Neighbors.* New York: Appleton-Century-Crofts.

32. Michaux, W.W., et al. (1970). *The First Year Out: Mental Patients After Hospitalization.* Baltimore: Johns Hopkins Press.

33. Mechanic, D. (1966). "Response Factors in Illness." *Social Psychiatry,* **1:**11–20.

34. Kadushin, C. (1969). *Why People Go to Psychiatrists.* New York: Atherton.

35. Mechanic, D. (1972). "Social Psychological Factors Affecting the Presentation of Bodily Complaints." *New England Journal of Medicine,* **286:**1132–1139.

36. Kadushin, C. (1962). "Social Distance Between Client and Professional." *American Journal of Sociology,* **67:**517–531.

37. Hollingshead, A., and F. Redlich, (1958)., op. cit.

38. Mechanic, D. (1968). *Medical Sociology: A Selective View.* op. cit.

39. Shepherd, M., et al. (1971). *Childhood Behavior and Mental Health.* London: University of London Press.

40. Dohrenwend, Bruce, and Barbara Dohrenwend (1969). *Social Status and Psychological Disorder*, op. cit.

41. Srole, L., et al. (1962). *Mental Health in the Metropolis: The Midtown Study.* New York: McGraw-Hill.

42. Leighton, D., et al. (1963). *The Character of Danger.* New York: Basic Books.

43. Langner, T. S., and S. T. Michael (1963). *Life Stress and Mental Health.* New York: Free Press.

44. Crandell, D. L., and B. Dohrenwend (1967). "Some Relations Among Psychiatric Symptoms, Organic Illness, and Social Class." *American Journal of Psychiatry*, **123**:1527–1538.

45. Bradburn, N. (1969). *The Structure of Psychological Well-Being.* Chicago: Aldine.

46. Dohrenwend, B. P., et al. (1970). "Measures of Psychiatric Disorder in Contrasting Class and Ethnic Groups: A Preliminary Report of Ongoing Research." In E. H. Hare and J. K. Wing (eds.), *Psychiatric Epidemiology*, op. cit., pp. 159–202.

47. Robins, L. (1972). "Social Correlates of 'Antisocial Personality'." Paper presented at the Annual Meetings of the American Sociological Association, New Orleans, Louisiana, August, 1972.

48. Cooper, J. (1970). "The Use of a Procedure for Standardizing Psychiatric Diagnosis." In E. H. Hare and J. K. Wing (eds.), *Psychiatric Epidemiology*, op. cit., pp. 109–131.

49. Wing, J. K. (1970). "A Standard Form of Psychiatric Present State Examination: And a Method for Standardizing the Classification of Symptoms." In E. H. Hare and J. K. Wing (eds.), *Psychiatric Epidemiology*, op. cit., pp. 93–108.

50. Merton, R. (1957). *Social Theory and Social Structure.* New York: Free Press.

51. Clinard, M. (ed.) (1964). *Anomie and Deviant Behavior.* New York: Free Press.

52. Sewell, W. H. (1961). "Social Class and Childhood Personality." *Sociometry*, **24**:340–356; and Sewell, W. H. (1968). "Mental Health: Social Class and Personal Adjustment." *International Encyclopedia of the Social Sciences*. New York: Macmillan, pp. 222–226.

53. Kohn, M. (1969). *Class and Conformity: A Study in Values.* Homewood, Ill.: Dorsey.

54. Dohrenwend, Bruce, and Barbara Dohrenwend (1969). *Social Status and Psychological Disorder*, op. cit.

55. Kohn, M. (1968). "Social Class and Schizophrenia: A Critical Review." In D. Rosenthal and S. Kety (eds.), *The Transmission of Schizophrenia.* Oxford: Pergamon, pp. 155–173.

56. Dunham, H. W. (1965). *Community and Schizophrenia: An Epidemiological Analysis.* Detroit: Wayne State University Press.

57. Turner, R.J., and M. Wagenfeld (1967). "Occupational Mobility and Schizophrenia; An Assessment of the Social Causation and Social Selection Hypotheses." *American Sociological Review*, **32**:104–113.

58. Mechanic, D. (1972). "Social Class and Schizophrenia: Some Requirements for a Plausible Theory of Social Influence." *Social Forces*, **50**:305–309.

59. Kohn, M. (1972). "Class, Family, and Schizophrenia: A Reformulation." *Social Forces*, **50**:295–304.

60. Hollingshead, A., and F. Redlich (1958). *Social Class and Mental Illness*, op. cit.

61. Sampson, H., et al. (1964). *Schizophrenic Women: Studies in Marital Crisis.* New York: Atherton.

62. Wing, J.K., and G. W. Brown (1970). *Institutionalism and Schizophrenia.* Cambridge: Cambridge University Press.

63. Rutler, M. L. (1972). "Relationship Between Child and Adult Psychiatric Disorders." *Acta Psychiatrica Scandinavica*, **48**:3–21.

64. Robins, L. (1966). *Deviant Children Grown Up*. Baltimore: Williams and Wilkins.
65. Robins, L. (1972). "Social Correlates of 'Antisocial Personality'," *op. cit.*; also L. Robins, et al. (1971). "Adult Psychiatric Status of Black Schoolboys." *Archives of General Psychiatry*, **24**:338–345.
66. Scheff, T. (ed.) (1967). *Mental Illness and Social Processes*. New York: Harper.
67. Spitzer, S., and N. Denzin (eds.) (1968). *The Mental Patient: Studies in the Sociology of Deviance*. New York: McGraw-Hill.
68. Goffman, E. (1963). *Stigma: Notes on the Management of Spoiled Identity*. Englewood Cliffs, N.J.: Prentice Hall.
69. Brown, G., et al. (1966). *Schizophrenia and Social Care*, op. cit.
70. Rosenberg, M. (1965). *Society and the Adolescent Self-Image*. Princeton, N.J.: Princeton University Press.
71. Coopersmith, S. (1967). *The Antecedents of Self-Esteem*. San Francisco: W. H. Freeman.
72. Bradburn, N. (1969). *The Structure of Psychological Well-Being*, op. cit.
73. Lazarus, R. S. (1966). *Psychological Stress and the Coping Process*. New York: McGraw-Hill.
74. Mechanic, D. (1962). *Students Under Stress: A Study in the Social Psychology of Adaptation*. New York: Free Press.
75. McGrath J. (ed.) (1970). *Social and Psychological Factors in Stress*. New York: Holt, Rinehart, and Winston.
76. Coelho, G., and D. Hamburg (eds.) *Psychological Stress and Coping Processes*, in press.
77. Scheff, T. (1966). *Being Mentally Ill: A Sociological Theory*, op. cit.
78. Gove, W. (1970). "Societal Reaction as an Explanation of Mental Illness: An Evaluation." *American Sociological Review*, **35**:873–884.
79. Dohrenwend, Bruce, and Barbara Dohrenwend (1969). *Social Status and Psychological Disorder*, op. cit.
80. Langer, T. S., and S. T. Michael (1963). *Life Stress and Mental Health*, op. cit.
81. Holmes, T. H., and R. H. Rahe (1967). "The Social Readjustment Rating Scale." *Journal of Psychosomatic Research*, **11**:213–218.
82. Brown, G. W., and J. Birley (1968). "Crises and Life Changes and the Onset of Schizophrenia." *Journal of Health and Social Behavior*, **9**:203–214.
83. Brown, G. W., et al. (1973). "Life Events and Psychiatric Disorders: Some Methodological Issues." *Psychological Medicine*, **3**:74–87.
84. Lazarus, R. (1966). *Psychological Stress and the Coping Process*, op. cit.
85. Mechanic, D. (1970). "Some Problems in Developing a Social Psychology of Adaptation to Stress." In J. E. McGrath (ed.), *Social and Psychological Factors in Stress*, op. cit., pp. 104–123.
86. Cohen, A. (1966). *Deviance and Control*. Englewood Cliffs, N.J.: Prentice-Hall.
87. Sykes, G. (1958). *The Society of Captives*. Princeton, N.J.: Princeton University Press.
88. Etzioni, A. (1964). *Modern Organizations*, Englewood Cliffs, N.J.: Prentice-Hall.
89. Thompson, J. (1967). *Organizations in Action*. New York: McGraw-Hill.
90. Perrow, C. (1965). "Hospitals: Technology, Structure and Goals." In J. March (ed.), *Handbook of Organizations*. Chicago: Rand McNally.
91. Pasamanick, B., et al. (1967). *Schizophrenics in the Community*. New York: Appleton-Century-Crofts.

92. Davis, A., et al. (1972). "The Prevention of Hospitalization in Schizophrenia: Five Years After an Experimental Program." *American Journal of Orthopsychiatry.* **42**:375–388.

93. Rosenthal, D., and S. Kety (eds.) (1968). *The Transmission of Schizophrenia,* op. cit.

94. Rosenthal, D. (1970). *Genetic Theory and Abnormal Behavior.* New York: McGraw-Hill.

95. Gardner, E. A. (1970). "Emotional Disorders in Medical Practice." *Annals of Internal Medicine,* **73**:651–652.

96. Fink, R., et al. (1969). "Changes in Family Doctors' Services for Emotional Disorders after Addition of Psychiatric Treatment to a Prepaid Group Program." *Medical Care,* **7**: -209–224.

97. Goldensohn, S., et al. (1969). "Referral, Utilization and Staffing Patterns of a Mental Health Service in a Prepaid Group Practice Program in New York." *American Journal of Psychiatry,* **126**:689–697.

98. Shepherd, M., et al. (1966). *Psychiatric Illness in General Practice.* London: Oxford University Press.

99. Mechanic, D. (1972). "Social Psychological Factors Affecting the Presentation of Bodily Complaints," op. cit.

100. Balint, M. (1957). *The Doctor, His Patient, and the Illness.* New York: International Universities Press.

101. Davis, M. (1966). "Variations in Patients' Compliance with Doctors' Orders: Analysis of Congruence between Survey Responses and Results of Empirical Investigations." *Journal of Medical Education,* **41**:1037–1048.

102. Leventhal, H. (1970). "Findings and Theory in the Study of Fear Communications." In L. Berkowitz, (ed.), *Advances in Experimental Social Psychology,* Vol. 5. New York: Academic Press, pp. 119–186.

103. Duff, R., and A. Hollingshead (1968). *Sickness and Society.* New York: Harper.

104. Belknap, I. (1956). *Human Problems of a State Mental Hospital.* New York: McGraw-Hill.

105. Caudill, W. (1958). *The Psychiatric Hospital as a Small Society.* Cambridge, Mass.: Harvard University Press.

106. Stanton, A. H., and M. S. Schwartz (1954). *The Mental Hospital.* New York: Basic Books.

107. Davis, K. (1938). "Metal Hygiene and the Class Structure." *Psychiatry,* **1**:55–65.

108. Szasz, T. (1970). *The Manufacture of Madness.* New York: Harpers.

109. Henry, W., et al. (1971). *The Fifth Profession.* San Francisco: Josey-Bass.

110. Halleck, S. (1971). *The Politics of Therapy.* New York: Science House.

111. Mechanic, D. (1969). *Mental Health and Social Policy,* op. cit.

112. McCarthy, R. (ed.) (1959). *Drinking and Intoxication.* New York: Free Press.

113. Pittman, D., and C. Snyder (eds.) (1962). *Society, Culture and Drinking Patterns.* New York: Wiley

114. Cooperative Commission on the Study of Alcoholism (1967). *Alcohol Problems: A Report to the Nation.* New York: Oxford University Press.

115. Fox, B., and J. Fox (1963). *Alcohol and Traffic Safety.* Washington D.C.: National Institute of Mental Health.

116. Bales, R. F. (1944). *The 'Fixation Factor' in Alcohol Addiction: An Hypothesis Derived from a Comparative Study of Irish and Jewish Social Norms.* Doctoral Dissertation, Harvard University.

117. Kornhauser, A. (1965). *Mental Health of the Industrial Worker.* New York: Wiley.

118. Blauner, R. (1964). *Alienation and Freedom: The Factory Worker and His Industry.* Chicago: University of Chicago Press.

119. Back, K. (1972). *Beyond Words: The Story of Sensitivity Training and the Encounter Movement.* New York: Russell Sage.

120. Hamburg, D. (ed.) (1970). *Psychiatry as a Behavioral Science.* Englewood Cliffs, N.J.: Prentice-Hall.

CHAPTER XIII

Issues in the Sociology of Organizations and the Administration of Mental Health Services*

In recent years there has been a major shift in the provision of mental health services from the hospital to community facilities. Most prominent among new features of mental health services was the establishment of community mental health centers with building and staffing funds from the federal government. Although eligibility for funding required all community mental health centers to make provision for certain services, the centers themselves developed a variety of personalities and priorities. Some developed useful services for chronic mental patients and gave considerable attention to their needs, while others serviced mainly patients with less incapacitating problems in living. Some centers focused mainly on their clients—offering personal services to assist them with their difficulties—while others developed an ambitious agenda to attack community problems which they felt were a major cause of distress in the population. Some utilized relatively conventional approaches to the delivery of personal services, while others began to experiment with new systems of care and new forms of mental health manpower.

It is very difficult to obtain a comprehensive picture of the ferment and chaos characteristic of the varying programs developed around the country. Careful evaluation of these centers is an important priority in the mental health field, but it will probably take some years before the appropriate questions are formulated and adequate data are collected. The phasing out of fed-

* Adapted from a chapter appearing in S. Feldman (ed.), *The Administration of Mental Health Services*, 1973. Courtesy of Charles C. Thomas, publisher, Springfield, Ill.

eral support for mental health centers also makes their future less clear. The emphasis in the 1960's on community mental health centers was a major shift in philosophy and practice, and involved the expenditure of large sums of money. An assessment of the costs and benefits of following these priorities rather than others is, therefore, of considerable importance.

This chapter examines the organizational problems inherent in delivering community mental health services. It considers the manner in which the work of varying professionals and paraprofessionals delivering mental health services can be coordinated and the problems inherent in working within a community context with a variety of other social agencies that have different tasks and varying perspectives. The discussion is analytic rather than evaluative and raises issues that are pertinent to a variety of human services agencies, not only to mental health facilities.

Models of Organization and Approaches to their Study

Organizations are social groupings developed around the pursuit of specific goals. They can be characterized by a planned division of labor, distribution of powers and responsibilities, and specified lines of communication. They differ from families, tribes, and other social collectivities in the extent of their planning, the more limited scope of their goals, and the degree of substitutibility of their personnel.[1] Organizations as entities are social instruments that are less tied to particular individuals in contrast to other social collectivities, and appear to have an identity independent of its personnel who may change from one period to another. Thus, the identity of hospitals, corporations, universities, and government agencies transcends the individual orientations and characteristics of the doctors, businessmen, professors, and politicians who play a crucial part in the shaping of organizational activities.

Much of current thinking about organizations derives from the clash of two very different perspectives. The scientific management perspective has been concerned with the efficiency of organizations and has placed the greatest emphasis on their formal characteristics. Constructed around the study of industrial organizations, scientific management emphasized the fit between man and machines, the most rational organization of tasks and their interrelationships, and the incentives that produced the highest productivity. Considerable emphasis was given to the formal plans of organization, schemes for designating the hierarchy of authority, appropriate lines of communication, and the rules and procedures through which goal-directed tasks were to be performed.

As a response to this highly formalistic approach, the human relations perspective developed, which emphasized how noneconomic aspects of the work context profoundly influenced workers' orientations to their tasks, how subgroup formations developed, and how informal cultures became influential in affecting the motivation of workers. Particularly influential were the "Hawthorne" studies, a series of investigations carried out at the Western Electric Company's Hawthorne Works from 1927 to 1932.[2] These studies began with various changes in lighting conditions, and it was assumed that improved lighting would increase worker productivity. The investigators were surprised to find that altering lighting—by increasing or decreasing it—had similar effects, and that the manner in which workers defined changes in working conditions was perhaps as important as the objective effects of the physical changes themselves. This led to a whole series of inquiries, which documented the variety of ways in which informal work groups developed and affected the conditions of work and rates of worker productivity. Thus, the human relations school emerged with an appreciation that human outcomes were the product of more than merely physical manipulations of the environment.

It was through the development of the human relations perspective that it became commonplace among sociologists and other social scientists to appreciate that activities in an organization frequently depart from the formal plan, that goals are pursued that may be irrelevant or even destructive to the major functions of organizations, and that an elaborate informal organization may develop which, in its operation, may significantly modify the aims and activities of organizational personnel. James Thompson[3] in describing approaches to informal organization has noted that:

> Here attention is focused on variables which are not included in any of the rational models—sentiments, cliques, social controls via informal norms, status and status striving, and so on. It is clear that students of informal organization regard these variables not as random deviations or error, but as patterned, adaptive responses of human beings in problematic situations . . . In this view the informal organization is a spontaneous and functional development, indeed a necessity, in complex organizations, permitting the system to adapt and survive (p. 7).

Over the years there has been a good deal of debate and interchange among proponents of each of the two perspectives I have described. The proponents, in pushing their own line of argument, have at times exaggerated the relative influence of the variables of major interest to them, but most organizational researchers borrow liberally from both perspectives, and current organizational thinking forms a synthesis of both points of view. With growing sophistication in the study of organizations, new problems have been given increasing attention, such as the relationship between organizations and the external environment, intra- and interorganizational linking and comparative organizational studies.

In considering organizations, researchers have usually classified them in terms of their particular functions, such as industrial organizations, schools, hospitals, and prisons. However, this kind of classification, fails to take into account the similarities and differences among organizations performing varying functions. A more ambitious classification was attempted by Etzioni,[4] who grouped organizations by their compliance structures. He distinguished between predominantly coercive organizations, such as prisons, concentration camps, and custodial mental hospitals; predominantly utilitarian organizations, such as white-collar and blue-collar industries; and predominantly normative organizations, such as religious organizations, hospitals, colleges, and voluntary associations. Etzioni hypothesizes that clients in coercive organizations have an alienative affiliation, clients in utilitarian organizations have a calculative orientation, and clients in normative organizations have a moral orientation. He argues further that the use of power in these organizations will be related to client orientation.

Other students of organizations tend to focus on particular aspects, such as size, complexity, type of technology, and degree of centralization, for example. One of the most persistent problems in organizational theory and research concerns the growth of bureaucracy, and a great deal of attention has been directed to the theory of bureaucracy elaborated by Max Weber. Weber specified these aspects of bureaucratic structure: (1) a continuous organization of official functions bound by rules; (2) specific spheres of competence; (3) the hierarchical organization of positions; (4) the technical specification of rules that regulate the conduct of positions; (5) separation of administration and ownership; (6) freedom from outside control and manipulation; and (7) the formulation of administrative acts, decisions, and rules in writing.[5] Many students of organizations have used these specifications as a guide in studying various types of organizations to see to what extent they approximated Weber's criteria and, in this way, different descriptions of bureaucratic variations became elaborated. Weber's concept of bureaucracy was an "ideal-type," a model that was not based on any particular reality, but that attempted to portray reality in an abstract sense.[6] Weber believed that the "ideal-type" was a powerful model to use in studying organizational phenomena and, indeed, there are various studies, such as those of hospitals, indicating in what ways particular types of organizations deviated from Weber's specifications. In recent years, a somewhat different approach to the study of organizations has become predominant, which emphasizes the empirical relationships among variables. Blau and Scott[7] maintain that:

> To exploit Weber's insightful analysis, it is necessary, in our opinion, to discard his *misleading* concepts of the ideal type and to distinguish explicitly between the conceptual scheme and the hypotheses. The latter can then be tested and refined rather than left as mere *impressionistic assertions.* We can ask, for example: does tenure promote efficiency? Under what conditions does it have this effect, and under what conditions does it not? Only in this way can we hope to progress beyond Weber's *insights* to the building of systematic theory (italics mine) (p. 34).

The Focus of This Chapter

At present it is not very productive to summarize empirical propositions on the functioning of organizations that are relevant to the administration of mental health services, although I shall mention such propositions when they are pertinent. Instead, I shall discuss the observation, noted earlier, that organizations frequently develop an elaborate informal organization that significantly affects the goals and directions of organizational activity. Although this observation may seem commonplace, it is one of the major insights of organizational theory and offers the keen administrator an important focus from which to begin to understand his own activities. Like many generalizations, this observation appears to be of little pragmatic utility but, through an understanding of the conditions under which such organizational modifications develop and persist, one begins to grasp how people come to terms with the human problems that every worker must confront on the job in concrete form. Informal structures and culture frequently arise in adapting to such human problems.

Organizations, of course, vary in the extent and importance of their informal structures. Professional organizations, and particularly the ones that are service oriented, tend to develop rich and varied informal networks that may be more indicative of daily activities than the usual descriptions of these organizations would suggest. This does not mean that the formal organization has a small impact or that administrative planning is futile. Administrative planning, however, must take place within the context of such considerations as the way in which the particular functions of the organization affect how people work, how professional norms and culture modify authority and other relationships, how interagency contacts require forms of relationships not specified by formal structures, and how outside social and political forces limit organizational activities.

Mental health agencies, by their very character, bring into sharp focus many of the complexities of organizations. The goals of such organizations—whether they are a hospital, mental health center, rehabilitation center, outpatient clinic, or some combination of these—are usually multifaceted and ambiguous. They normally encompass some concept of treatment, rehabilitation, and consultation. They frequently combine such functions as providing service to clients, training of professionals and other personnel, and some research. In addition, they are ordinarily expected to perform various tasks for the community, such as the detention and evaluation of persons disruptive to the community, consultation with the courts and other community agencies, and a variety of other functions. Moreover, the organization may become involved in efforts directed toward community education, prevention, and social amelioration.

These functions would be difficult enough under the best of circumstances, but problems are compounded at almost every point by the absence of agreed-upon technologies, by differences in ideologies among varying professional groups, by disagreements on basic intervention approaches, and by continuing situational pressures involving community support, funding, and staffing. These problems and difficulties would ordinarily require considerable administrative direction and control, but the nature of professional organizations—and mental health agencies are dominated by professionals—confronts the administrator with personnel who are jealous of their rights, protective of their autonomy, and closely committed to particular ideologies about the nature of their work. The administrator thus must exercise his authority rather lightly, mediating jurisdictional and professional disputes, nurturing enthusiasm for new organizational directions, building commitment and loyalty to the organization's goals, and in general developing a sense of mission around some coherent set of viable functions. If an administrator wishes to have influence on anything more than the physical plant and financial aspects of his enterprise, he must have the capacity to command the loyalty and commitment of his personnel. But to the extent that he exercises authority instead of influencing individuals to share his goals, he is unlikely to gain their loyalty or commitment, and may even have difficulty retaining them in the organization.

Mental health agencies require considerable discretion and flexibility on the part of their major personnel. In the absence of clear and effective technologies,[8] the worker must depend on his judgement and professional experience in dealing with the array of problems that he faces. The nature of these activities makes them almost impossible to control through formal mechanisms, and when such mechanisms are developed they are reasonably easily subverted or ignored. It is almost impossible to effectively control a professional who offers a client service when there are limited criteria for evaluating the service and disagreement about how the service is most effectively delivered. The exercise of ineffective controls only erodes the professional commitment and creativity of the worker, and may be conducive to making him a disgruntled member of the team.[9]

Conditions Affecting the Development of Informal Structures

Despite ideal definitions of organizational goals and the formal structures through which such goals are to be achieved, organizations must make continuing adaptations to the conditions of their environment—whether this involves changing political demands, modifications of technology, scarcity of manpower or resources or changing interagency relationships, for instance.[10,11] Moreover, in the area of human services it is inevitable that people in key roles will face problems or contingencies that have not been anticipated or for which there are no agreed-upon solutions. Or they may find that the prescribed solutions in the form of bureaucratic procedures are inadequate or ineffective, and these solutions will tend to be abandoned. Individual members of organizations may also work toward facilitating their own personal goals and aspirations, which may be more or less consonant with formally defined goals of the organization; and, since organizations have multifaceted goals or goals that are often intangible, it becomes easier for individuals to subsume their own goals within such diffuse organizational definitions.[12]

Mental health agencies are particularly vulnerable to the incorporation of personal goals. Since the structures of such organizations tend to be new or changing (as in the community mental health centers), the possibilities abound for new role definitions of various workers. Indeed, with the growth of new types of mental health professionals, one can expect to find a great deal of role construction and modification going on.[13] Unlike more traditional hospital settings, mental health workers in community mental health centers are testing new relationships relative to clients and professionals and, since such roles are frequently not clearly defined, each of the professional groups attempts to stake out its work territory relative to other groups, new forms of cooperation, and new definitions of its scope of work, autonomy, and authority.[14]

The manner in which such definitions develop is a relatively open process, particularly in its early stages. Factors such as the personality and aggressiveness of various workers, the nature of their training and professional experience, and the character of personal relationships within the organization all play a part. Although this process goes on in both the mental hospital and the more traditional mental health agency, authority relationships are more established, and the medical model prescribes the basic framework within which such adaptations will occur. But as the community mental health center moves away from the traditional medical model and involves a larger proportion of nonmedical and nonnursing personnel, an authority vacuum may develop that provides a wider field for attempts at role-construction and negotiations about the nature of work and relationships among workers. Such negotiations provide creative possibilities, but they also provide opportunities for chaos and conflict, and the particular outcome may depend on the extent to which there is coherence of administrative perspective and the nature of power relationships in the community.

The provision of administrative coherence is difficult because of the various pressures acting on the organization that may modify its course in the implementation of its defined goals. The extent of these influences was not fully appreciated in organizational theory, since much of the early work on informal structure came from the study of industrial work groups who were faced with relatively well-defined work tasks. Even here it was observed that a system of social norms developed that defined the appropriate rate of work and controlled output.[15] Although these studies documented the presence of an elaborate informal system, the contexts studied involved sufficiently specific goals so that there was only limited opportunity for workers to pursue their own personal goals or external group goals within work contexts. They could pace work and control output if they wished, but they could not easily initiate changes in the assembly line or the manner in which work processes were performed.

In mental health agencies, as in human service generally, work tasks are not so closely prescribed, and the outcomes achieved are difficult to evaluate. Thus, individuals and subgroups in such organizations can initiate their own goals that may or may not be compatible with organizational goals, or their goals may be irrelevant to the organization's definition of its environment. The imposition of such subgoals may originate for a variety of personal reasons. In its most simple form, it may be the product of the participant's desire to achieve status, recognition, or other rewards by working through his own professional framework and conforming to the values of his own professional group. Thus, many psychiatrists are reluctant to depart too drastically from what they perceive among their own peer group as the valued forms of treatment and treatment organization. Similarly, social workers may resist the establishment of a lay-therapist program or other organizational modifications because it challenges their status position and presumption of expert skills. Whatever the circumstances, it is clear that innovations in organization are likely to threaten the autonomy or status of particular persons or groups, and such changes—if they are to be effectively implemented and if they are not to tear the organization apart internally—require considerable loyalty, assurance, and commitment on the part of organizational personnel.

The dispersion of goals can occur, of course, within the organization as well. Each of several organizational components may respond to its own situation, emphasize its own needs, and promote its own agenda independent of the needs of the whole. The personnel in each unit will come to view organizational goals in terms of the conditions they face without full awareness of the whole picture. For example, mental health centers may subdivide their staff into neighborhood teams, which are responsible for a selected population area. These teams then may "follow" their clients through all center services. This form of organization allows a closer relationship between services and population groups and continuity of care, but if the subunit comes to think of its work only in terms of the interests of its own population area, and not in terms of the larger population that the health center serves, conflict can easily develop between the subunits and the health center. Although there is much to be said in favor of a subunit serving as ombudsman for its clients, resources are inevitably limited, and if one subunit pushes too hard it may divert a reasonable and fair allocation of resources. Administrative direction is particularly crucial in decentralized units, since each unit only tends to see "a piece of the action" and may come to define the crucial issues and priorities on the basis of a distorted picture of the whole.

The difficulty of maintaining internal equilibrium often stems from the problem of controlling external pressures on the organization itself. The community often imposes demands on mental health agencies that are unrealistic in terms of time, resources, and available technology and knowledge. Thus, the community expects to turn to mental health agencies to manage community deviance and other problems that become manifest, independent of the demands that such agencies can realistically meet. Ideally, the agency would define its goals and its realistic limitations of knowledge and expertise, and expect support for its activities. But, in competition for resources and community support, the agencies usually must accept external definitions and, indeed, they often encourage even more unrealistic expectations. Since such organizations usually seek to widen their scope of activities and the number of · clients they deal with, organizational representatives are frequently unwilling to advertise their limitations and, instead, encourage further demands. One does not often find a mental health administrator—or, for that matter, any other kind of administrator—reporting to community funding agencies, in detail, his limitations of knowledge and efficacy. If anything, administrators tend to provide optimistic estimates of their accomplishments and possibilities for future contributions, since they consider that their budget and support are dependent on such declarations. The competition for resources thus encourages a cycle of exaggeration and counter exaggeration that feeds public expectations and places such organizations under greater pressure to achieve the impossible. It is not surprising that personnel within the agency often tend to become cynical and develop roles for themselves which are comfortable and which they protect. Having been disillusioned too often, they resist innovation and seek to maintain the adjustments they have worked out for themselves.

The demand for particular kinds of task performance comes not only from clients and the public but also from other community agencies that have formal and informal links with a particular organization. Regardless of how social organizations are defined legally and administratively, it is the nature of informal networks to encompass the regions within which work must be done rather than the formal boundaries of organizations. The activities of mental health agencies bring them into close contact with other community agencies and groups with whom they must deal on an ongoing basis, and an informal system develops that binds them together. Thus, mental hospitals, community mental health centers, and the like become part of a particular social network that makes demands on them that cannot be ignored. These demands may come in the form of suggestions from Washington, D.C., influence from the

County Board, pressures from a local judge, or complaints from the local police. Since the mental health agency must depend on all of these agencies for support and possible assistance, and is part of a larger system involving these organizations, social arrangements may develop that place considerable restraints on organizational work. Since these agencies must work together to facilitate their own efforts and goals, the failure to conform to informal arrangements may become costly.

Arrangements of this kind are, of course, pervasive in the community, and would pose no special problem except that such external demands may come into conflict with the needs and interests of the client. Personnel responsible for therapeutic care may feel that a patient should be returned to the community, but the resistance of a local judge may cause problems. To the extent that the agency accedes to the judge's wishes, it may alienate its therapeutic staff who feel that political considerations are being given weight over the needs of the client; to the extent that the agency alienates the judge or other influential persons, it may face opposition in the future. Although sociologists have not made definitive studies mapping out such intraorganizational linking, there are growing indications that social agencies that have public ideologies of protecting the client often become intimately linked with organizations that may have interests opposed to the interests of the agency's clients. For example, members of regulatory agencies tend to become more closely associated with the groups they regulate than with the groups they represent, and they come to share many of the attitudes and definitions of the regulated groups. Similarly, public defenders, and parole and probation officers tend to become part of the court system and, on a day-to-day basis, they must work more closely with district attorneys and judges than with civil liberties groups and rehabilitation groups.[16,17] This results in certain attitudes and behaviors that become necessary to sustain continuing cooperative relationships, which may be costly to certain clients. Since clients tend to pass through the organization—while agency relationships must persist through time—it is unusual to strain such relationships in the interests of particular clients except under very special circumstances. These typical processes raise grave issues concerning who are the clients of mental health agencies.

The processes of intraorganizational linking, described above, have as their key element the principle of reciprocity. Favors done must be repaid by various forms of cooperation and a willingness to protect one's colleagues in related agencies. The informal networks that develop, therefore, not only facilitate organizational tasks and the survival of the organization itself, but also may set up extraorganizational demands and expectations that participants can violate from time to time (but not in any persistent fashion). Any continuing attempt to challenge such community relationships, to undermine the power of particular community groups, or to support one community group against others—whatever the merits of the case—will soon lead the persons responsible to be labeled as troublemakers and deviants. If they manage to survive at all, they will soon find it difficult to sustain sufficient cooperation to do their jobs.

I do not wish to imply that naturally occurring community processes are just; indeed, they tend to maintain existing power relationships and frequently are disadvantageous to particular community groups. The life of social agencies tends to be characterized by continuing transactions and negotiations, where various groups are allowed to define certain issues of crucial importance, to them in return for allowing others similar privileges when their major interests are at stake. However reasonable such understandings may appear to be, the ability to play this particular game depends on what rewards one can mediate for others, and this, of course, depends on the distribution of power.[18] Clearly, there are constituencies who tend to be excluded from these understandings because they have no power. A mental health agency that views its mission as one involving a more just distribution of power may develop procedures that build the power potentialities of specific groups—as, for example, may occur in developing mechanisms for community control. To some extent this is possible to achieve on a modest scale in respect to the delivery of services, but it also involves dangers; and if the agency comes to threaten seriously other community groups, they usually have the power to destroy or reconstitute it. The potentialities of community agencies are limited by the larger system of which they are a part, and although they may take a leadership role, they do not have the power by themselves to establish new priorities, except in a very limited sphere.

As an interested community becomes conscious of how an agency operates relative to its environment, the agency becomes readily susceptible to the charge that it is corrupt and nonresponsive to the needs of particular community groups. When the larger conceptions and values are attacked—as they are by militants in battles involving community control—the organization is then exposed to a variety of disputes that may threaten its existence. Critics may demand that rules and operating procedures be explicit and standard but, at the same time, they insist that flexibility and discretion be protected. They may demand more community involvement and cooperation but, in the process of the confrontation, animosities and feelings may be so aggravated that such cooperation becomes impossible. They may demand protection of individuals but also insist on open meetings and disclosures that violate such protections. They may insist on a deep examination of issues and priorities, but the context of such discussions often develops so that it becomes impossible for people to feel they can speak honestly, and they may be attacked if they do so. Unfortunately, these confrontations frequently become so threatening that the organization becomes even less responsive to disenfranchised groups.

Frequently when administrators feel sufficiently threatened, they tend to develop protective devices that make their organizations less accessible and less democratic. Pressures mount to abuse discretionary privilege, to cover up administrative activities, to withhold information and engage in propaganda against opponents, and to engage in closed and informal decision making. Thus these pressures result in organizations departing more profoundly than ever from their ideals and usual operations, and such pressures feed the cycle of distrust and recriminations. Trust and legitimacy are the glue that holds organizations together; in its absence, administrators tend to place greater dependence on subterfuge and coercion, which in turn undermines the commitment of participants.[19]

Internal Adaptations to Problems of Work

In a great variety of organizational contexts, people respond as much to the contingencies affecting their daily work as they do to matters of general public policy. The pressures of daily activities and the needs to overcome barriers to action lead to many ingenious mechanisms through which organizational participants pursue their work. Organizational rules may be violated because participants often feel that the end result could be achieved as well or better through less time-consuming shortcuts. The violation of procedural norms tends to be justified in terms of work saved and other advantages.[20]

Such adaptations are particularly characteristic of professional workers who tend to resist bureaucratic regulations. These workers have acquired particular professional orientations that emphasize autonomy and flexibility of decision, and they resent rules and regulations that close their options or require behavior that they do not view as goal-directed. Generally, professional workers are more satisfied with tasks that maximize their flexibility; and militancy and independence of such workers tend to be associated with their degree of professionalism.[21]

Professional workers have strong commitments to their clients, and often resent legal restrictions or rules that interfere with what they regard as proper management in the clients' interests. Consequently, they may readily violate regulations or make false certifications with respect to disability, indications for abortion, involuntary commitment, or other matters to achieve "optimal outcomes."[22] When personnel engage in actions of this kind, they do not conceive of themselves as violators but, instead, they view the rules as inhibiting their proper activities and the needs of their clients. This short-circuiting of rules and procedures can be used to assist a weak and relatively powerless client, or it can be used to manage him for the community. The dilemma in granting discretion is that there is always the danger that it can result in evil as well as good.

Developing and Maintaining Direction in Mental Health Agencies

Until very recently, mental health agencies have been characterized as dreary, routinized institutions—bereft of sufficient resources and staff to do an adequate job—and characterized by an atmosphere of hopelessness and apathy.[23] Typically, the staff had drifted into comfortable routines that made them reluctant to participate in innovations that would result in more work or disruptions in their established network of relationships. Administrators frequently found these institutions to be immovable and difficult to reorganize, and they either drifted away or fell into a rather routinized existence. Such agencies often served the community more than the patients by isolating and detaining deviants whom the community did not wish to tolerate; the patients in these institutions deteriorated as much from institutional routines as from their problems.[24]

Since the middle 1950's, the situation has shown considerable improvement.[25] A variety of changes—including the introduction of psychoactive drugs, new administrative attitudes, growing community support for community care, and an infusion of funds from governmental sources—resulted in a growth of enthusiasm and confidence on the part of mental health personnel. With government support, considerable strides were made in the training of mental health professionals, in the building and staffing of community mental health centers, and in the upgrading of state and county mental health institutions. There was also a wide appreciation that institutional living and prolonged inactivity could lead to a significant deterioration of skills and attitudes that made rehabilitation extremely difficult.

The question of just which of the many components involved were most important in stimulating new attitudes and efforts will be argued for many years. No doubt, psychoactive drugs stimulated hope and confidence, encouraged changing administrative attitudes, and made it more possible to manage patients in the community. But there is also evidence that similar changes were noted prior to the introduction of psychoactive drugs in some English hospitals, where there was strong administrative leadership and encouragement for new forms of community treatment for the mentally ill Whatever the specific impact of particular forces, it is reasonably clear from experience in other countries as well as our own, that the momentum of treatment institutions and the attitudes of personnel have pervasive effect on the performance of patients. Whether we consider the history of moral treatment in psychiatry,[26] or review the differential impact of the introduction of psychoactive drugs in hospitals where the staff had varying attitudes toward them,[27] it becomes clear that the communication of efficacy and hope is an indispensible aspect of an effective mental health facility. A major problem in all forms of therapy is the patient's poor self-image and history of failure, and if staff cannot communicate optimism to the client, it is difficult to see how the client can sustain it himself and persist in attempting to cope with his problems and the external environment.[28] Without hope, he is likely to sink into a state of apathy and inactivity, and there is no better measure of failure than evidence that the patient is doing nothing and making no serious attempt to struggle against adversity.

In one of the few comparative studies of mental hospitals over time, Wing and Brown[29] have traced the developments in three English mental hospitals between 1960 and 1968 and the effects of such changes on the clinical state and performance of schizophrenic patients. One of their significant findings was that the most important factor associated with the improvement of primary handicaps was the reduction of inactivity. In tracing the developments in these hospitals, these authors report considerable change in patient performance and clinical state following the implementation of modifications of hospital regimens and the initiation of a more developed rehabilitation perspective. Most improvement took place early in the study period but, by 1968, there was strong evidence in two of the three hospitals studied that the rate of improvement had declined as compared with the earlier period. In accounting for these changes, the investigators point out that there are several alternative explanations. It is possible, for example, that as patients get older, the staff turn their attentions to younger and newer patients, but the researchers did not find sufficient age effects in their analyses to make this a very likely explanation. Moreover, the researchers do not believe that their study spurred the staff to greater efforts, since the staff knew relatively little about the details of the investigation. Still another hypothesis is that, with developing community care, a lesser proportion of clinical time was devoted to long-stay patients. In the context of our discussion, still another alternative that Wing and Brown offer merits attention:

> The second kind of explanation is, in some ways, more disheartening; that the therapists (doctors, nurses, occupational therapists, and supervisors) began to feel, at different turning points in different hospitals, that they had done as much as they could; that expenditure of further time and energy would prejudice the chances of other patients, or simply enough was enough (p. 191).

Wing and Brown speculate further that the loss of certain key administrators, who left these hospitals during the study period, would also have to be taken into account. For example, Dr. D. H. Bennett, who had done much to build up the rehabilitation and resettlement services at Netherne Hospital, left in June 1962 to become a consultant at the Maudsley. Anyone who has seen Dr. Bennett in action can appreciate his boundless energy and ethusiasm, his optimism and patience, and his abilities to nurture involvement and enthusiasm among the people who work with him. Although I am not a great believer in great-man theories of social organization, I have no doubt that these qualities are immensely significant in administrators who have, as a prime responsibility, the coordination of a network of services, and who must depend on a wide variety of therapeutic workers for success. Major aspects of the task include developing cohesiveness and a cooperative spirit, and underplaying the status and ideological differences that may separate such workers.

Community mental health centers and other mental health institutions operate in a great sea of uncertainty. In the presence of diffuse goals and the lack of clear standards of performance, it is not difficult to gravitate to traditional and familiar forms of delivering services to the least disabled and most attractive clients, thus neglecting the clients who are most difficult to work with and the ones who are most impaired. Similarly, it is easy to neglect the maintenance of a complex web of relationships that increase service potential or that allow flexibility in care. Moreover, it is not difficult to lose unattractive clients, to neglect those who appear less cooperative, or to pass them off on other agencies. In short, there is considerable incentive to fall into the old patterns—that is, following the easy, routinized way of caring for patients who most vigorously and aggressively seek help, and of neglecting the rest. The major deterrents to falling into the old patterns are a strong sense of commitment and mission, and an organizational network that can provide meaningful services to the more difficult and disabled patients.

How, then, does an organization ensure a continuing sense of mission? In part, one sets the conditions for enthusiasm by recruiting able and energetic personnel. The personnel, if they have initiative, will want to participate and share in policy formation and implementation, and will desire considerable autonomy in pursuing organizational tasks. To the extent that directions and rules come from administrators without consultation, they will be resented and resisted. A major way of involving personnel in the goals of the organization is to make them feel a part of it and influential in its directions. This is inevitably time consuming and may even be annoying, but it is usually a worthy investment. Administrators often become defensive and angry when the staffs they have recruited oppose them on particular decisions, but a staff that is first-rate will inevitably do so; and a successful administrator accepts such decisions with good grace. If he pushes decisions against the wishes of his staff, he will only alienate the staff, and he may find that his decisions are not being implemented anyway.

Frequently, "old hands" in organizations resist changes in procedures or insist that this or that innovation was tried in the past without success. Yet, one frequently will find that new and younger personnel are committed to change and wish to try it. They usually are not convinced by the advice of more experienced persons that all sorts of problems will become manifest, and that the innovation will not work as smoothly as imagined. The "old hands" may be technically correct, but the resistance of innovation when there are strong feelings in support of it can be extremely costly. There are many ways to pursue a particular goal and, very often, the particular procedures followed do not have a great impact, one way or the other. What does have impact is the involvement and enthusiasm of the staff; and, if they have a sense of innovation and movement, this often encourages their energies and instills hope and enthusiasm in others as well. Mental health agencies probably help patients as much by instilling hope and confidence as in any other way, and a staff that is enthusiastic and hopeful is an invaluable asset. Maintaining this enthusiasm and movement is one of the major tasks facing a good administrator, and it is often the key to successful performance.

In pursuing innovation, initiation usually comes from the professional staff; yet, frequently, modifications of procedures require other personnel—such as clerical workers, attendants, and aides—to assume new and perhaps more time-consuming tasks. Since these persons often must do the work, they frequently resent changes in their routines about which they have had no voice. Although such personnel can rarely initiate changes, they have the capabilities to resist and divert changes and to frustrate new programs.[30] All workers, at whatever level, need to be appreciated and respected; and all workers resent changes that they feel are capricious or that fail to take into account the difficulties they have in doing their jobs. These workers have their own informal associations of friendship and work relations, and they may do much to retard change if the administration fails to enlist their loyalty and to give them a sense of importance with respect to the success of the enterprise. An administrator who neglects his subordinates is bound to find himself in considerable difficulty.[31]

The Corrupting Effect of Rules

Bureaucracies tend to proliferate rules that standardize procedures throughout the organization. These regulations are developed to ensure that certain standards of performance and functioning exist, and to protect against abuses and irregularities. Individual units of an organization and its personnel, however, have different functions. They operate in varying environments and face different needs. Rules that appear rational in general may create real obstacles to individual departments. These departments will face the alternative of subverting organizational rules or allowing efficient performance to suffer. Where performance is highly valued, rules are frequently violated; but, in violating rules, personnel feel vulnerable and, in being forced to violate the rules, their loyalty becomes eroded. Unfortunately, many large organizations invest more money in enforcing trivial rules than they could lose through the termination of the rules. Rules serve a specific purpose and, like other investments, should be judged in terms of an overall cost-benefit assessment. Too frequently, administrators fail to see the tremendous costs of unnecessary rules, both in terms of resources and the commitment of organizational participants.

The enforcement of standardized rules, which are not viewed as instrumental by the persons who are guided by them, often leads to cynicism and tendencies toward violation of the rules. In the process, both important rules and trivial rules tend to be violated. This leads to an informal atmosphere of expediency. Many organizational participants come to recognize that if they conscientiously conform to all the rules, they may achieve a certain security, but they know that their performance will suffer. Therefore, they violate rules but, in doing so, they become vulnerable to criticisms that can later be used against them. There are a few fearful persons who are extremely reluctant to violate rules and thus suffer in their work;[32] there are others who violate rules so liberally that they call into question the integrity of the organization. Some administrators use rules as a device to control their personnel. William Westley[33] described a police chief who developed a series of unreasonable regulations that he encouraged his men to violate. He could then use these regulations to control his men when they became too enthusiastic in performing their duty in situations where the chief felt that such performance was undesirable (arresting gamblers, for example).

The function of rules, of course, is to define expected behavior under ordinary circumstances. The rules serve as deterrents to behavior that exploits the organization, its personnel, its clients, or that compromises the organization's public stance. When problems arise, it is usually preferable to negotiate a resolution, and rules become a part of the currency of the negotiations.[34] It is better for organizations to operate on trust and the informal resolution of disputes rather than on the formal invocation of rules. The major function of rules is not enforcement but, instead, guidance and deterrence. When rules proliferate thoughtlessly and deal with every triviality, they tend to lose their power of guidance and may even encourage deviant and ineffective behavior. When persons are required to violate numerous rules to do their ordinary work, the rules themselves may become debased, and the respect for rules is undermined. Moreover, rules that are often established as minimal standards come to be viewed as standards of adequate performance, and they may even encourage a low level of performance. It is always difficult to specify the conditions under which rules are and are not necessary. A rule is a form of investment and, like other investments, it must be evaluated in terms of what it can and cannot achieve. The positive gain, as measured by likely deterrence or incentive, must be weighed against the losses resulting from alienation, violation, disrespect for rules in general, and resulting limits on spontaneity and innovation.

The need to protect flexibility of response is so important in many activities that organizations frequently develop an informal code that protects rule violators from external criticism. The unwillingness of professional and service organizations to take punitive action against their own members helps to maintain an atmosphere in which flexible action and risk-taking remain possible. For example, police departments are extremely reluctant to discipline their officers who violate due process; mental hospitals rarely punish nurses and attendants who illegally restrain patients; and organizations generally function by ignoring most rule violations. Since organizations must deal with rule violation selectively, they usually punish offenders when violations are clearly contrary to the welfare and goals of the organization, when the violator has incurred the wrath of persons in the organization for other reasons, or when the violations become sufficiently visible to the community so the organization requires sacrificial lambs for its own survival. Rules become only one element of a complex negotiation process, which involves consideration of the circumstances of rule violation, the "character" of the rule violator, and external pressures to respond in particular ways.

Professional organizations often face external criticisms of alleged abuses because they give their personnel considerable discretion. Community organizations and clients, more and more, insist on control mechanisms and a review of the work of personnel. In dealing with external demands, these organizations frequently develop mechanisms that are recognized as ineffective by persons within the system, but that exist primarily to subdue criticism from outside and to protect discretion. Most medical societies, police departments, universities, and hospitals, for instance, have disciplinary committees and procedures. However, these measures are rarely strict or effective. They function primarily to assure outsiders that the organization has the will and the capacity to police itself. Recently, there has been growing awareness of the ineffectiveness of such controls, and there have been growing demands for stronger disciplinary procedures in professional organizations. Although protections against significant abuse are necessary, any mechanisms developed must protect a wide range of discretion if they are to facilitate innovation and constructive risk-taking.

Notes on Organizational Power

The source of power in organizations is the ability to control persons, information, and resources, thus making others dependent. Ordinarily, the persons who have formal power also have considerable real power, because their formal position gives them ready access to control over the important elements of organizational life. However, persons with little formal power also may achieve access to information, persons, and resources through their strategic location in the organizational structure, their expert information, and the reliance of the organization on their skills and cooperation, for example.

As long as organizational participants recognize the legitimacy of the rights and powers of the persons in formal positions of authority, power may operate as expected. However, in complex organizations where subunits are competing among themselves and share varying goals, organizational participants have opportunities for a variety of alliances, and they may use the advantages of their location in the organizational structure and their access to information and people to further one set of objectives or another. Although such participants may use what power they have to protect their own goals and patterns of work, they may also form coalitions to further particular organizational programs outside of their own unit or to retard particular policies that they view as undesirable.

All organizations also have various groups that assume leadership on matters that are important to the organization. To be effective, these leadership groups must form alliances at various levels of the structure to ensure that the policies developed will be translated into a true action potential. As persons in powerful positions have noted over and over again, it is one thing to give directions and quite another to have them implemented. Each leadership group must seek from its possible constituency various persons among whom it can distribute tasks and privileges and from whom it can seek information and advice. Although, theoretically, the possible population from which such persons might be chosen is very large, generally the persons chosen are the ones about whom the leaders have direct knowledge or are aware of through trusted associates. Thus, within each leadership group there is a tendency for a "leadership circle" to emerge, which may become intimately involved in the decision-making processes of the organization.[35] As the persons in the leadership circle prove themselves in performing certain tasks and come to be trusted by one another, they tend to seek each other's assistance as new tasks emerge.

There is a tendency for the persons in the leadership circle to perpetuate their influence in various aspects of organizational life since they have closest knowledge of members within their own social group and tend to distribute tasks among them and to share information. However, if the social circle from which participants are chosen is too limited or is restricted to only one social segment of the organization, then the leadership group endangers itself because it might become isolated from the main currents of organizational activities, information flow, and personal transactions.

Defining a Coherent Mission

A mental health facility, like any effective organization, must have some sense of its priorities and commitments. In light of the extent to which the term "mental health" incorporates a vast spectrum of psychological, social, and even cultural problems, certainly no single facility, or even a complex of facilities, can attack the entire array effectively. Many of these problems are manifestations of the dilemmas and contradictions in society generally, and are not amenable to effective intervention without vast modifications in the social and cultural fabric, and greatly improved knowledge. Priorities in the mental health field should be set in terms of criteria of need and assessment of the efficacy of intervention strategies. This implies that any mental health facility must have a population perspective that is alert to the manner in which disorders present themselves in the population, how they develop, and the techniques that most effectively help to manage the problems.[36] Such an agency must also be receptive to the evaluation of its programs and must not become committed to specific efforts to such an extent that assessment and change become threatening to its personnel. This, of course, presents a dilemma, since the process of nurturing enthusiasm and involvement also is likely to cause personnel to become committed to certain programs and to protect them. Administrators, to the extent possible, should nurture commitment to goals or outcomes as compared with processes, since processes must change with the advance of knowledge and understanding.

One way of making priorities clear and salient is to develop a theory or set of perspectives about what the agency is supposed to be doing. It is helpful in constructing such models to develop an understanding of the limitations and constraints under which the agency must work and the aspects of the problem that are reasonably amenable to intervention. For example, in recent years, a growing interest has been evident in nonmedical approaches to mental patient care in the community. One approach is the educational model that attempts to improve patients' coping capacities through retraining and rehabilitation experiences, or that makes an effort to help relatives deal with inevitable problems that arise in living with a handicapped patient. In pursuing these goals, the agency may require a variety of services: partial hospitalization or transitional institutions such as half-way houses, sheltered workshops, and employment assistance, for instance. The success of such ventures is likely to depend not only on the efficacy of the interventions but also the existing conditions in the community and the family. The efficacy of job training or retraining will depend on the job market; the success of family adjustment will depend on the attitudes of family members who may support or oppose the program of care. Mental health agencies, when they operate in the community, must work within a range of options which the community will at least tolerate if not accept, and they must be sensitive to the realities of what they can and cannot influence. The realities are themselves changing, and the agency must be perceptive to such changes and to new opportunities as they occur. It is highly unlikely, as I mentioned previously, that the formal definitions of relationships will be responsive to conditions as they change, and agency personnel must have the flexibility and opportunity to develop new patterns of service that are adaptable to changing need.

As community mental health develops, services will occur outside of the physical confines of a single facility, and these services will require significant coordination among various agencies. The concept of a community mental health center is basically a concept of an available array of services in special institutions and in the community. By its very nature it presents certain inconveniences to workers who, if they do their jobs well, cannot as easily settle into established routines as in some other kinds of service organizations. Yet, there is a strong tendency in all social organizations for people to attempt to develop a niche for themselves which presents them with a certain degree of predictability and security in their daily routines. When such needs become pervasive, coordination among agencies, coping with the complex and difficult client and the unresponsive family, or attack on the deeper and more resistent human problems, may be compromised. I strongly believe that when the task is not routine, and goals are uncertain or difficult to establish precisely, there is no force more important than a deep commitment to the job and a sense that one's agency has the capacity to do it. Established routines, rules, clear lines of authority and function, and other bureaucratic devices may help to smooth the processes by which work in the organization is accomplished, but if the rules become too elaborate and deal with trivialities rather than instrumental needs, they may become significant barriers to successful performance. In the final analysis, bureaucratic mechanisms are nothing more than instruments that facilitate desired performance. When they become ends in themselves, or consume great time and effort, the organization can no longer maintain a mission or momentum.

Notes

1. Etzioni, A. (1964). *Modern Organizations*. Englewood Cliffs, N.J.: Prentice-Hall, p. 3

2. Roethlisberger, F., and W. Dickson (1939). *Management and the Worker*. Cambridge: Harvard University Press.

3. Thompson, J. (1967). *Organizations in Action*. New York: McGraw-Hill.

4. Etzioni, A. (1961). *A Comparative Analysis of Complex Organizations: On Power, Involvement, and Their Correlates*. New York: Free Press.

5. Etzioni, A (1964), op. cit., pp. 53–54.

6. For a discussion of ideal types and alternate methodologies, see Mechanic, D. (1963). "Some Considerations in the Methodology of Organizational Studies." In H. Leavitt (ed.), *The Social Science of Organizations: Four Perspectives*. Englewood Cliffs, N.J.: Prentice-Hall.

7. Blau, P., and W. R. Scott (1962). *Formal Organizations*. San Francisco: Chandler Publishing.

8. Perrow, C. (1965). "Hospitals: Technology, Structure and Goals." In J. March (ed.), *Handbook of Organizations*. Chicago: Rand McNally. This paper uses a concept of technology that strictly excludes social devices, which may have therapeutic effect. I see no good rationale for excluding social and educational interventions from the concept of technology. But Perrow's basic point—that in mental health work the interventions are for the most part of uncertain efficacy—still pertains.

9. Scott, W.R. (1969). "Professional Employees in a Bureaucratic Structure: Social Work." In A. Etzioni (ed.), *The Semi-Professions and Their Organization*. New York: Free Press.

10. For a classic analysis of how organizations may respond to external constraints, see Selznick, P. (1949). *TVA and the Grass Roots*. Berkeley: University of California Press.

11. For some views of what may happen to an organization in the face of a breakthrough in technology, see Sills, D. (1957). *The Volunteers: Means and Ends in a National Organization*. New York: Free Press.

12. Warner, W. K., and E. Havens (1968). "Goal Displacement and the Intangibility of Organizational Goals." *Administrative Science Quarterly*, **12**:539-555.

13. The basic perspective taken here is outlined in greater detail in Strauss, A. (1963). "The Hospital and Its Negotiated Order." In E. Freidson (ed.), *The Hospital in Modern Society*. New York: Free Press; and Bucher, R., and J. Stelling (1969). "Characteristics of Professional Organizations." *Journal of Health and Social Behavior*, **10**:3-15.

14. Rushing, W. (1964). *The Psychiatric Professions: Power, Conflict, and Adaptation in a Psychiatric Hospital Staff*. Chapel Hill, N.C.: University of North Carolina Press.

15. Roethlisberger, F., and W. Dickson (1939), op. cit.

16. Sudnow, D. (1965). "Normal Crimes: Sociological Features of the Penal Code in a Public Defender Office." *Social Problems*, **12**:255-276.

17. Blumberg, A. (1967). *Criminal Justice*. Chicago: Quadrangle.

18. For an elaboration of this point of view, see Thibaut, J., and H. Kelly (1959). *The Social Psychology of Groups*. New York: Wiley.

19. For a theoretical discussion of the relationships between forms of involvement and forms of control, see Etzioni, A. (1961), op. cit.

20. Various studies of the police illustrate these processes clearly. Police work has many similarities to community mental health. The policeman has great autonomy and discretion in dealing with various problems that he confronts, and it is particularly difficult to audit such encounters. See Skolnick, J. (1966). *Justice Without Trial*. New York: Wiley; and Westley, W. (1970). *Violence and the Police: A Sociological Study of Law, Custom, and Morality*. Cambridge: The MIT Press.

21. Corwin, R. (1970). *Militant Professionalism: A Study of Conflict in High Schools*. New York: Appleton-Century-Crofts.

22. For a discussion of the dynamics of such processes, see Mechanic, D. (1969). *Mental Health and Social Policy*. Englewood Cliffs, N.J.: Prentice-Hall, pp. 121-145.

23. Belknap, I. (1956). *Human Problems of a State Mental Hospital*. New York: McGraw-Hill. Perhaps the most influential treatment of this subject was Goffman, E. (1961). *Asylums: Essays on the Social Situation of Mental Patients and Other Inmates*. New York: Doubleday-Anchor, particularly pp. 3-124.

24. For a review of such issues, see Mechanic, D. (1968). *Medical Sociology: A Selective View*. New York: Free Press, pp. 369-403.

25. For an excellent review of recent developments in psychiatry and some future directions, see Hamburg, D. (1970). *Psychiatry as a Behavioral Science*. Englewood Cliffs, N.J.: Prentice-Hall.

26. For a brilliant historical analysis of the social forces affecting forms of treatment, see Grob, G. (1966). *The State and the Mentally Ill: A History of Worcester State Hospital in Massachusetts, 1830–1920.* Chapel Hill, N.C.: University of North Carolina Press; see also Bockoven, J.S. (1957). "Some Relationships Between Cultural Attitudes Toward Individuality and Care of the Mentally Ill: An Historical Study." In Greenblatt, et al. (ed.), *The Patient and the Mental Hospital.* New York: Free Press.

27. Frank, J. W. (1961). *Persuasion and Healing.* Baltimore: Johns Hopkins Press.

28. Mechanic, D. (1967). "Therapeutic Intervention: Issues in the Care of the Mentally Ill." *American Journal of Orthopsychiatry,* **37**:703–718.

29. Wing, J.K., and G. W. Brown (1970). *Institutionalism and Schizophrenia: A Comparative Study of Three Mental Hospitals, 1960–1968.* Cambridge: Cambridge University Press.

30. Mechanic, D. (1962). "Sources of Power of Lower Participants in Complex Organizations." *Administrative Science Quarterly,* **7**:349–364.

31. Scheff, T. (1961). "Control Over Policy by Attendants in a Mental Hospital." *Journal of Health and Human Behavior,* **2**:93–105.

32. For a discussion of the relationship between personality and bureaucratic behavior, see Merton, R. (1957). "Bureaucratic Structure and Personality." In *Social Theory and Social Structure* (rev. ed.). New York: Free Press.

33. Westley, W. (1968). "The Informal Organization of the Army: A Sociological Memoir." In H. Becker, et al. (eds.), *Institutions and the Person.* Chicago: Aldine.

34. Gouldner, A. (1954). *Patterns of Industrial Bureaucracy.* New York: Free Press.

35. Kadushin, C. (1968). "Power, Influence, and Social Circles: A New Methodology for Studying Opinion Makers." *American Sociological Review,* **35**:685–699.

36. It is essential for any administrator to appreciate that the pathways into his facility or pattern of services are affected by a wide variety of cultural, social, psychological, and situational variables, and that those who seek help may not be those most in need of the particular services available. For a review of this general literature, see Mechanic, D. (1968), op.cit., pp. 115–157.

CHAPTER XIV

The Right to Treatment: Judicial Action and Social Change

The decision of the United States district court in *Wyatt v. Stickney* constitutes the frontier of a continuing battle to insure that the mentally ill will have decent and humane care in public institutions. It maintains (as in some previous decisions) that involuntary commitment for the mentally ill, allegedly for their own protection or treatment, is a form of imprisonment and "preventive detention" if the institutions involved do not provide a humane social environment and a specific treatment regimen. The decision puts public officials on notice that the misuse of involuntary commitment for the mentally ill, for the convenience of the community under the guise of treatment and rehabilitation, is an infringement of constitutional rights. Persons who have been involved and concerned with the treatment provided in public institutions over the years will applaud those who brought the case to court, the involvement of *amici curiae*, and the court's decision. Nothing in this discussion can detract from the contribution of this decision to the ideals of decency and justice.

My discussion will consider *Wyatt v. Stickney* within a larger social and historical perspective, and will explore the relevance of such legal challenges for mental health developments. I will examine, in a tentative way, how the movement toward the right to treatment relates to other trends and I will speculate on its possible effects.

Movements in the mental health field have always had a strong ideological thrust, although careful examination of their underpinnings suggests more pragmatism than is generally appreciated. Even a cursory history of mental institutions and a brief examination of social processes affecting the mentally ill indicate that there is no stronger combination than ideology and pragmatism. In early colonial history, when mental illness resulted in dependency not

227

attributable to a flawed moral character, the community assumed responsibility for the maintenance of the mentally ill. But the limitations were clear; no matter how worthy the outsider, he was excluded from care or support, and when he appeared he was escorted to the nearest county line.[1]

During the Jacksonian period there was concern with individualism and the growing stress in society, and conceptions of the origins of mental illness shifted from those based on God's will and individual failings to the turbulence of society itself. Since society was the villain, it had a special responsibility to deal with its victims.[2] Insanity was now viewed as treatable by environmental manipulation, and the insane asylum was seen as a model community, protecting the inmate from the turbulent society outside.

By 1860, 28 of the 33 states had established insane asylums. In the preceding years, there was considerable optimism about treatment as great claims were made about curability, and inaccurate and unreliable statistics were promulgated. Later, the basis of these claims was shattered when it was shown that institutions were counting the same patient as multiple cures each time he was released from the asylum. In retrospect, of course, it is difficult to assess the true effects of these institutions; and, in any case, there was enough diversity among them to suggest that what may have been true of one institution may not have pertained to another. Yet, it is reasonable to suspect that the effects of the institutions and the form of treatment some provided (moral treatment) were quite helpful to patients. As Rothman observes, "Medical superintendents designed their institutions with eighteenth century virtues in mind. They would teach discipline, a sense of limits, and a satisfaction with one's position, and in this way enable patients to withstand the tension and the fluidity of Jacksonian society."[3]

Moral treatment had a variety of precepts that sound strangely familiar today. The object of this care was to provide discipline and regularity to the inmate's life in a humane and considerate fashion. It was to be neither brutal nor indulgent, but was meant to induce tranquility and order. Inactivity was considered sinful, and these asylums kept patients busy with a great variety of tasks. Habits of industry and regularity were to be encouraged, and useful work endeavor was the vehicle through which the regimen was accomplished. Work efforts were viewed as both economical and rehabilitative. There was, of course, a thin line between exploitation of patient labor and healthful activity, but it was one of those useful devices that appeared to serve both the institution and the inmate.

In the better institutions there is reason to believe that moral treatment and the organizational regimens associated with it were modestly effective. The basic ideology, whatever its emphasis on discipline, was humane; and, in its early stages, staffing was reasonable. The relationships reported between patient and staff were sympathetic, and the cause of mental illness was seen as a product of the environment rather than as a consequence of the worthlessness of the patient. But all this changed rapidly with growing industrialization and urbanism in the last half of the nineteenth and early part of the twentieth century. With changes in social structure, tolerance for the chronic patient and alien foreigners (who were well represented among them) decreased substantially. Institutionalism was now a convenient way to cope with deviants of all sorts who were difficult to contain in a rapidly growing and dynamic community. Although legislatures provided for asylums, they were not sufficient to cope with the increasing number of inmates incarcerated. With overcrowding and change in the social characteristics of the clientele, an era of custodialism began to emerge. Abuses in these institutions became more prevalent, the social characteristics of persons sent to the institutions were increasingly seen as less desirable, and the persons who had options began to avoid the institutions whenever they could. Thus, asylums became warehouses for the hopeless, the impoverished, and persons with little power and discredited social status.

The growth of custodialism was concomitant with growing skepticism concerning the rehabilitative effects of asylums. Yet the institutions continued to be subsidized and built because they performed important functions for an increasingly industrialized and urbanized society, which was less able than before to tolerate deviance. With the demise of the cult of curability and growing pessimism concerning the intractibility of mental disorder, less and less attention was given to the environmental conditions of care. This was justified by a growing feeling that mental disorders were organic and unresponsive to environmental treatment, and was reinforced by the growing number of chronic patients sent to asylums from other types of institutions. Thus, institutions developed techniques to manage masses of patients with limited personnel and facilities and at minimum cost.

The product of these forces was a sense of hopelessness and a need for regimentation and control over patients. How else could a small staff deal with hordes of patients destined to a hopeless future? Legislatures faced other needs, and the clients of the asylums were hardly a group to affect political decisions. The reformers who played an important role in the earlier history of the asylum were pushed out by the growing professionalization of the psychiatric profession.[4] The irony was that the new professionals had so little to offer in their stead.

Although there were outcries from time to time against existing conditions in mental hospitals, the age of custodialism was dominant until very recently. Not only was there little treatment and supportive care for patients, but there was also evidence of physical deprivation, abuse, and a regimented, destructive psychological environment. Whatever attention was available was devoted to new patients. Patients who were resistant to early care were relegated to back wards to waste their lives in idleness and despair. Although exposés of the shocking conditions in mental hospitals created attention and concern, other events soon pushed this awareness to the background, and the majority of the mentally ill made few gains. The most influential of these movements in the early part of this century was the organization of the National Association for Mental Health, initiated by Clifford Beer's autobiographical account of his experiences in a mental hospital. Although this movement had considerable influence, it was largely rooted in middle-class values and concerns[5] and had only a marginal effect on the vast numbers of impoverished mental patients.

Like the mental hygiene movement, many of the other developments in the mental health field had little effect on mental hospital operations. The child guidance movement was largely preventive in orientation and was predicated on the assumption that early treatment of deviance could limit later morbidity. The influence of psychoanalysis and its popularity in the United States directed attention away from the mental hospital and the mass of mentally ill, and drew the professional community largely into therapeutic work with less-incapacitated and better-educated clients.

Sociological studies of the mental hospital in the 1950's demonstrated its character.[6,7] The public hospitals were organized to allow a limited staff to direct and control the activities of large numbers of patients. Life in the hospital was organized around its maintenance, and patients were used to insure that essential work functions were performed. Particularly effective workers were kept in hospitals, since their useful labor was highly valued, while patients who were more impaired or less effective were left alone as long as they caused no disturbance. The average ward was inactive and apathetic, and if patients were vigorous enough to cause a disturbance, a variety of restraints and controls was readily available. Regardless of whatever feelings the staff might have had, the magnitude of numbers forced a custodial ideology and behavior consistent with it.

But even custodial treatment was expensive and, following the Second World War, it was apparent that state legislatures were troubled by the growing costs of incarceration of large numbers of patients who occupied more than half of the hospital beds in the United States. As sensibilities required that the most brutal aspects of hospital wards be eliminated, money was necessary; and the total number of resident patients was also increasing. The states, therefore, were looking for federal leadership and some relief from what appeared as a growing economic burden.[8] In the middle 1950's the introduction of psychoactive drugs had a dramatic impact on the confidence of personnel to deal with the mentally ill. Since pharmaceutical control was now more possible, the reliance on restraints and seclusion was less necessary, and hospitals began to open their doors. Drugs also facilitated the return of patients to the community, since families and the community could more readily cope with patient behavior.

The development of the community mental health movement has received wide attention. In our present captivation with this ideology, however, we neglect certain elements that are of interest to the issue before us, and I shall emphasize these aspects. Although the psychoactive drugs were dramatically effective in alleviating some of the most difficult problems of patient management, there is a tendency to attribute more direct significance to drugs than they really had. There is evidence from particular institutions that the open-door policy and administrative change could be accomplished prior to drug introduction.[9] The availability of drugs probably contributed most importantly by giving hospital personnel and the public at large some confidence that community care was feasible, and drugs provided control over the aspects of behavior that were most frightening and disruptive to the community. Thus, drugs facilitated attitudes that eased radical alterations in administrative policy. Also, by the late 1950's, the thinking about the origins of mental illness had once again shifted significantly. Mental disorder was seen mainly as reactive to social conditions and life environments, and there was growing appreciation that the regimen of the custodial hospital had detrimental effects on social functioning and potentialities for future social adjustment.[10] Moreover, evidence linking social inequality to mental health care[11] had a major impact on a profession and a society that were becoming more and more sensitive about this issue. But what made the community-care movement particularly viable was its parallel direction with the needs of the states to find some way of coping with the growing burden of providing care for the mentally ill and the mentally retarded. The economic motivation of the localities was not a trivial aspect of the entire picture and provided the fuel for what was described as a revolution in psychiatric practice.

Many of the states probably would have settled for major federal support to mental hospitals, but they did not prevail in Washington when the details of federal investment were hammered out. Thus, much of the funds came in the form of community programs and construction grants for mental health centers and, later, in money for staffing. Although states and counties were anxious to obtain what funds they could by turning toward programs of community care, they were much slower in spending dollars to provide necessary services for the mentally ill within the community or for helping families and other institutions that were now taking on the burden that had previously been primarily dealt with in hospitals. The administrative action of returning patients to the community occurred quite rapidly, and the trend of mental patients, resident in mental hospitals, showed a sharp decline. The long and hard process of building adequate community services occured more slowly, and there is evidence that much is still lacking.

Even a cursory examination of the present state of affairs shows an enormous gap between the ideology and realities of community care. While it has been relatively simple to alter administrative policies to avoid hospitalization and to release hospitalized patients as quickly as possible, the development of an adequate framework of community services to assist the mentally ill or their families has been very slow. As economic pressures have mounted for federal and state governments, as well as for localities, there has been less willingness to invest the resources to meet, even minimally, the needs of patients in the community, and the new neighborhood health centers have frequently avoided the most impaired patients. Disturbed and disabled patients are kept in the community under the banner of community care only to suffer community "institutionalism." Various agencies, each attempting to protect its budget, shift the responsibilities to others, leaving many patients greatly in need, unattended and living under appalling conditions.

It is only now becoming apparent to what extent greatly impaired patients have been "dumped" in the community without adequate financial and social resources. In the big cities—like New York—many impaired patients live with other deviants in "welfare hotels" in disorganized areas where they are frequently intimidated and frightened. With poor community care, these patients frequently experience an exacerbation of symptoms and insecurities and, in view of their limited coping capacities, they face horrendous life problems. Although living situations in smaller communities expose the former patient to less disorganized and frightening conditions, similar problems prevail. In the case of schizophrenic patients, it is recognized that aggressive care is required if they are not to regress; but under most community circumstances, this care is not available and former patients simply become lost in the community.

In directing our attention to the conditions of hospital care, we must keep in mind that the responsibilities for patient care in the community are equally important. The fact that a patient is released to the community in no way lessens the responsibility of mental health authorities to insure that there is adequate provision for care. In putting pressure on hospitals, it is possible to encourage the dumping of patients which, under some conditions, may greatly exacerbate their difficulties. In focusing our attention on improved standards of hospital care, we must keep in mind what the state of community facilities is, or we may be in danger of displacing difficult problems from one context to another.

There is no question that many conditions prevailing in mental hospitals and institutions for the retarded are horrible, and that the standards for involuntary hospitalization are extremely lax. No matter how important it is to improve hospital conditions, this improvement should not serve as an excuse to give less attention to due process in involuntary hospitalization procedures. Similarly, if involuntary hospitalization is enforced only as a last resort—which I believe it should be—then there is a special obligation to insure that impaired persons living in the community have adequate opportunities to receive assistance. An adequate conceptualization of the legal problem must, I believe, give considerable attention to the social difficulties of retaining bizarre and impaired persons within the community.

The Problem of Standards and the Mental Hospital

In *Wyatt v. Stickney* the court held that involuntarily committed patients "unquestionably have a constitutional right to receive such individual treatment as will give each of them a realistic opportunity to be cured or to improve his or her mental condition."* The court found that the defendant's treatment program was deficient because it failed to provide a humane psychological and physical environment and a qualified staff in sufficient numbers to administer adequate treatment and individualized treatment plans. The court concluded that "whatever treatment was provided was grossly deficient and failed to satisfy minimum medical and constitutional standards." After hearing evidence from involved parties and *amici curiae*, the court proposed detailed standards, which it defined as "medical and constitutional minimums." The judge emphasized that "a failure by defendants to comply with this decree cannot be justified by a lack of operating funds."

There can be no legal (or moral) justification for the State of Alabama's failing to afford treatment—and adequate treatment from a medical standpoint—to the several thousand patients who have been civilly committed to Bryce's for treatment purposes. To deprive any citizen of his or her liberty upon the altruistic theory that the confinement is for humane therapeutic reasons and then fail to provide adequate treatment violates the very fundamentals of due process.

The court emphasized that "the unavailability of neither funds, nor staff and facilities, will justify a default by defendants in the provision of suitable treatment for the mentally ill."

The major precedent for right to treatment is found in *Rouse v. Cameron*.[12] Judge David Bazelon, in reviewing various criticisms of his decision in that case, accepts them as appropriate:

(1) Courts are not as competent as hospitals to make treatment decisions;
(2) The evaluation of standards of adequacy and suitability may be next to impossible in the present state of psychiatry, where "treatment" means different things to different psychiatrists;
(3) No matter how much compulsory treatment is afforded, compulsory hospitalization is itself generally based on ill-conceived standards and goals and ought to be reformed radically or discontinued altogether;

* A similar case was decided differently in Georgia. These cases have been consolidated and as of August 1973 were under appeal in the United States Court of Appeals for the Fifth Circuit.

(4) The real problem is one of inadequate resources, which the courts are helpless to remedy—the question posed is one for the legislature and is a basic policy judgment involving overall priorities in the allocation of scarce resources.[13]

Before exploring these points, it is useful to consider the larger context of the right-to-treatment decisions.

It is commonly accepted that right-to-treatment decisions expose the hypocrisy of commitment procedures and injustice in society. The guise of care and treatment frequently becomes the justification to remove disturbing members from the community without due process and with only the most shabby care. By exposing these processes for what they really are, it is conceivable that influential members of the community and legislators have their sense of justice aroused and may take steps to remedy the situation. Moreover, it is possible that court-set standards of treatment may at least temporarily make unjust practices more salient, achieve improvements in particular situations, and indirectly encourage authorities to be less abusive of involuntary procedures because it becomes more costly for the authorities to make use of them.

The issue in *Wyatt v. Stickney* arises from the fact that the patients concerned are involuntarily incarcerated for the alleged purpose of treatment and cure. If civil commitment insured due process and adequate protection of patients' rights, the right-to-treatment issue would be a much more minor one and one that could be readily resolved. Since only a fraction of the patients who are presently civilly committed would continue to be involuntarily institutionalized, the cost of providing a humane environment would be more limited and, hence, conceivably less painful to the taxpayer and the legislature. What makes right to treatment a central concept is that mental hospitals—particularly in the backward states—remain as warehouses for second-class citizens, for the chronically ill, the aged, the retarded, and a host of other poor unfortunates. Certainly, a reasonable criterion for attacking the conditions in many of these institutions is the constitutional standard protecting against cruel and unusual punishment. But even if this problem did not exist, the lack of entitlement to adequate care among the handicapped and needy would present problems that the legal approach by itself could not cope with.

The need for treatment and care does not diminish by improving the processes of civil commitment. A great many persons in the population require medical care and support and, with the increasing trend toward community care and away from civil commitment, there are growing numbers of needy mentally ill in the community, functioning at very low levels and suffering from a variety of personal and social troubles. Community agencies, including welfare services, face cutbacks and limited budgets, and make efforts to avoid assuming responsibilities for the mentally ill. One possible unanticipated consequence of treatment standards for involuntary patients is a tendency to return the patients to the community without adequate provision for their care and maintenance.

It is well known that the patients who receive least services in mental hospitals are the most chronic patients. Frequently, the disturbing behavior for which they were originally hospitalized has not been evident for some time, and they are viewed as neither a danger to themselves nor to others. Their residence in hospitals stems from the difficulties of providing suitable living and maintenance arrangements within the community, and it is frequently felt that such patients who have adapted to hospital life might find continued hospitalization of greater comfort than the realities that face them in the community. The right-to-treatment decisions do not protect patients who may be returned to the community without adequate resources or minimal comfort and support. These patients may suffer in the community or they may return to institutions as voluntary patients without having the protections of the new standards.

Having raised the broader issues, let us consider the specific points referred to by Judge Bazelon. Although I do not believe, in the long run, that court standards can insure appropriate treatment and care, they draw attention to the enormous gap between the legal forms and the realities. As such, they constitute part of the consciousness necessary for social reform.

The Problem of Inadequate Resources

The standards ordered by the Court in Alabama require what, in effect, is a redistribution of benefits among its citizens. This can be appreciated by examining the minimum staffing ratios established by the court: that there be 28 physicians, 48 registered nurses, 8 psychologists with graduate training, and 28 social workers per 1000 patients. However, the state of Alabama had 2827 nonfederal physicians in 1970, 5685 registered nurses employed in nursing in 1966, and 65 psychologists—only 39 of whom were clinical—in 1968.[14] The doctor-to-patient ratio in Alabama has been one of the lowest in the nation, approximately 75 to 80 physicians for every 100,000 patients. Even if we assumed that the mental hospitals could recruit the professional personnel required (a highly dubious assumption), it does not follow that meeting these standards would be the most reasonable allocation of such resources.

Americans have grown to regard access to health care as a right, but many citizens of Alabama receive inadequate medical care or none at all. Many of these patients have treatable diseases that can clearly benefit from prompt medical attention. Is it reasonable, then, to insure the kinds of ratios mandated by the court for mental hospitals when it is dubious that many of the patients concerned are treatable by medical intervention? From more humanistic considerations it may be reasonable to reallocate medical services to mental hospitals if for no other reasons than to ameliorate the degrading conditions that presently prevail. But if, indeed, medical staffing is only one of many ways to improve the conditions of the mentally ill, should a solution that is cost-ineffective be the one chosen?

The state of Alabama is one of the most deprived areas in the United States, and its social and educational services would be deficient on the basis of national comparisons. The court, in searching for an appropriate standard for treatment, could not reasonably use services for Alabamans generally, since such a comparison would hardly insure meaningful care and treatment. Thus, the court established standards on the basis of evidence from experts and national organizations concerned with the quality of mental health services. The theory underlying these standards is one of advocacy for the mentally ill rather than one based on consideration of how society can put its limited resources to best use. I have not checked the data, but I would not be surprised if one cannot make a similar case for deficiencies in Alabama in educational expenditures, class size, teacher preparation, welfare payments, access to primary medical care, social services, county hospital services, and garbage collection.

Since I believe that a national minimal standard is reasonable, then how do Alabama, Mississippi, and other deprived areas achieve the standard? I maintain that the achievement of such a standard is a federal responsibility, and this implies important modifications in how federal health, education, and welfare programs are funded. Birnbaum[15] has argued that financing for the mentally ill in public institutions could be substantially improved by including such patients under Medicare and Medicaid, and insuring that the funds go to the mental hygiene agencies rather than to general revenues. Mental patients in state hospitals are presently largely excluded from these programs. Whatever the weaknesses of recent legislative proposals for federal assumption of direct responsibility for a guaranteed income program, one of its greatest virtues is its ability to bring all areas of the country up to a uniform minimum standard. Matching programs (the more usual mode of federal financing in the health and welfare service area) inevitably come to favor the areas that have the most progressive programs and are most willing to invest their own resources in such programs. Thus, matching-funds programs frequently favor the rich against the poor and sometimes allow the rich to reallocate expenditures already made to new concerns with the initiation of federal programs. However, as the battle in the United States over welfare reform has illustrated, such shifts in the philosophy of funding threaten a variety of vested interests, including the richer states that can be expected to oppose any program of redistribution that diminishes their share. Thus, a viable program probably requires both an increase in overall benefits and redistribution at the same time.

Matching programs have frequently established minimal guidelines and standards for participation—whether in health, welfare, or education. The history of the relationships between the federal government and the various localities gives one little confidence that the federal government has the will or is ready to sacrifice political benefits to insure that recipients adhere to the criteria for participation.[16] Civil rights issues have been the most controversial battleground in the enforcement area, but similar failures are evident in welfare administration, Medicare standards for nursing homes and extended care facilities, housing standards, and the like.

Standards of Adequacy and Suitability

Assuming that it is appropriate for courts to mandate changes in staffing and other resources and in treatment, the issue remains as to whether it is possible to develop reasonable standards and whether the standards established in *Wyatt v. Stickney* are wise. Conformity with them would surely provide a more humane physical and psychological environment for the patient, but the questions remain whether such standards can be reasonably interpreted and monitored, what their long-term effects on mental health policies and practices are likely to be, and their bearing on the untreatable patient and the patient who wishes to refuse treatment.[17]

Although the court was obviously aware of the uncertainties of treatment for the mentally ill, the right-to-treatment cases are based on the assumption that a technology for cure and rehabilitation exists. Judge Bazelon, both in *Rouse v. Cameron* and in his later writings, was clear about the limitations of psychiatric practice. As he noted, however, " . . . it is nevertheless essential to ensure that the patient confined for treatment receives some form of therapy that a respectable sector of the psychiatric profession regards as appropriate— and receives enough of that therapy to make his confinement more than a mockery."[18] In contrast, Thomas Szasz has maintained that:

The idea of a "right" to mental treatment is both naive and dangerous. It is naive because it considers the problem of the publicly hospitalized mental patient as a medical one, ignoring its educational, economic, religious and social aspects. It is dangerous because its proposed remedy creates another problem—compulsory mental treatment—for in a context of involuntary confinement the treatment too shall have to be compulsory.[19]

Szasz' view is extreme, but it should alert us to real dangers intrinsic to all involuntary treatment. When the psychiatrist is an agent of a voluntary patient, then whatever the uncertainties of psychiatric ideologies and practices, the relationship is one established at the agreement, convenience, and interests of the parties concerned. Since psychiatric ideologies can justify almost any practice under the rubric of treatment, institutional psychiatry not only has enormous power over the patient but also becomes almost impossible to monitor in any specific sense. The psychiatrist comes to utilize *ad hoc* theories, which he changes and justifies at his convenience. Moreover, it is no secret that mental hospitals of the kind we are considering attract many incompetent physicians and psychiatrists who frequently lack elementary knowledge and understanding of patients' rights. Not infrequently these hospitals recruit foreign physicians who have difficulty speaking and understanding English and who have no grasp of the cultural assumptions that govern their patients' lives.

In his book, *Prisoners of Psychiatry*,[20] Bruce Ennis describes his participation in *Wyatt v. Stickney* and other mental health litigation as part of a New York City Civil Liberties Project. Throughout his book he dramatically illustrates what is so well known by those who have had any sustained contact with psychiatry—that psychiatric concepts are as fluid and changing as the motivation of the psychiatrist using them. In this light, his hopefulness about the effects of *Wyatt v. Stickney* impresses me as unduly optimistic:

> Those standards, if followed in other states, would cause a revolution in institutional health care services. Under those standards, for example, Willowbrook would have to employ eighty-seven psychologists; it now has five. In order to meet the standards, states would be forced to discharge vast numbers of inappropriately hospitalized patients. Those who remained would live in a normally furnished homelike environment, retaining all the rights of privacy, communication, and human dignity enjoyed by other citizens. And they would be given individualized programs of treatment, job training, and assistance designed to return them quickly to their communities.[21]

It is not as clear as Ennis would have it that the standards would be enforceable. Moreover, it is not apparent that those patients who would be forced back in the community would have decent and adequate lives, that even minimal services would be provided for them or to assist those who assumed custody for them, and that privacy and dignity would become the institutional norm. Although one can readily identify with such commendable aspirations, it is sobering to consider another revolutionary change initiated by Judge Bazelon and to ponder its course and outcome.

In 1954 Judge Bazelon, in *Durham v. United States*, declared a new test excluding criminal responsibility in cases where the unlawful act was the product of mental disease or defect. The course of Durham case law, in expanding the concept of exculpatory mental illness, eventually came full circle when the Court of Appeals found:

> As an example of this causal connection or relation, if a person at the time of the commission of the crime is so deranged mentally that he cannot distinguish between right or wrong, or, being able to tell right from wrong, he is unable by virtue of his mental derangement to control his actions, then his act is a product of his mental derangement.

Richard Arens reports in his book, *Make Mad the Guilty*,[22] on a project involving litigation applying the Durham rule to nonpsychotic conditions. In accounting for the rule's failure, Arens maintains that both psychiatrists and the courts basically destroyed its potential. In particular, psychiatrists at Saint Elizabeth's hospital managed their courtroom testimony so as to send unattractive mentally ill persons to jail rather than to accept them on their already crowded wards. Others saw the new rule as a basic threat to the legal process and the presumption of accountability and did what they could to counteract it. The motivation to widen the insanity plea was based on the assumption that more humane care would be more available under this mechanism than through the criminal process. But it became evident that this attempt to bootleg rehabilitation to persons charged with criminal offenses by exculpating criminal responsibility was too radical for the society to accept at the time.

The right-to-treatment approach is one of many strategies used to circumvent our deplorable rehabilitation system and our more inhumane institutions. Whether such mechanisms can be effective is at best an uncertainty, but whatever hopes they have will depend on the ability of courts and the public to seriously audit and enforce specific standards that improve the lives of individual patients. Thus, the standards and their specification are central.

Although one would anticipate that psychiatrists of any persuasion would have welcomed any effort to improve the deplorable conditions in custodial institutions, it was reasonably clear that establishment psychiatry was not exactly euphoric over *Rouse v. Cameron*. The American Psychiatric Association saw this decision as potentially interfering with the psychiatrist's autonomy; and in issuing its official response on the question of adequacy of treatment, the Council of the APA began by asserting that, "The definition of treatment and the appraisal of its adequacy are matters for medical determination."[23] It later justified prevalent custodial practices as forms of treatment.

The conceptual contrasting of "treatment" on the one hand with "punishment" on the other sometimes obfuscates more than it clarifies the problem. Some Courts, attorneys, statutes, and judicial formulations reiterate, almost ritualistically, that hospitalization without treatment equates with punishment. This is not precisely the case.

Involuntary hospitalization clearly does imply restraint and may be properly viewed as a kind of punishment in a simple, unqualified context. But if such hospitalization is part of a treatment program aimed at interrupting a disease process (even though the treatment is refused or failed), it is not useful to dub it punishment any more than it would be useful to view depriving an addict of the narcotic of his choice as punishment. The utilization of this kind of involuntary restraint may be viewed in one sense as analogous to problems encountered in child rearing wherein there are no sharp delineations as between guidance and discipline or between discipline and punishment, all of which are directed towards putting internal and external limitations on unacceptable behavior. Restraints may be imposed from within by reinforcing a patient's inner defenses, or from without by pharmacological means or by locking the door of a ward. Either imposition may be a legitimate component of a treatment program. Only if the patient were restrained and did not receive any of the treatments cited above could the restraint properly be called punishment. Furthermore, it is unsound to dismiss a procedure as "purely custodial" or "purely punishing" without assessing the total circumstances in which it has been prescribed. The procedure is often of therapeutic value.[24]

As the statement of the Council makes clear, almost any practice seen by some authority in the interest of the patient becomes treatment by definition, and there is very little that cannot be so justified. Erving Goffman's classic descriptions of these processes are even more relevant today than they were when he made them because institutional psychiatry has increased the sophistication of the theories by which it justifies control practices under the guise of medical treatment.

Regimentation may be defined as a framework of therapeutic regularity designed to allay insecurity; forced social mixing with a multitude of heterogeneous, displeased fellow inmates may be described as an opportunity to learn that there are others who are worse off....The punishment of being sent to a worse ward is described as transferring a patient to a ward whose arrangements he can cope with, and the isolation cell or "hole" is described as a place where the patient will be able to feel comfortable with his inability to handle his acting out impulses. Making a ward quiet at night through the forced taking of drugs, which permits reduced night staffing, is called medication or sedative treatment....Reward for good behavior by progressively increasing rights to attend socials may be described as psychiatric control over the dosage and timing of social exposure. . . . Some of the verbal translations found in mental hospitals represent not so much medical terms for disciplinary practices as a disciplinary use of medical practices.[25]

In light of the above considerations, it becomes essential to consider what standards are reasonably enforceable, prudent, and effective. In general, standards referring to a humane physical and social environment are more amenable to court action than those pertaining to individualized treatment regimens. Of the various standards, those relating to staff-patient ratios, physical standards of the institution, and care of the person are most easily specified and enforced.

There is a growing feeling in the health services field that rigid assignment of functions and restrictions on the efforts of nonprofessionals hampers effective and efficient delivery of health services. The standards, as specified, tend to reinforce existing stratification of work in "psychiatric" tasks and conceivably can have the effect of bureaucratizing treatment and hampering innovation relative to alternative standards. Although the use of the concept of "qualified mental health professional" guards against a medical monopoly, the conditions for allocating "professional" functions to nonprofessionals appear somewhat restrictive. Although I am fully aware of the abuses that this is meant to guard against, I am similarly cognizant of how difficult it will be to achieve the mandated staffing ratios, and an effective program will require the innovative use of nonprofessional staff members.

In *Wyatt v. Stickney* the court also developed specific and enforceable standards concerning physical facilities and amenities. These standards, applied seriously to many state institutions, would require considerable expenditure for rebuilding and remodeling. It is not fully clear what the costs would really be or whether such expenditures, relative to other investments for the mentally ill, would be to their utmost benefit. It is conceivable that such investments, if made, might solidify unwillingness to abandon dependence on such facilities relative to alternate community facilities. Assuming that the application of all new standards involves a specified expenditure of some magnitude, is it not reasonable to have the state reconsider its entire system of mental health care and the alternative levels of care and treatment necessary for a satisfactory program? Standards imposed on one aspect of the system may result in disproportionate resources allocated to mental hospitals relative to newly emerging models of community facilities. Whether the court has any authority beyond the involuntary patient is not clear, but certainly in the case of the retarded population, consideration of alternate facilities would appear to be a reasonable course to encourage.

The difficulty with standards that pertain to actions that are undefinable is that it becomes hard to establish whether the institution is conforming. Often, the conscientious professional will make an effort to meet the spirit of the requirement, and the requirement may interfere with optimal application of his efforts; while the less conscientious professional easily subverts the rule. Having spent a fair amount of time on psychiatric units both good and bad, I am still at a loss to understand how a court will determine that medication is not used as punishment or for the convenience of staff, or that it is unnecessary or excessive. Such standards probably can guard against the most blatant abuses, but they are probably not very useful in regulating more usual excesses.

It is generally maintained that the establishment of an individualized treatment plan is the basis for a rational and humane therapeutic approach. It implies the consideration of the patient's needs, an examination of alternative approaches to meeting them, and it insures a certain degree of planning for each patient. In principle, the establishment of such a program and its continuing review are an essential mechanism; in reality, it can become a farcical ritual that has little to do with the daily conditions affecting the patient and, indeed, if staffing is limited, it may reallocate whatever staff time is available away from contact with patients. It is quite conceivable that professionals come to spend all of their time formulating and reviewing paper plans, while nonprofessional staff continue to run the institution and to have almost exclusive contact with patients. One has only to review the present practice of many institutional psychiatrists to become aware of the large proportion of their time spent on administrative and legal matters. As the staff come to view certain activities as rituals, they sometimes begin rejecting particular patients who by law require certain services. For example, many state hospitals are required to perform physical examinations on newly admitted patients with each admission. Since this is a time-consuming task, medical personnel find patient recidivists (such as alcoholics) a nuisance. To cope with such patients, the staff begin to develop special release and admission policies for them to limit unnecessary work. The long-term consequences of such adaptations may be more dysfunctional than abandoning specific requirements that have their own rationale.

The standards mandated by the court appear to require considerable documentation and review of treatment and control measures. One develops the impression that much professional time would be spent on maintaining proper records that can be useful in court reviews of hospital behavior. But the various standards—no matter how commendable they seem to be—tend to work against one another. We begin with the premise that patients require more attention from mental health professionals. We realize that they are difficult to recruit and are unlikely to be drawn to mental hospital practice, but we forbid one of the major recruiting devices by specifying that all such professionals "shall meet all licensing and certification requirements . . . for persons engaged in private practice of the same profession. . . ." We then specify that those recruited will be required to spend much of their time making entries in records. Each of these requirements, by itself, in a context of adequate recruitment and staff would be reasonable. But are we any better off if we set standards so high that we insure that the institution cannot possibly meet them?[26] If we start by assuming a condition of scarcity and consider how one might use available resources and staff most creatively and effectively, it is likely that we would develop a somewhat different set of standards.

The Competency of Courts and Treatment Decisions

I do not believe that anyone seriously advocates that courts should make treatment decisions, and thus I find this issue a false one. To the extent that rules are carefully specified so that judgments are possible, I assume that courts can be an appropriate vehicle for reviewing contested judgments by hearing from relevant experts on the issue of appropriateness of care. Courts appear to undertake similar functions in areas equally complicated,[27] and the notion that courts have no business reviewing the contested behavior of physicians is one to which I do not adhere.

Indeed, my experience in the mental health field has convinced me that one of the major difficulties in protecting patients is the awe that many judges have for physicians and the lack of confidence they appear to have in their own judgment. Courts frequently have allowed physicians to make judgments that should be the province of the court, because the judge was unwilling to consider whether the determination required was properly a medical judgment. The abuses of civil commitment are attributable partly to the failure of courts to seriously hear the evidence and their tendency to accept whatever medical advice is given to them. Questions such as "competence to stand trial," "dangerousness," "legal insanity," and the like frequently have not been examined as social issues involving considerations beyond medical ones. Such decisions are properly community decisions that take into account medical knowledge and behavioral research but involve other considerations as well. Instead, courts have frequently accepted unexamined and unreliable assertions often reflecting little more than personal bias as medical truth and as a basis for decision making.

In my view, courts must develop more competence in making judgments concerning mental illness on the basis of the facts with greater awareness of the appropriate bounds and limits of medical and psychiatric evidence. The willingness to blandly accept such evidence and to shift responsibility from the court to the physician has caused much injustice. I can think of no greater contribution the courts can make to the involuntary patient than to take their claims seriously and to give them their day in court with full due process.

One of the issues left unresolved by the court in its standards in *Wyatt v. Stickney* was the case of patients who wish to refuse treatment, and I am not convinced that in this area the judge made the most appropriate determination. Although the standards specify that "patients have a right to be free from unnecessary or excessive medication," the patient's right to refuse involuntary medication is not protected. Patients are protected against experimental research without consent, against major physical treatments (such as ECT) against adverse reinforcement conditioning, and "other hazardous" treatment. Although patients' rights to be free from physical restraint and isolation are guaranteed except in emergencies, medication is treated as an exception. This exception, therefore, deserves inspection.

Today, drug therapy is the most significant treatment modality available to psychiatry. There is considerable evidence of its usefulness in treating depression and in the maintenance of schizophrenic patients. Medication, however, has been one of the most frequently abused means of ward maintenance and patient control. Although most of the mandated standards are consonant with the viewpoint that mental patients can reasonably exercise judgment in their own behalf, the right to refuse medication—one that is available to almost any other kind of patient—is denied. In my view, this treatment power of the hospital is in conflict with a humane hospital environment. In a busy and active ward the availability of involuntary medication becomes a substitute for the time-consuming efforts to achieve voluntary consent through persuasion and trust. I am not maintaining that extending this right would not create some problems, as do many of the other mandated standards: there may be occasions where involuntary medication is justified and sensible. But one must consider both the benefits and costs, and I believe that the extension of the right to the patient to refuse medication would do more to insure his integrity than almost any other standard.

The dilemma of the patient who refuses treatment exists only in respect to the standards relevant to individualized treatment programs. Certainly such patients, regardless of what course they choose, would benefit by improved physical conditions, the protection of their rights, and a more humane physical, psychological, and social environment. A prudent application of the right-to-treatment standard should require no more than that the hospital unit on which the patient resides have sufficient facilities, staff, and treatment modalities to provide a minimal acceptable standard of care. In my view, all that a unit would have to demonstrate to meet this requirement is that facilities are available and that a reasonable effort was made to extend them to the person involved. It would be unfortunate, indeed, if the right to treatment became a new form of tyranny that limited the patient's options.

The above position presents some problems relative to the patient who refuses treatment but who finds the new hospital environment a comfortable and attractive place. There is evidence that, for some patients with longterm chronic disabilities who face difficult and impoverished community conditions, a decent hospital environment can become a refuge from the outside world.[28] To the extent that such patients are involuntary and are extended the right to refuse treatment, there are few options. Under some conditions such involuntary patients can be released and be readmitted voluntarily, contingent on their acceptance of certain types of treatment. For patients who cannot be released, we may have to accept their lack of cooperation as the price society must pay for continuing to depend on involuntary commitment procedures. Since this issue is the key to the larger problem, let us examine it.

The Reform of Involuntary Procedures

In one sense, right to treatment is an indirect attack on the current abuses of involuntary procedures, such as in civil commitment and in incompetency to stand trial. But in another sense, the right-to-treatment approach encompasses an endorsement of the medical model in contrast to competing views of the conflict between patient and community. Although the right-to-treatment approach attacks commitment procedures where they are perhaps most vulnerable, by exposing how little treatment is made available, there is danger of implicitly accepting the idea that the provision of treatment is the only issue at stake. This approach potentially is harmful if it implies that even superb treatment lessens the obligations of the community to provide rigorous due process in commitment procedures, or if it suggests that the patient is obliged to accept specific treatments for either a limited or prolonged period. If we create the illusion that because the services offered in mental hospitals are appropriate by the standards of "a respectable sector of the psychiatric profession" that there is less need to be vigilant in protecting the civil liberties of the patient, then the right to treatment can become a retrogressive step in the development of a more humane social policy.

Although I believe the intention of right-to-treatment advocates is to fundamentally recast mental hygiene approaches and to maximize patients' dignity, there is always the danger that the community in its incremental approach to social change will adopt the posture, but not the substance, of the position. It is conceivable that, by improving some aspects of hospital care, public officials may deflect criticism of the processes that violate patient rights and inadvertently may help to sustain the existing pattern of removing bizarre and disturbing persons from the community even when they pose no great threat. Let us make no mistake about it; communities will continue to insist that bizarre and annoying members be removed. The pressures for incarceration are considerable, and it is only through concern and vigilance that abuses can be minimized. Also, if community pressures are to be resisted, mental health programs in the community will have to be sophisticated and attuned to possible difficulties.

The right-to-treatment issue alerts us to a fundamental difficulty—the failure to insure an adequate level of treatment entitlement to citizens as a whole. For if the courts act to protect the treatment rights of the involuntary patient, it is hard to imagine that legislatures will not insist that voluntary patients receive at least comparable services. If successful, then, these suits will create societal dissonance that will contribute to social reforms. The question of how successful such suits can be in the long run is a difficult one. Even small gains are not to be minimized, and in conjunction with other challenges to some institutional psychiatric practices and involuntary care, real improvements are possible.

Recent litigation in the area of patients' rights, taken as a whole, must be seen as attempts to undermine existing mental hygiene legislation and its role in society. Bruce Ennis has stated the matter quite candidly, "So much is wrong with involuntary hospitalization that a reasonable tightening up of commitment standards and a modest extension of patients' rights would cripple the enterprise beyond recovery."[29] It is not so clear, however, that the courts and the legislatures are prepared to allow such a useful mechanism of social control to suffer such injury. It is more likely that they will attempt to adapt to external attack by modifying the most abusive practices, by providing greater opportunities for review, and by attempting to improve those most visible conditions that arouse public concern. It is essential for those who attack such injustices by litigation to be ambitious but also realistic about possible achievements and dangers. The mental hygiene bureaucracies of the various states have enormous resources and advantages. They can deplete the energies and resources of their antagonists without undergoing fundamental change. Although litigation creates temporary discomfort, it is difficult without constant surveillance to insure that gains achieved can be maintained in the future. Perhaps what worries me most is that in the event new standards can be sustained, hospitals will increasingly unload their less attractive patients to other institutions that are even less humane or release them to the community without decent care and attention. Already there is considerable indication that such practices are being followed under the pressures of funding and under the guise of the new community psychiatry ideology. While it may be true that many hospital patients are not appropriately amenable to civil commitment and would not be commitable if the process had greater integrity, many suffer from significant handicaps that require assistance.[30-32] I fear that it is not unlikely that they will find themselves back in the community with few benefits and supports, and the new pressures on mental hospitals will make them less willing to accept these patients voluntarily or as part of their community programs. We should not forget the fate of the well-intentioned Durham rule.

The existing conditions in our institutions and procedures for handling persons who violate community norms are deplorable. However, it is not evident that the litigation approach, by itself, can have a lasting effect. A just and effective rehabilitation system must exist within a larger context of justice for the deviant, the impoverished, the disenfranchised, and the sick; and there must be a greater understanding of how to deal more effectively and equitably with such persons. No matter how astute the litigants or how passionate the court, the long-term quality of our hospitals, our rehabilitation institutions, our schools, and our society generally depends on more fundamental decisions made through the legislative process. The fact that litigation may arouse the conscience of the legislature and the concern of the public is evident. But in the long haul, the fate of the mentally ill, like all other unfortunates, is in the hands of the people who make and administer the laws and the persons who elected them. It seems, then, that the rights of the mentally ill must ride the crest of other waves that entitle all citizens to certain benefits to enhance and protect their health. These benefits should be considered as property[33] to be used on one's own volition.

Notes

1. Deutsch, A. (1949). *The Mentally Ill in America.* New York: Columbia University Press, p. 45.
2. Rothman, D. (1971). *The Discovery of the Asylum: Social Order and Disorder in the New Republic.* Boston: Little, Brown, pp. 109–129.
3. *Ibid.,* p. 154.
4. Grob, G. (1966). *The State and the Mentally Ill.* Chapel Hill, N.C.: University of North Carolina Press.
5. Davis, K. (1938). "Mental Hygiene and the Class Structure." *Psychiatry,* **1**:55–65.
6. Belknap, I. (1956). *Human Problems of a State Mental Hospital.* New York: McGraw-Hill.
7. Goffman, E. (1961). *Asylums: Essays on the Social Situation of Mental Patients and Other Inmates.* New York: Anchor-Doubleday.
8. Mechanic, D. (1969). *Mental Health and Social Policy.* Englewood Cliffs, N.J.: Prentice-Hall, pp. 57–61.
9. Mechanic, D. (1968). *Medical Sociology.* New York: Free Press, pp. 383–385.
10. Joint Commission on Mental Illness and Health (1961). *Action for Mental Health.* New York: Science Editions.
11. Hollingshead, A., and F. Redlich (1958). *Social Class and Mental Illness.* New York: Wiley.
12. 125 U. S. App. D. C. 366, 373 F. 2nd 451 (1966).
13. Bazelon, D. (1969). In D. Burris (ed.), *The Right to Treatment.* New York: Springer.
14. National Center for Health Statistics (1971). *Health Resources Statistics—1970.* Public Health Service Publication 1509:134, 153, 198. Washington, D.C.: U.S. Government Printing Office.
15. Birnbaum, M. (1972). "The Right to Treatment—Some Comments on Implementation." *Duquesne Law Review,* **10**:578–608.
16. Handler, J. (1972). *Reforming the Poor: Welfare Policy, Federalism, and Morality.* New York: Basic Books.
17. Katz, J. (1969). "The Right to Treatment—An Enchanting Legal Fiction?" *University of Chicago Law Review,* **36**:755–783.
18. Bazelon, D.(1969), op. cit., p. 2.
19. Szasz, T. (1969). "The Right to Health." In D. Burris (ed.), *The Right to Treatment.* New York: Springer.
20. Ennis, B. (1972). *Prisoners of Psychiatry.* New York: Harcourt Brace Jovanovich.
21. *Ibid.,* p. 108.
22. Arens, R. (1969). *Make Mad the Guilty: The Insanity Defense in the District of Columbia.* Springfield, Ill.: Thomas.
23. Council of the American Psychiatric Association (1967). "Position Paper on the Question of Adequacy of Treatment." *American Journal of Psychiatry,* **123**:1458.
24. *Ibid.*
25. Goffman, E. (1961), op. cit. pp. 380–382.
26. See Friedman, L. (1968). *Government and Slum Housing: A Century of Frustration.* Chicago: Rand McNally.

27. Bazelon, D. (1969). "Implementing the Right to Treatment." *University of Chicago Law Review*, **36**:742–754.

28. Ludwig, A. (1971). *Treating the Treatment Failures: The Challenge of Chronic Schizophrenia.* New York: Grune and Stratton.

29. Ennis, B. (1972), op. cit., p. 230.

30. Pasamanick, B., F. R. Scarpitti, and S. Dinitz (1967). *Schizophrenics in the Community.* New York: Appleton-Centruy-Crofts.

31. Brown, G. W., et al. (1966). *Schizophrenia and Social Care.* London: Oxford University Press.

32. Davis, A., et al. (1972). "The Prevention of Hospitalization in Schizophrenia: Five Years After an Experimental Program." *American Journal of Orthopsychiatry*, **42**:375–388.

33. Reich, C. (1964). "The New Property." *Yale Law Journal*, **73**:778–787.

PART FIVE

NEW DIRECTIONS IN THE ROLE OF HEALTH CARE SYSTEMS

CHAPTER XV

Social Issues in the Study of the Pharmaceutical Field*

The solo practice of medicine sets limits on the potentialities for developing new health manpower roles and on using new personnel effectively and efficiently in the provision of health care. Although solo practitioners have frequently developed ingenious sharing arrangements and affiliations to insure access to technological aids and ancillary assistance, this form of practice restricts very severely innovations in the effective use of manpower. It is inevitable, in the long run, that there will be a greater aggregation of practitioners in groups and other arrangements as well as a specification of responsibility for defined populations. Such aggregation will be accompanied by bureaucratization and by a variety of other problems, resulting from larger-scale and more complicated organizational arrangements. But it will also offer great opportunities for innovations in the use of existing and new health manpower and for a scale of operation that makes possible supporting types of manpower that are impractical under the current dominant organizational auspices of medical care.

In this chapter I will consider the role of the pharmacist—an occupational role that has suffered considerable erosion in recent decades. With changes in the manufacture and distribution of drugs, the pharmacist's role has become more limited, and he has been slow in adopting new functions. Much of the difficulty results from the problems of integrating pharmacy services into current modes of outpatient medical practice. In this sense, the pharmacist might be seen as a proxy for the social worker, the nutritionist, the public health nurse, and the health educationist, for example. Each of these roles is

* Adapted from a paper that appeared in the *American Journal of Pharmaceutical Education,* **34:**536–543 (November 1970).

important to overall health services, but it is difficult to integrate these functions into the delivery of ambulatory services by large numbers of unattached physicians from their own practice premises. Thus, the structure of care profoundly affects the scope of care that patients are likely to receive, the coordination of varying aspects of health services, and the potentialities of a variety of health occupations.

Pharmacy as a profession finds itself in the midst of a crisis of purpose. In some early forms of medical practice the apothecaries were practitioner-tradesmen. Although under some circumstances they could not charge for their advice, they were viewed as having special information on medication and they could charge for it.[1] As medical practice developed, and the use of drugs increased, the pharmacist provided an essential service through his role in purifying and compounding medications. Increasingly, however, with manufactured drug combinations the technical role of the pharmacist has eroded and, despite his training, the typical American pharmacist appears to be more of a businessman than a professional, and he provides the consumer a limited technical service.

If schools of pharmacy are to meet their social responsibilities, then they must seriously grapple with the problem of developing new and significant roles for the pharmacist, roles which have relevance to modern medical care. It is ironic that, at a time when persons knowledgeable about pharmaceuticals are more needed than ever before in a wide variety of roles in the medical care field, the profession of pharmacy has not become more fully engaged in the provision of health care services. Given the number and variety of drugs, the varying potencies in which they are manufactured, their significant dangers to life and health, the number of contingencies under which such dangers may become manifest, the confusing designations attached to medications, and the need to understand the safety and effectiveness factors in drug action, the significant possibilities for new pharmaceutical roles become obvious.

Such roles might include: the maintenance of drug information centers; advising doctors on alternative drugs, appropriate dose, possible adverse effects, and contingencies under which they are most likely to occur; development of adequate drug histories on patients which provide the doctor with greater information including past adverse experiences with drugs; general advice on the efficacy and safety of various categories of drugs; advice to patients on the proper use of prescribed drugs and proper regimen; follow-up of patients' drug regimens to insure conformity with advice; better counseling on drug use generally including better labeling of individual prescriptions; advice to patients on proper disposal of drugs prescribed for previous illnesses; advice on the relative costs of possible alternative drugs; general education on drug effects; and many similar functions of this sort.[2]

Studies of the Effects of the Structure of Medical Care on the Structure of Pharmacy

The scope and potentialities of pharmacy depend very largely on how medical care is organized generally, and different forms of pharmaceutical practice will fit varying forms of medical practice. The erosion of the pharmacist's role is in no way predetermined by the technical changes which have occurred in medical care. To the contrary, the changes which have taken place in the scientific basis of medical care and its developing technology demand a more rather than a less central role for the pharmacist. The irrelevant character of much that the pharmacist does today is as much a result of the antiquated models of medical care current today as it is a product of the development of the pharmaceutical industries. The vast proliferation of drug combinations, the potent and dangerous side effects of drugs, the rapidity with which drugs are introduced onto the market and the manner in which they are introduced, the varying costs of drugs having the same chemical composition—these and many other complexities accompanying changes in medical care argue for the substantial importance of the pharmaceutical profession as part of the larger health care approach.

In view of the pressures on physicians, it is unlikely that they will be fully informed on drugs, their proper use, and relative cost. Even if they are aware of the general problems, the rapidity with which they must work and the demands on their time make it difficult for them to inform themselves adequately on these matters. As a consequence, risks and dangers which could and should be avoided are commonly taken. It would be proper for every medical team to have as one of its members a specially trained pharmacist who is available for consultation and information. Such assistance, if properly provided, would vastly improve the quality of medical care and greatly contribute to the integrity of the pharmacist's role.

To some extent, the role described is already being tried in the context of hospital treatment, but for the most part hospital pharmacies are operations giving greatest attention to management concerns. In outpatient practice the pharmacist has almost no health role at all. In part, this is a simple product of the organization of medical care where the large bulk of medical practice is provided by solo practitioners or by practitioners practicing in small groups. The economics of such practices make it difficult, if not impossible, for doctors to make use fruitfully of the pharmacist, although larger group practices and health centers can more readily integrate such a person into the health team. Here I refer to more than the operation of a pharmacy as we know it today, but rather one where the pharmacist has a direct informational and consultative role, where he comes into contact with patients in the clinical setting, and where his role is defined specifically in terms of the needs and welfare of patients.

Social and Cultural Attitudes Toward the Use of Drugs

There is a wide variety of attitudes and behavior relevant to the use of drugs.[3] These views and practices can substantially condition how people use drugs, the conditions under which they use them, the extent to which they conform to medical regimens, their conceptions of drug action, and the like. In the ordinary practice of medicine doctors frequently do not provide patients with sufficient information on why they have prescribed medications, the proper mode of taking medications, the results and side effects likely from drugs, how long to continue the medication, and many other kinds of information important to patients. Given the ambiguities of prescribing, it is not surprising that cultural beliefs, folk knowledge, and situational contingencies affect the patient's behavior. We have all heard about some of the errors patients make under such circumstances such as eating suppositories, distributing dangerous medications to friends and relatives who are believed to have similar problems, using drugs which have decomposed on recurrent occasions when symptoms develop, and the like. A more relevant pharmaceutical practice may not eliminate all such abuses, but it may provide a context at least where some of the most serious dangers are alleviated.

The inadequacy of present practice is clear from studies which demonstrate the relatively low level of conformity with medical regimens.[4] We know that the more demands doctors make on patients the less likely they are to conform to them. We also know that various inconveniences and feeling-states following drug use frequently lead patients to discontinue their medication. With proper instruction of patients and more appropriate choice of medication, taking into account not only the patient's illness but also his necessary life regimen, the gap between instruction and conformity may be somewhat narrowed. It is unlikely that the medical profession under present demands can carefully do this, and thus the opportunities for the pharmacist should be clear. It follows that the pharmacist must have some awareness of varying cultural and social attitudes towards illness and the manner in which they may manifest themselves in response to drugs.

It would also be central for the pharmacist to understand the psychological components of drug use in motivating the use of drugs, in affecting drug action, and in response to drug action.[5] The placebo effect in drug use is well known, and, indeed, the effect is sufficiently strong in some areas to require controlled trials which take such effects into account. Similarly, not only do patients often feel better after taking placebos, but also a wide variety of side effects is reported following the administration of placebos. In short, the manner and context in which drugs are prescribed are likely to affect the patient's response to drugs, and this fact suggests that this area is central in pharmacy and pharmaceutical practice.

The Sociology of the Pharmacist

Although there are abundant data on doctors, nurses, and several other health workers, the literature is bereft of studies of pharmacists, their modes of work, their values and life orientations, and their career patterns. We know very little about the kind of students drawn to pharmacy, their values and motives, their reactions to their educational experiences, the effects of such experiences on their career patterns, and similar matters. We similarly know little about how pharmacists view themselves, how they see their place in medical care, how they relate to other health professionals, how they view their responsibilities, and a host of related matters.

It is clear that in more recent times the pharmacist's role has fallen between that of a professional guided by certain universalistic standards and ethics and that of a businessman whose primary orientation is the maximization of profit. The community pharmacy as a unit has increasingly diversified its functions so as to be part of a more general enterprise. The multiplication of nonpharmaceutical products sold by pharmacies has helped insure the economic viability of neighborhood pharmacies in an increasingly competitive environment. To some extent, the difficulties of pharmacies have been contributed to by the large capital investment necessary to stock the tremendous variety of combinations and brand-name products characteristic of modern pharmaceuticals. In this context there are frequent occasions when the profit motive or economic viability clashes with the professional behavior of the pharmacist and legal restrictions affecting his role. When economic pressures are strong, either because the pharmacist has a businessman's orientation or because the economic viability of his business is threatened, he is more likely to violate various ethical and legal requirements of his position.[6] Those who see their roles in a more professional light are more likely to resist such behavior. In any case, it is reasonable to assume that the location of the pharmacist's role in the medical care network affects not only his potentialities for making an important contribution to health care but also the extent to which professional standards and ethics govern his behavior. There are indications, for example, that in group practice where doctors must work in close proximity to colleagues they are more attentive to professional standards of colleagues and less subject to client controls and extraneous influences.[7]

Although we have many conceptions of what pharmacists presently do, we really have very little information which corroborates these views. Indeed, how much communication takes place between doctors and pharmacists in a community? How frequently do pharmacists become aware of errors in prescriptions and make inquiries of doctors before filling the prescription? Do doctors seek advice from pharmacists, and on what kinds of questions? How much advice do pharmacists give patients on the proper use of drugs? I would suggest that the amount of contact is probably less than most people ordinarily believe and that other pressures and concerns among both doctors and pharmacists lead to minimized collaboration.

The Organization of the Pharmaceutical Industries

Social scientists have given little attention to the organization of the pharmaceutical industries in the United States and in other countries. Much of our information comes from various congressional committees which have inquired into such matters as drug pricing, safety, and effectiveness.[8] Moreover, we know relatively little concerning the complex interactions within the industry and between the industry and government agencies. These are matters of great importance which require enlightened social science analysis.

The organization of the pharmaceutical industry is particularly interesting because companies frequently find themselves in a context where their values are in opposition, and there are always costs in terms of one or another set of values. Since the industry operates in an economic context where profit is a central value, companies must frequently weigh opportunities for profit against margins of safety and therapeutic effectiveness.[9] The manner in which pharmaceutical companies relate to other components of the health field—such as doctors, hospitals, government agencies, political organizations, and the like —also deserves attention. The form in which their products are researched, manufactured, advertised, and distributed also raises a variety of issues.

One can trace changes in the industry by inquiring into changes in various roles. The detail man in the past, for example, frequently had considerable scientific background and education relevant to pharmaceutical products. Many detail men had training in pharmacy. Increasingly in recent years, pharmaceutical concerns have been recruiting detail men with business and marketing backgrounds who have very limited understanding of the products they promote. As a consequence, detail men are probably less reliable than in the past, although the needs for reliability have increased. Perhaps pharmacy schools should be training information officers who are guided by a strong scientific background and a set of professional ethics, and we should know more than we do about the extent to which personnel are exposed to conflicts between commercial and scientific values, how they are resolved, and the outcomes in terms of treatment and costs. It might be useful to have a categorical tax on the production of pharmaceuticals which is allocated for the training and maintenance of information officers unattached to any particular company.

In viewing interrelations within the pharmaceutical industry itself, it might be informative to have a better grasp of the interrelationships among firms, the negotiations among dominant and small suppliers, the modes of setting standards and prices, and the like. From the perspectives of individual companies themselves, one might inquire as to the forces affecting innovation, factors affecting the manner in which innovations are distributed and accepted, forces affecting the maintenance of an adequate informational system, factors influencing the wise and appropriate use of drugs by physicians and patients, and so on. A key question concerns the conditions under which the industry is either more or less likely to serve the public interest.

These are but a few of the issues which can be illuminated through the application of the social sciences to pharmacy. Since most of the discussion has been at a general level thus far, it would be useful to go into some detail on two examples of social science studies which have direct relevance to the pharmaceutical field and which raise a variety of interesting issues beyond the results of the studies themselves.

The first study, financed by a pharmaceutical company, focused on the characteristics of doctors and their social networks related to the time of introduction of a new member of a family of frequently used drugs.[10] The main variable in the study—the time of introduction of the new drug by a particular physician—was arrived at through a sample audit of prescriptions on file at local commercial pharmacies in the four midwestern cities in which the study was undertaken. The drug in question was adopted relatively rapidly. Sixteen months after it was first introduced on the market a large proportion of doctors in the sample had tried it, and half of them were prescribing it more often than any of the other drugs in the same family. Doctors who adopted the new drug early were more cautious in its use than those who did so later. Those who attended specialty meetings, who received more than three journals, who were professionally oriented as compared with patient-oriented doctors, who participated in the medical community, etc., were more likely to use the drug and to adopt it earlier than their counterparts. Similarly, doctors who had regular staff appointments, who attended four or more hospital meetings, who shared their offices with other doctors, and who were named by other doctors as advisors, discussion partners, and friends adopted the new drug earlier.

258 SOCIAL ISSUES IN THE STUDY OF THE PHARMACEUTICAL FIELD

Such studies can be viewed in a variety of ways. They probably have some practical value in that they may aid a company in planning how to market a drug. They also can be used to test certain social science hypotheses; in this particular case the investigators used the data for the purpose of trying to build a mathematical model of the diffusion of innovations generally. This study is also a useful and provocative teaching aid in that it raises a variety of new issues either through its results or through examination of certain assumptions made by the researchers. One of the puzzling findings in this study was that, although doctors believed that detail men were important in coming to know about the drug, the number of detail men seen does not correlate with the time of adoption. The researchers conclude that, although detail men may help the doctor become aware of the drug, legitimation of the use of the drug must come from other sources—mainly professional channels and colleagues. This is indeed an important question. Just how much are doctors influenced by detail men and in what ways? But we must also consider whether some of the results of this study are a product of the marketing practices of the pharmaceutical concern itself. Is there a strategy used by companies relating to how they approach doctors and who are the key people to be influenced? And what is the relationship between such strategies and results?

This study raises other educational issues as well. The researchers implicitly assume that the more quickly a new drug is adopted by the medical community, the better. This view is certainly one consistent with the interests of pharmaceutical concerns. There are obvious circumstances under which rapid adoption of innovations is important and desirable, but is it really in the public interest to achieve rapid adoption of new drugs before we have had an opportunity to evaluate more fully the experience with them? The thalidomide tragedy would suggest that this is not always the case. Considering the adoption of drugs in general, would similar results on diffusion have occurred more slowly if it had not been part of a well-known and commonly used family of drugs; if it had a different pattern of adverse effects; or if the medical system were more bureaucratically organized in contrast to a system based on solo practice? Even the simple question of drug diffusion becomes relatively complex when examined carefully.

The second study which I shall briefly comment on is one by Zborowski[11] on the reactions of different ethnic groups to pain. In his study he found that Jews and Italians were more likely to express their concern about pain than Irish or "Yankee Americans." He also found, however, that, although the expression of pain among Italians and Jews had the same external manifestations, they were derived from very different underlying attitudes. The Italians appeared to be primarily concerned with the experience of pain itself and responded well to pain medication. In contrast, the Jews in the sample were concerned more with the significance of pain for their health than with pain itself. Thus, pain medication was insufficient to satisfy their basic anxieties and concerns.

Now what relevance does such a study have for the pharmacist? If we assume the results are reliable and generalizable, then it might be a consideration in determining the proper regimen for different patients. If the health worker responds directly to a complaint without understanding underlying attitudes, then it would appear that those who continued to complain of pain require more pain medication. The appreciation of cultural differences, however, may lead the health worker to pose varying hypotheses about the nature of the complaint and how it might best be handled. Despite cultural differences, there are very large variations within groups and, thus, knowledge of cultural differences does not suggest a specific approach. But sensitivity to such variations may help the health worker avoid needless mistakes. Indeed, such studies suggest even further the importance of the kinds of communication which accompany prescribing medication, and different circumstances require varying information. Drug-taking is influenced profoundly by the meanings patients attribute to their illness and how they define the context in which they are treated. For example, in a comparative study of pain, Beecher[12] asked a group of wounded soldiers and a group of male civilian patients undergoing major surgery the same questions about their desire for pain medication. While only one-third of the soldiers wanted medication to relieve their pain, 80 percent of the civilians wanted pain relief, although they were suffering from far less tissue trauma. He explains the variation in terms of different definitions of pain in the two circumstances. The soldier's wound, Beecher explains, was an escape from the battlefield and the possibility of being killed; to the civilians, surgical pain was viewed as a depressing, calamitous event. Beecher reports that the civilian group reported strikingly more frequent and severe pain, and he concludes that there is no simple, direct relationship between the wound per se and the pain experience. It may be that an appreciation of the patient's attitude may even resolve an issue of which of two drugs to use—one more potent in relieving pain but more dangerous, the other less effective but safer. Finally, knowing that all drugs have some potentiality for harm, the properly trained pharmacist should see as part of his role the responsibility to discourage needless use of drugs.

In short, I believe that the social study of pharmacy is an important area to be developed. There is a great deal of work crying to be undertaken and, indeed, part of training in this area should be devoted to impressing the student with how little we know about this field and to providing the tools for systematic inquiry of important questions. As pharmacy begins to forge new roles for itself in the health field, it seems clear that it will more frequently face problems and alternatives which can be illuminated through a social science approach.

Notes

1. Abel-Smith, B. (1964). *The Hospitals: 1800–1948*. London: Heinemann.
2. Deno, R. A. (1967). *Proceedings, Pharmacy-Medicine-Nursing Conference on Health Education*. Ann Arbor: University of Michigan.
3. Mechanic, D. (1968). *Medical Sociology: A Selective View*. New York: Free Press.
4. Davis, M. S. (1966). "Variations in Patients' Compliance with Doctors' Orders: Analysis of Congruence Between Survey Responses and Results of Empirical Investigations." *Journal of Medical Education*, **41**:1037–1048.
5. Mechanic, D. (1968). *Medical Sociology: A Selective View*. op. cit.
6. Quinney, E. (1963). "Occupational Structure and Criminal Behavior: Presciption Violation by Retail Pharmacists." *Social Problems*, **11**:179–185.
7. Freidson, E. (1963). "Medical Care and the Public: Case Study of a Medical Group." *Annals of the American Academy of Political and Social Science*, **346**:57–66.
8. Mintz, M. (1965). *The Therapeutic Nightmare*. Cambridge, Mass.: Houghton Mifflin.
9. Mintz, M. (1969). "FDA and Panalba: A Conflict of Commercial, Therapeutic Goals?" *Science*, **165**:875–881.
10. Coleman, J., et al. (1966). *Medical Innovation: A Diffusion Study*. Indianapolis, Ind.: Bobbs-Merrill.
11. Zborowski, M. (1952). "Cultural Components in Responses to Pain." *Journal of Social Issues*, **8**:16–30.
12. Beecher, H. (1959). *Measurement of Subjective Responses*. New York: Oxford University Press.

CHAPTER XVI

Promotion of Health, Health Maintenance, and Health Education

As the debate on the future of medical care in America continues, more and more statements are made about the need to give greater emphasis to health promotion, health maintenance, and health education. These statements stem from the realization that much of the morbidity evident in the population is the result of environmental forces and harmful patterns of behavior, and that a curative system of medical care—no matter how elaborated or sophisticated—can have only a limited impact on patterns of health and disease in society at large. Although much of this new emphasis is relevant to current needs, there is a tendency toward superficial statements that reflect little realization of the complexity of health behavior or the difficulties in successfully altering behavior patterns. Before rushing ahead with expensive national programs in health education and health promotion, we must assess more carefully what we know about changing health behavior and make more fundamental inquiries about the behaviors that we wish to alter.

Since most concepts of health promotion and health education are vague, diffuse, and cover a wide scope, it is very difficult to develop a coherent set of principles or even to examine their many facets in a comprehensive and organized way. Thus, we must begin with the concept of "health" itself and the implications of varying conceptions. As René Dubos[1] has wisely warned us:

> [Man's] self-imposed striving for ever-new distant goals makes his fate even more unpredictable than that of other living beings. For this reason health and happiness cannot be absolute and permanent values, however careful the social and medical planning. Biological success in all its manifestations is a measure of fitness, and fitness requires never-ending efforts of adaptation to the total environment, which is ever changing (p.25).

Health is only one of many salient priorities, and illness tends to come to the forefront only after it has occurred. When persons are healthy, thoughts about illness are not usually prominent; thus other valued priorities frequently have the greatest influence on behavior. Moreover, many patterns of behavior, potentially detrimental to health, are deeply ingrained in social and cultural patterns and in the structure of social and economic activities. Preventive action is often possible at several levels of intervention, and in weighing alternatives we have to consider both the efficacy of individual interventions and the barriers to their implementation.

Automobile accidents serve as an adequate illustration of both the possibilities for intervention and the complex barriers to their implementation. The automobile has become one of the major hazards to health and longevity in modern life: it not only kills and maims many and contributes heavily to disability and medical care costs, but it also has an indirect effect on health through environmental pollution and the encouragement of physical inactivity. The cause of automobile accidents and possible interventions may be seen from the perspective of the individual driver, from the technical construction and capacity of the automobile to respond to threat, and from the larger physical and social environment in which auto accidents take place.

From a personal viewpoint, it is clear that the protection of health depends on the skills and attitudes of the driver, and this in turn depends on the social preparation he has had. Since the automobile is an important symbol in Western society, various attitudes may be reflected in driving patterns, as in the risk-taking that is characteristic of many adolescents. Driving also reflects various psychological traits such as aggression and anxiety, although research in this area is very limited.[2] Most dangerous, of course, is the association between drinking and driving;[3,4] most drivers in single-vehicle accidents have been drinking.[5] The alcohol-driving pattern is implicitly encouraged by social and recreational patterns that are relatively forceful as compared with the admonition not to drink and drive. Protections against injury in the case of accidents, such as the use of seat belts, are frequently ignored.

When we think of intervention at the individual level, driver education is usually given high priority. It is not clear, however, that education is a particularly powerful tool in affecting either the driver's attitudes or behavior. Other resources at the individual level include more restrictive licensing or harsher penalties for violations, but these remedies are either relatively limited in effectiveness or face serious political difficulties in enactment. More and more, public health experts are urging the adoption of technical solutions to individual behavior problems. They seek technical innovations that bypass the need to motivate persons to follow suggested behaviors. Such inventions as the inflatable air-bag, or fortified foods in the nutrition area, are attempts to achieve outcomes without changing individual behavior. To the extent that such inventions are possible, they offer potentialities for preserving health and preventing injury, but technical solutions cannot solve all of our potential health problems and, under some circumstances, they may create new ones.

In the past public health practitioners underestimated the value of technological approaches to health prevention, but it is now widely appreciated, for example, that auto design, structural road conditions, and traffic control can incorporate major safety features. These include the ability of the automobile to successfully contain persons without injury during collisions[6] and other features such as maneuverability, steering, braking, and skid potential. Alteration of the larger driving environment includes the provision of controlled access roads, highway construction and repair, traffic control, lighting and visible markings, and so on. Although investments in structural and community conditions may initially require much larger expenditures, such allocations may be more cost-effective than interventions carried out at the individual level.

Once we come to view the promotion of health as requiring various levels of intervention, it becomes necessary to consider the types of barriers encountered in each instance. At the individual level, the problem most frequently experienced is the uncertainty of the technologies of behavior change and in our ability to achieve desired effects. Many behaviors detrimental to health bring other rewards or are deeply ingrained in personality or behavior patterns. Health promotive behaviors may also be costly for the individual in terms of time, money, effort, inconvenience, or in terms of their conflict with social values. At the level of structural change economic and political considerations become more salient. The implementation of technological innovations conducive to health and safety is embedded in a complex economic system which involves weighing health considerations against many other priorities. Similarly, the willingness of communities to use their resources and powers to promote safety is influenced by many considerations including cost, public sentiments, political processes, and the like. Few community actions are totally free of costs. Thus, decisions involve considerations of who will bear the cost of one policy or another conducive to health promotion. Moreover, as we move into greater concern for regulation of the environment such questions of cost allocation become a prime concern.

As we begin to look more carefully at preventive and promotive health behavior, it becomes clear that the problem has a variety of dimensions as well as alternative levels of intervention. First, there is a wide range of preventive health services that are of known efficacy— immunization, for instance—but have uneven penetration among varying subgroups in the population. Here the major concern is how to bring such services to groups who are presently not receiving them. In large part, this involves the question of entitlement to services and their accessibility. It may also involve, to some extent, consumer knowledge and motivation. Second, we have various services and screening procedures that are presently being used or are feasible but whose efficacy is not fully determined. Here we require a careful assessment of the value of each of these procedures and their costs relative to the prevalence of the conditions to which they are directed. If there is evidence that they are effective, then the issue remains of how best to organize such services to serve the population or specific subgroups who are most vulnerable to that particular condition. Finally, there is a great variety of health practices that are not necessarily pertinent to the delivery of services, but do promote health and longevity. These behaviors involve a broader consideration of sociocultural and technological influences, and concern the problems of health education and behavior modification. Since these are issues on which there is considerable confusion at the present time, I turn now to a discussion of some of the gaps in our knowledge and the complexities in understanding this area.

Health Knowledge and Behavior

We all appreciate the uncertain relationship between health knowledge and health behavior. We know that knowledge about the consequences of smoking, drinking, use of drugs, physical inactivity, failure to use seat belts, and other matters relevant to health has only a limited relationship to the occurrence of the appropriate health behavior. It is thus necessary to become aware of the environmental, personal, and behavioral factors that intervene between knowledge and behavior. The area dealing with the discordance between attitudes and actions has been studied by a variety of social scientists for many years and is, in no sense, a new area of concern. The degree of discrepancy is dependent on a variety of intervening conditions that relate to an individual's social context and goals, the social influences to which he is exposed, the gains and costs of enacting his attitudinal dispositions, and many other factors.

In considering the role of knowledge on health actions, it is important to distinguish circumstances in which there is a readiness toward action, few barriers, and a lack of information in contrast to situations in which a desired health action comes into conflict with other personal needs and dispositions. For example, a person may have a considerable readiness to obtain a particular health service—such as birth control information, an abortion, or child health services—but may not know where to seek the service. Here, information on the availability of services may be an important factor in triggering their use. In contrast, information on appropriate physical exercise, driving after the use of alcohol, and the dangers of smoking may have only a very small impact on desired behavior. It is difficult to believe that there are many smokers in the United States who are not aware of the dangers inherent in smoking. The achievement of significant change obviously requires a great deal more than information programs.

Information programs oriented toward people with established patterns of behavior, such as smoking, must be differentiated from programs directed at persons who have not as yet adopted the behavior pattern. It is likely, for example, that information programs on smoking have a greater effect on youngsters who have not yet begun to smoke than they have on persons who have developed the habit. But even in the case of youngsters, information will be only one of many conditions affecting the behavioral outcome, and it is unlikely to have much influence in the absence of other reinforcing factors.

The health knowledge-behavior area can be fruitfully analyzed within the model used for explaining diffusion of innovations.[7] Many of the health practices urged by public programs are dissonant with other valued behavior patterns and routines. The adoption of such patterns of behavior, therefore, is likely to depend on the credibility of the communication, the trust in the communicator, the extent to which the desired health pattern can be integrated into other behavior patterns, the informal reinforcement from family, peer groups, and the community, and the models set by significant others. Providing information about some health practice without reinforcing the conditions of its acceptability is usually ineffectual.

When there are barriers to adopting particular patterns of desired health behavior, inconsistencies in the messages or contradictions among communicators result in low credibility not only in relation to the specific message but also in respect to related messages. There have been few areas that have received as much recent propaganda and community concern as drug use, and much emphasis has been put on marijuana. It appears that the target audience (students) has been influenced very little by such drug information programs in part because it has not found them to be particularly credible. Frequently, in attempting to discourage drug use, programs have used fear appeals that students recognized as inconsistent and erroneous. Once the credibility of the communicator is challenged in a particular area, potential influence in respect to other patterns of behavior may be undermined.

Is There a Global Promotive or Preventive Health Pattern?

A large number of behaviors are believed to be directly relevant to health maintenance and, indeed, if the concept of relevance is stretched a bit, almost all behavior is pertinent in one fashion or another. In some cases, harmful consequences of a particular behavior pattern are demonstrable: as in smoking, poor nutrition, physical inactivity, use of many drugs, overeating, and consumption of alcohol, for instance. Other types of behavior patterns that are encouraged—such as obtaining medical examinations at regular intervals, visiting the dentist every six months, regularity in eating and sleeping, and patterned leisure—are believed to have some effect on health, but are of much less demonstrated importance. Still other health promotive behaviors may be performed explicitly for the purpose of enhancing health but may be uncertain, irrelevant, or even possibly harmful: food fads, taking heavy doses of vitamins D and E, and frequent preventive X rays to detect disease of low prevalence, for example. Thus, it is important to distinguish between behaviors that objectively promote health status from those that do not; it is conceivable that persons who are responsive to most healthful activities are also responsive to less effective fads.

The question of efficacy relates to practices advocated by health experts and to practices adopted by various cultural groups in the population. Some physicians urge all sorts of preventive diagnostic procedures that have an unproved relationship to preventing morbidity. Some screening practices are quite useful and are based on evidence showing the value of preventive care. But many of the advocated preventive screening procedures are uncertain, and it is not clear that anything can be done, once a particular condition has been identified.[8] Indeed, it is conceivable that the identification of conditions that cannot be effectively treated is harmful to the individual's functioning and even to his social status, and it might be better not to identify the conditions.

It is apparent that there is imperfect generality from one preventive health practice to another. The person who drives carefully does not necessarily exercise; and the individual who uses his seat belt may have a poor diet. We currently lack a clear idea of the extent of generality among different types of behavior meant to protect health or the degree to which health behaviors in general can be encompassed within a limited number of behavioral dimensions. Even within the same general area of behavior—for example, driving behavior—we have little reason to believe that such varied specific actions as obeying speed limits, using seat belts, properly maintaining one's car, and avoiding drinking and driving are highly correlated. Each of these behaviors may be differentially affected by personal, social, and situational factors. At present data that allow estimates of the extent of generality from one type of healthful behavior to another are very limited.[9]

Jean Langlie,[10] who is working on a doctoral dissertation dealing with the generality of preventive health behaviors, has suggested four aspects of behavior that may have greater consistency within each dimension. These include risk-taking (the propensity to engage in behavior having high risk probabilities); illness-avoiding behaviors (such as obtaining immunizations and avoiding contact with contagious persons); health-promotive behaviors (conscious efforts to engage in behaviors to stay healthy, such as proper diet, exercise, and getting sufficient rest); and illness-detection behaviors (seeing one's doctor and dentist regularly, propensity to identify symptoms and seek help, for instance). These groupings may help to arrive at more unitary dimensions.

The manner in which health behavior is usually discussed implies a global personality disposition influencing a wide range of behavioral activities relevant to health. To the extent that such a predisposition exists and can be encouraged in child development, the potentialities for teaching an adaptive health pattern in early life are enhanced. Experience in developmental psychology provides little encouragement, however, since few general orientations toward such complex patterns of behavior have been successfully identified, and situational factors have effects of considerable magnitude on performance. To some extent, the failure to demonstrate generality may be a product of measurement difficulties peculiar to development studies—the most difficult one being in obtaining comparable measures for particular concepts at different stages of the life cycle.

Rosenstock[11] has suggested a general model of preventive health behavior that includes the psychological readiness to take specific action and the extent to which a particular course of action is believed to contribute to reducing the threat of illness. Psychological readiness is defined by the extent to which an individual feels vulnerable to a particular condition and the extent to which he feels the condition would have serious consequences in his case. Other factors that Rosenstock deals with are perceived barriers to taking action and cues that trigger appropriate behavior. The Rosenstock model, applied in a variety of research endeavors, has yielded relatively consistent but weak support. We are still a long way from defining clear-cut and significant behavioral orientations toward health maintenance, and we know even less about how to shape development to achieve health promotive behaviors. In the long run, the most productive course might be to attempt to shape each behavior separately, concentrating efforts on those of greatest importance to society. But location of general orientations that are modifiable would make educational efforts a great deal easier.

Since working with specific behaviors allows the targeting of communications and audiences, it presently offers greater opportunities for success. Moreover, persons are more susceptible to communication when they have a desire to know, and effective and responsive communication and behavior modification approaches can be more easily developed in a targeted fashion. Of course, it would be more advantageous to nurture orientations receptive to new health information and flexibility in adapting to new environments. There is a tendency for responses to persist beyond the time they are adaptive, and many people tend to retain certain practices that were once believed to be conducive to health but are now obsolete.

Social Policy and Health Education

With the realization of the extent to which life patterns affect illness, there has been increased emphasis on health education and activation of the health consumer through communication appeals. Despite the fact that the technology for effective health education is poorly developed and of uncertain effectiveness, there is relatively little support for research that seeks a basic understanding of the mechanisms of behavior change. Although there is a willingness to invest large sums of money in communication appeals on a variety of problems, there is much less interest in experimental and evaluative work on health education.

Much of the faith in health education comes from observation of commercial advertising and the belief that companies would not invest such large sums in the media if it were not effective. But this analogy is a poor one, since most commercial advertising is intended to achieve the visibility and recall of particular products in situations where one assumes that the consumer is motivated to make a certain type of purchase but must select among many competing products. Advertising may also create needs by introducing consumers to new products or variations of products but, generally, there is an assumption of a motivated consumer.

Health education programs may be most effective when there is a felt need for information or instruction. It is also possible that such programs contribute toward awareness and toward a threshold for action, but this has not been generally demonstrated. Most health education programs, however, are oriented toward changing complex behaviors, such as smoking, drug use, the use of alcohol, and driving. In such cases it is highly unlikely that most of the population are not aware of the dangers, and it seems farfetched that information programs alone can have a major impact except perhaps with targeted audiences such as children. Since most health education programs are oriented toward complex behaviors and hard-to-reach populations, it is hazardous indeed to anticipate that they will have intended effects. Frequently, such campaigns produce outcomes that are quite different from the ones intended, and it is essential to develop the communications carefully and to test their impact on varying audiences.

Possibly, the most fruitful opportunities for health education occur within the medical context when patients seek help for a particular problem and when they are experiencing a certain degree of anxiety. Instructive media presented at this point, when patients are motivated for information about a particular problem, may be extremely helpful to them. This instructive health information might also be provided by community health information centers to persons who seek instruction on particular matters. This, too, requires study because we know that persons who seek preventive programs are frequently not the persons who need them most. However, self-selected audiences who wish to know more about particular health matters may be the audiences most amenable to change through a media approach.

The use of instructional and audiovisual materials may be particularly useful in medical practice, where physicians and other health personnel find themselves repeating certain information and routines again and again for both patients and their relatives. But if such materials are used, it is important that the patient be given an opportunity to question the physician about matters not covered, about matters they do not fully understand, or about issues that require further detail. These aids could be extremely helpful in a variety of medical and rehabilitation circumstances, but they must not be used mindlessly as a way of saving the time and efforts of health personnel.

Although health education is an important aspect of an overall approach to health maintenance and disease prevention, there is a tendency to imply that more can be achieved than the facts presently warrant. Most diseases are not preventable in any specific sense at this time, and attempts to change complex forms of behavior are fraught with difficulties. For the most part, we lack the technology and understanding to bring about changes through health education approaches, and a good deal of basic research is necessary to provide a basis for more effective programs. If health education, as an approach, is not to be discredited in the future, advocates should temper the exaggerations and overstatements that are now so characteristic of the field.

Finally, most of the destructive health behavior patterns that we are concerned about reflect the way in which we have chosen to live as individuals and as a society. They derive from our forms of social organization and social life, and from the types of economic and social patterns that we have encouraged. Thus, to put excessive emphasis on individual responsibility for various preventive health behaviors is to misgauge the conditions from which they arise. As a society we must confront the issue of how important health maintenance is relative to other social commitments, and how far we are willing to go to promote conditions that facilitate a healthful pattern of living. There is no particular reason why health should be the highest of values or the most central of social goals. But for those persons who particularly value health and who seek to promote it, it is important to recognize the realistic constraints and opportunities for change.

Notes

1. Dubos, R. (1959). *Mirage of Health*. New York: Harper.
2. Selzer, M. (1969). "Alcoholism, Mental Illness, and Stress in 96 Drivers Causing Fatal Accidents." *Behavioral Science*, **14**:1–10.
3. Haddon, W., Jr., et al. (eds.) (1964). *Accident Research: Methods and Approaches*. New York: Harper and Row.

4. Selzer, M., et al. (eds.) (1967). *The Prevention of Highway Injury.* Ann Arbor: Highway Safety Research Institute, University of Michigan.

5. Haddon, W., Jr., and V. Bradess (1964). "Alcohol in the Single Vehicle Fatal Accident, Experience of Westchester County, New York." In W. Haddon, Jr., et al. (eds.), op. cit.

6. Nader, R. (1965). *Unsafe At Any Speed: The Designed-in Dangers of the American Automobile.* New York: Grossman.

7. Rogers, E., and F. F. Shoemaker (1971). *Communication of Innovations: A Cross-Cultural Approach.* New York: Free Press.

8. McKeown, T., et al. (1968). *Screening in Medical Care: Reviewing the Evidence.* Fair Lawn, N.J.: Oxford University Press.

9. Williams, A. F., and H. Wechsler (1972). "Interrelationship of Preventive Actions in Health and Other Areas." *Public Health Reports,* **87**:969–976.

10. Langlie, J. Ph.D. dissertation in progress. University of Wisconsin.

11. Rosenstock, I. (1969). "Prevention of Illness and Maintenance of Health." In J. Kosa, et al. (eds.), *Poverty and Health: A Sociological Analysis.* Cambridge: Harvard University Press, pp. 168–190.

CHAPTER XVII

A Plan for the Geographic Distribution of Physicians

A frequent concern, expressed about medical care, is the lack of accessibility of medical services in various parts of the United States, despite the fact that the ratio of physicians to the population is higher than in most other countries. Problems of accessibility result largely from a maldistribution of available physicians, geographically and by activity. Physicians concentrate in urban and suburban areas, and serious shortages exist both in urban ghettos and rural areas. Also, the physicians available are disproportionately concentrated in medical and surgical specialties in contrast to primary care activity. Even taking into account internists, pediatricians, and obstetricians—who are not fully substitutes for family physicians or general practitioners—it is clear that in recent decades we have taken a very sharp turn away from primary care activities.

There is wide agreement that the maldistribution problem is largely a product of uneven geographic concentration of physicians and of growing specialization of functions. The geographic maldistribution, however, is often confused with the question of whether there is a doctor shortage; and this question is hotly contested. Much of the debate stems from a reluctance to accept the kinds of measures necessary to redistribute physicians. Thus there are few options left except to try to increase the number of physicians in the hope that some of them will move into underdoctored areas. In recent years we have increased substantially the available medical school places by starting new schools and expanding enrollment in existing ones. Although it is difficult to assess how added numbers of doctors might assist a redistribution policy, it is reasonably clear that a simple increase in the number of physicians, by itself, is unlikely to alter fundamentally the existing pattern of geographic distribution or the allocation of functions. Barring a vast excess of physicians or dramatic changes in government reimbursement policies, most communities can absorb a large number of physicians before economic conditions force relocation of practices.

The problems of locating physicians in rural areas and urban ghettos are different and require varying remedial measures. Moreover, in considering the need for primary care services, the difficulty in providing physicians for certain areas has caused some analysts to encourage a variety of physician substitutes, such as nurse practitioners, physician assistants, and the use of sophisticated computer and cable television technologies. I maintain that it is possible and feasible to achieve geographic redistribution of physicians although, to achieve lasting effects, it would be desirable to buttress such attempts with supportive manpower and technology systems.

The most frequent means used to attempt redistribution of physician manpower to rural areas are loan forgiveness programs. Many states have these programs, and some programs have been in effect since the 1940's. Mason reports that in 11 states that provide data on these programs 60 percent of students repay such loans by doing some rural practice.[1] Settlement rates are, of course, considerably lower.

In evaluating Mason's data, several cautions are necessary. First, several states, not included in the analysis, discontinued the program because it was a failure (although one, Mississippi, despite obvious distributional difficulties, gave as its reason for discontinuance that the program was no longer necessary because of its success). Thus, the 60 percent rate of some service repayment is probably based on the most successful programs. Second, most of the states with high success rates are largely rural states, and it is conceivable that many of the students who entered the forgiveness program would have settled in rural areas anyway. Third, it is clear that only a very small number of students enter forgiveness programs, and it is doubtful whether these programs can be vastly expanded. In view of the existing economics of medical practice, it is rational for the student to pay off loans and retain full freedom of selecting a practice site.

In 1971 and 1972, more than 29,000 students applied for approximately 12,000 medical school places,[2] and it is reported that significant numbers of Americans are studying medicine overseas. Many other eligible and talented students interested in medicine probably did not apply because of the difficulty of gaining admission to medical school. Thus, the potential pool of qualified students is much greater than the available places, and average grades and Medical College Admission Test (MCAT) scores of entering medical students have gone up in recent years. How, then, can one draw on this pool to insure the training of physicians who will practice in underdoctored areas?

A Modest Plan

One of the difficulties in changing practice location is that economic incentives contained in forgiveness programs are weak in contrast to the earning capacities of the physician. The magnitude of the incentive could be greatly increased if the incentive were not only a loan or scholarship but the *opportunity to attend medical school*. Since the pool of qualified students is very large, one can require service commitments from students in exchange for the opportunity to attend medical school.

The feasibility of this proposal depends on the willingness of medical schools to hold fixed proportions of its available places for qualified students who are willing to enter into service commitments. This can be achieved through a program offering attractive financial incentives to medical schools that undertake to develop such admission policies. At the same time, economic support for the students who enter into the program can also be provided.

Is the Proposed Program Consistent with American Values?

As the pool of qualified students has increased in recent years, the entry into medical school has been dependent on small differences in grades and MCAT scores. There is no evidence that these small distinctions are indicative of different probabilities of becoming good physicians. Medical students, even in private medical schools, only incur a small proportion of the cost for their medical education, while the largest proportion comes through federal and state support. Since the support for medical education is intended to subsidize the fulfillment of community need, it is not unreasonable for the public to require a certain commitment from the student that is consistent with public goals.

Since our social and political values support the idea that students should have maximal opportunity to choose their occupational specialty and practice location, it is necessary to avoid coercion in balancing public need against individual choice. Limitations on choice probably should be no greater than in other occupational spheres. In making this comparison, it is clear that physicians claim the right to choices that few other Americans have. Salaried workers face limitations of choice determined by the employment market, and few salaried professionals have unlimited choice of where to practice their professions. By developing some functional equivalent of an employment market, it would be possible to redistribute physicians without coercing any physicians to work in a particular location.

The simplest way of achieving this kind of redistribution would be to establish an employment market for physicians, such as would occur if physicians were salaried in a national health system. A nationalized system is highly unlikely in view of existing social and political realities, and thus a possible substitute would be the development of contractual service obligations which are fulfilled in terms of a national system of designating needy areas. If areas of national need are drawn widely enough, young physicians would have a very wide choice of practice locations, which might involve as much as 50 percent of the United States including cities and rural areas. Thus, in fulfilling his obligation, no physician would be forced into any area that he finds personally unattractive, although certain options (i.e., overdoctored areas) would not be permitted for the duration of the contract. In short, redistribution would occur by enforcing a contractual agreement with the student, but one that offers him the widest possible range of choice within the intent of the agreement.

The mechanism of joining the availability of a medical school place with a service commitment offers advantages beyond redistribution itself. It is more likely to select young physicians with a service orientation; it would probably attract a wider representation of students in terms of racial, social class, and geographic background; and it would probably encourage a diversification of the practice models taught by medical schools.

Are Excellence and Flexibility in Medical Education Assured?

Any program that allocates medical school places on criteria other than academic standing inevitably raises issues concerning the quality of the student and the excellence of training. To repeat: in no sense does this plan suggest that unqualified or partially qualified students receive preference. It argues that the pool of potential applicants be selected on the basis of academic factors, but that, among these, it is more appropriate to introduce new criteria for selection than small and unreliable differences in grades and test scores. Since only a part of the total medical school class will be filled on the basis of a service commitment, sufficient places would remain for students training for academic careers in medicine, research, or other possible roles. In any case, nothing in this plan would restrict students in the program from entering research or academic medicine, but they would be expected to complete their contracted commitment after a liberal but limited period of postgraduate education.

Legal Aspects of the Proposal.

The contractual arrangements implied in this plan are legally viable, and enforcement of such an agreement has considerable precedent in employment contracts. Some of the possible approaches to enforcement (such as injunction against practice in an overdoctored area) may raise legal issues but, barring such extreme measures, there is a variety of deterrents against failure to comply with the agreement. Professor Clark Havighurst, of Duke University School of Law, has developed a model contract in which the student agrees that, during the period of five years following his training, he will not practice a medical specialty except in a geographic area that, at the time, is identified as a health service scarcity area. Guidelines for these definitions have already been established by the Department of Health, Education, and Welfare to be used in their own programs such as the National Health Service Corps.

The contract is developed to achieve the intended goal with limited restriction on the student's choice. Within a limited range, it allows him to practice in a number of needed specialties and to move from one area to another if he wishes. On entering the contract, the student would be able to designate one underserviced area in which he would be allowed to practice even if the area was no longer underserviced on completion of his training. Also, once a doctor has established practice in an area, he may stay to complete his obligated service even if the area does not remain classified as an underserviced area. Thus the contract makes it possible for students from particular underserviced areas to plan to return to their home areas following their medical education, and it also maximizes stability once a practice has been established.

It is not necessary to elaborate here on the enforcement powers of such a contract or to consider the likely response of the courts to a variety of possible options for enforcement. These matters have been worked out, and it is reasonably clear that teeth can be put into the program. For example, the student who wishes to release himself from the obligation can be required to repay the entire cost of his education, which would be considerably more than the possible penalties under forgivable loan programs. The use of injunctions barring physicians who entered the contract from practicing in overdoctored areas until they have completed their obligated service might raise the most legal difficulties, but it is unlikely that such an approach would be necessary for enforcement. There are other viable enforcement options consistent with precedent in other areas and constitutional standards.

Encouraging Permanent Practices in Underdoctored Areas.

Service commitments under the contract would have to be for a limited period of time. Ideally, one would like to achieve more stable and permanent conditions of practice in many underdoctored areas, although there may be some areas that are so isolated and energy-consuming that a certain amount of rotation may be desirable. Under such conditions, a limited period of practice (as in the Health Service Corps) may be a model to follow and, indeed, credit toward the contracted obligation can be given for service in the Health Service Corps.

In most underdoctored areas, however, it would not be unreasonable to develop stable and effective health services, and thus attention must be given to the conditions that are conducive to physician tenure and practice stability.* Physicians are more likely to remain in underdoctored areas if they have acquired techniques of medical practice consistent with the types of practice required in such areas. This would depend on the models of practice characteristic of the medical schools and residency programs in which they were trained. As medical schools develop community models for training students in both urban and rural areas, using paraprofessional health teams effectively, young physicians will be better prepared for dealing with the types of problems they may confront in underdoctored areas. The development of such teaching models can be encouraged through financial incentives to medical schools interested in developing these areas.

Medicine, of course, is no longer a solitary activity, and sustaining a practice without supporting facilities is extremely frustrating for the physician. Doctors are more likely to remain in underdoctored areas if they are supported by adequate facilities and ancillary manpower. These areas cannot support the facilities characteristic of the urban medical center, but they must be sufficiently developed to allow a reasonable translation of modern medicine to the population. Also, attention must be given to means to alleviate the tremendous work load that doctors in underserviced areas are likely to face. Here, such paraprofessional support as nurse practitioners, physician assistants, and technicians may be the difference between a hopeless and viable medical situation.

The problems of locating doctors in many underserviced areas go beyond the conditions of practice and involve the social and cultural amenities available to their families: the quality of schools and cultural opportunities, for instance. Often the families may feel more isolated than the physicians themselves. Here we have a good deal to learn from programs outside medicine that locate professional personnel in areas of need. They characteristically develop opportunities such as "home leave" to insure that such personnel do not become too isolated. A major program designed to service underdoctored areas might provide sabbaticals and a corps of physicians who substitute for such doctors while they attend postgraduate education courses or just get a breather. Also, it would be possible to use cable television, video tape, and other technologies to reduce the feeling of isolation; and it may be feasible to

* This discussion assumes that doctors practicing in underserviced areas have the potential to earn incomes comparable to those practicing in other areas. In most cases this assumption is reasonable, but in situations where there is inadequate income potential, it is possible to guarantee minimum incomes if necessary. The relative opportunities to earn a good income in underdoctored and other areas are likely to have some effect on the willingness of physicians to "buy out" their contractual obligations.

develop regional networks of physicians working in underdoctored areas and thus allow them opportunities for seminars, visiting one another's practices, and the like. There is a variety of possibilities for providing support, encouragement, and advice to the extent that this is needed.

In outlining the plan for redistribution, I have left out a variety of details that would support such a plan. I have neglected, for example, the issue of recruiting students from a wider range of geographic contexts and social and economic backgrounds. Also, I have ignored administrative matters such as how to insure that we reward more than existing inclinations to settle in underdoctored areas or how we administer compliance. These are important but not particularly difficult matters. Such incentive plans never work perfectly, and some problems are likely to develop. Thus, in evaluating any proposal, we must compare it to other options and not to some unrealistic ideal.

I must emphasize that as long as we follow our current course, there is no chance that we will make significant inroads in coping with the problem of geographic distribution of physicians. Indeed, as older physicians die and retire, it is likely that the maldistribution that presently exists will become even more pronounced. Similarly, it seems that in the foreseeable future the United States is unlikely to develop the type of national health program that will include forceful manpower distribution policies. The value of the proposed plan is that it offers an opportunity to achieve an important national goal without violating major values and in a manner consistent with the existing organization of the health sector. To fail to do even this much is to accept maldistribution of physicians as a permanent feature of health services in America.

Notes

1. Mason, H. (1971). "Effectiveness of Student Aid Programs Tied to a Service Commitment." *Journal of Medical Education*, **46:**575–583.
2. Dube, W., et al. (1971). "Study of U.S. School Applicants." *Journal of Medical Education*, **46:**837–857.

CHAPTER XVIII

Toward a Viable National System of Delivering Health Services

---

The major issues in health care delivery are usually described as access, quality, and financing. Each, however, can be understood only in reference to the others, and any attempt to alter one or another dimension carries profound implications for the total system. Thus far—because of the absence of any coherent national health policy—we have gone in all directions at once, pursuing policies that are inherently contradictory. For example, we are substantially increasing the number of physicians on the assumption that primary care largely will be delivered by physicians; at the same time, we are encouraging a wide variety of physician extenders on the premise that the substance of primary care is unlikely to be of interest to most scientifically trained physicians. If, indeed, the most appropriate model for primary care is to rely extensively on nonphysician manpower, then the projected increase in physicians is probably not warranted; however, if we take the position that a physician is the most appropriate person to deal with the ordinary medical complaint, then the new enthusiasm for extenders may be excessive. In any case, we have been quite unwilling to develop a national policy on this issue—as with so many others—and the policy of going in all directions at once is usually justified on the basis of diversity and pluralism.

This tendency to go in every direction at once and to avoid any unitary national policy has led many persons to refer to American medical care as a "nonsystem." This designation is a poor one because it fails to take into account the extent to which the current organization of medicine consciously reflects social and ideological priorities held by large numbers of decision makers in health care. Certainly there is a very strong feeling among those with more conservative economic views that an emphasis on diversity and competition enhances the quality of care and the responsiveness of health institutions to the persons who use them. It is also apparent, however, that the outcome of such priorities results in inequalities in care and other abuses. In considering the necessary direction for a coherent health policy we should keep in mind the abuses that are characteristic of our present system as well as a highly centralized one, and we should seek policies that best balance the advantages and risks of each approach.

Before considering these questions, in order to get a perspective, let us consider how, within the same ideological context, the thinking about human services institutions can go in opposite directions. As a professor at a large university, I am impressed with the extent to which students, the articulate public, and many faculty members have been rebelling against the use of professor extenders (i.e., teaching assistants). Increasingly, it has been maintained that the most experienced professors ought to spend more time with introductory students as compared with graduate students, and that they should teach basic as compared with more specialized courses. It has also been maintained that universities should depend on nothing less than "fully qualified" faculty. In contrast, in medicine and other helping professions, it is maintained that physicians are too expensive to provide many of the services that can be delivered by less qualified and less expensive personnel. It is impressive how frequently one meets persons rebelling against the use of professor extenders but urging the use of physician extenders. I believe that this contradiction goes quite deeply, and that much of the new enthusiasm for one or another solution is as much determined by fashion and the pressures of the times as by serious examination of the institutions involved and the advantages and liabilities of pursuing one approach or another.

In considering the use of extenders, it is clear that they allow a more efficient use of resources in a variety of settings. Indeed, specialization either across occupations or within professions usually results in each procedure being performed more expertly. As the specialization becomes more elaborate, problems in communication and coordination of varying services may develop. But perhaps the greatest difficulty with too elaborate an allocation of tasks is that each worker, in performing his part, loses sight of the whole and, indeed, he may have little expert knowledge outside his own area. The advantage of a physician generalist is that, presumably, he has had sufficient training and experience to develop competence as a problem solver. It is anticipated that he knows enough and has sufficient skills to adapt to changing knowledge and to know how to obtain information about new problems. To the extent that one trains extenders to do specific jobs, it is less likely that one will develop a group of professionals of sufficient experience and judgment to, respond effectively or flexibly to changing needs. Extenders may be used in a very fruitful way to increase the productivity of physicians or to supplement their usual activities. I am very skeptical, however, of the use of extenders as a substitute for physician services in the American context. Although this may be the only way in the foreseeable future to bring medical services to people in the underdeveloped countries, the United States has the resources and physician manpower to bring physician services to every American. I believe that a decent health policy would have sufficient direction to achieve this goal.

No system of health care in the world is willing to devote an unlimited amount of its resources to medical care as opposed to other needs. All systems must have some way of limiting the expenditure of its resources. In highly centralized systems, decisions are made as to how much to devote to the medical sector, and it is the limitation of resources that holds costs down. Other systems, like our own, allocate resources largely in terms of the market for medical services, and economic barriers are important filters that control the use of the health care system. The difficulty with such economic filters is that they affect both important and trivial instances of illness, and they encourage delay in seeking necessary treatment.

The persons who urge competition in the delivery of health services as a way of bringing down medical care costs believe that the market can very much increase equity by forcing greater responsiveness, more efficiency, and more rapid adoption of innovations that reduce costs. They have repeatedly pointed out that a cost reimbursement system of payment offers no incentives for a more effective application of resources.[1] It is highly unlikely that the assumptions of a free market system can be approximated in the health care system even with major modifications in licensing, the availability of information, and the like.[2] Yet, it is not unlikely that greater competition could bring prices down even in a market that is very imperfect. But other disadvantages might be incurred in achieving greater price competition.

If the health care market were corrected to allow greater competition among units delivering care, it is conceivable that, although the price per unit of service declines, the number of units of service delivered would substantially increase.[3] Since health units will require a certain scale of operations to remain viable—and each, therefore, will require a substantial income—one way of adjusting to such needs is to generate more work. Medical care is a highly discretionary activity, allowing for considerable latitude in the services performed, the amount of follow-up, and in a variety of other matters. Thus, a competitive situation may lead to a lower price per unit of service that may benefit some patients but a greater overall cost as each unit generates work to maintain its market situation.

In most areas of the economy the generation of additional demand is seen by many as reasonable or desirable. If competition among the airlines encourages proposals to stimulate travel and vacations—thus resulting in the airlines increasing their passenger miles—it is difficult to maintain that the outcome is harmful or undesirable. Or if people are encouraged to buy various consumer goods, the expenditures may not be particularly wise but neither are they particularly dangerous. In contrast, the generation of medical demand or unnecessary surgical care may have major undesirable consequences for individuals and society. Thus, in evaluating the economic argument, it is important to consider not only price but total expenditures; and total cost should have a reasonable relationship to careful assessments of the services that people need.

The industry most similar to medical care in this respect is the drug industry, and we can to some extent visualize the consequences for medical care resulting from the introduction of greater competitiveness among firms. A wide range of drugs is readily available to the population, although price is maintained at high levels for various drugs through different regulatory and monopolistic devices. Even though many useless drugs and combinations of drugs are produced, companies show little interest in nonprofitable pharmaceuticals for which the market is very limited. The more common drugs are produced in a variety of forms and are vigorously advertised to promote use. Although many drugs have undesirable side effects and are a major cause of disease, pharmaceuticals are promoted frequently in a promiscuous and irresponsible fashion in respect to both the consumer and the physician. The competitiveness of the industry and the desire to maximize profits result in a vigorous effort to encourage the use of drugs for almost any symptom, and drug advertising is highly prevalent in the media.

The issue of the promiscuous sales of drugs is sometimes confused with the related issue of whether the American public is too promiscuous or too stoical in its attitudes toward drug use. The question, as such, is a meaningless one, since the issue is not whether persons take too many or too few drugs, but whether the use of drugs is appropriate to need and whether, in a particular case, drugs offer a greater probability of relief of distress and symptoms than potential damage. There are clearly many Americans who could benefit from a particular class of drugs, but who are reluctant to use them for a variety of reasons including a certain stoicism. But knowing that such a group may exist hardly argues for promiscuous encouragement of dangerous drug use for dealing with ordinary types of daily distress. This is particularly true in the case of short-term, self-limited conditions and normal life stresses. In a context in which it is difficult for the consumer to make informed judgments about the benefits and risks of taking a specific action, competition in sales promotion can have perverse and pathological effects.

Much of the justification for regulation over medical care is that consumers are not in the position to make detailed choices, in view of the complexity of medical care services. More recently, economists have argued that with more information consumers can make reasonable choices, and they have encouraged greater competitiveness among providers and lesser public controls.

These economists maintain that, since quality of care is intangible and since physicians have difficulty in agreeing among themselves on such issues, the choice should be made by consumers.

In my view, this position is naive and discounts many essential questions. As some conservative economists would have it, the purchase of medical care is not essentially different than the purchase of a camera or television set. They maintain that most consumers know as little about these goods as they do about medical care, yet the market mechanism works quite well. It should be evident that in contrast to the purchase of these consumer goods, medical care potentially has greater importance for the person, is usually characterized by greater anxiety and emotional involvement, and is not a discrete purchase but may involve a complicated set of additional decisions contingent on the first. Instead of venturing assumptions about what decisions consumers can and cannot reasonably make on the basis of theoretical dogma, it is necessary to examine more carefully the many facets of medical care in its various stages in respect to possible consumer choice.

Various studies of consumers' views of medical care indicate that patients seek physicians who are "competent" and "interested in them."[4] When patients are asked to elaborate on the meaning of "interest," it becomes clear that they refer not only to demeanor but also the accessibility of the physician when he is needed. Varying dimensions of physician services seem to be important, depending on the circumstances and the persons involved. Some studies suggest that for routine needs, consumers frequently seek a physician sufficiently accessible to minimize their costs of time and effort in obtaining the necessary services.[5] Some persons also give greater importance to rapid accessibility than to continuity or other features of service. For illnesses of a life-threatening character or for those that have a high element of fear, such as impending surgery, confidence in the physician is a major consideration for many patients. This is reflected, for example, in the high rate of use of surgical services outside of prepaid health plans by members of such plans.[6] Thus, when an illness is sufficiently threatening, many consumers appear to be willing to pay a high price for alleged competence or the feeling of confidence in a particular physician.

In considering what choices might be open to patients in seeking medical care, it is necessary to consider the components of care involved in patient-physician interaction. When a patient seeks care from a physician, the physician must consider the complaint, must undertake necessary tests and other diagnostic procedures, must seek consultation if needed, and must decide on further care, hospitalization if necessary, therapy, and the like. When patients seek the assistance of a physician, the initial choice implies that they purchase an entire package of care, including the physician's services, his judgment about additional necessary care, and his hospital and colleague affiliations.

Once the basic choice of a physician is made, it is not clear how consumers can realistically have a great deal to say about the tests to be ordered, whether hospitalization is necessary, and how the condition should be treated, for example. At the margins, physicians should indicate possible choices to patients when reasonable options exist, but in general the patient must trust to the physician to make choices in his best interest. In view of the realities of medical practice and its organization, once the choice of a physician is made, patients have relatively little to say about additional services needed, the use of one or another hospital (unless the physician has a choice to offer), or the ultimate cost of treatment for a particular illness. They can, of course, change doctors, ignore medical advice, or even shop around for a doctor who will follow instructions, but these options really do not get to the core of decision making in medical situations.

The view that patients should make decisions because treatment is an uncertain process is unrealistic for a variety of reasons. First, as discussed earlier in this volume, distress is frequently associated with illness and seeking medical care. Persons who are anxious and upset are frequently not in a position to make complex and difficult decisions about their own care. Second, in complex situations with considerable uncertainty, one seeks the best judgment obtainable. It is because there is complexity and uncertainty that consumers require the physician's judgment and experience in making such decisions. If quality of care could be objectively formulated and precisely stated, it would be more simple. However, if the decisions are difficult for experienced physicians, how can we reasonably expect laymen to make wise choices? It is, of course, the physician's responsibility to consult the patient, to seek relevant information from him, and to communicate possible options. But the burden of such decisions cannot reasonably be placed on patients. Finally, we must recognize that when people are ill or greatly involved in a situation, decisions are frequently difficult to make. It is no accident that physicians ordinarily do not take care of their immediate families or treat serious illnesses of their own. An important component of the physician's role and his value to the patient is partly a result of the fact that he assumes responsibility that relieves the patient's stress.

On the assumption that consumers make detailed choices, many economists have placed emphasis on deductibles and coinsurance as mechanisms to limit "unreasonable demand" and to ration more generally the proliferation of service. The assumption is frequently made that if services are free at the point of entry, the system will be flooded by trivial conditions and hypochondriacs.[7]*

---

* The discussion of price rationing of medical services is not dependent on the assumption that those using more services at lower prices are more likely to be hypochondriacs. Economists, in focusing on cost problems, tend to concern themselves with developing mechanisms to control utilization. The main issue is the various costs and benefits of imposing barriors to the patient's access in contrast to incentives which affect the physician's behavior.

It is maintained that the cost barrier will serve as a sieve to screen out persons who are not "really sick," or who do not really need or value the service. The contention that medical care is a type of service that persons who are "not sick" will seek for its own sake is a dubious one, but since this is widely assumed, let us proceed on this basis. It follows from this argument that patients have the knowledge or expertise to understand when they are "really sick," and that economic barriers allow a rational selection into care.

Apparently economic barriers have varying effects on persons in different socioeconomic groups, and frequently they keep seriously ill persons from seeking care or encourage delay. Also, if determinations of who is "really sick" are as clear as some imply, why is it that physicians have great difficulty making determinations on such matters? The assumption that patients should be their own doctors and presume to know the meaning and consequence of symptoms is difficult to justify. It seems fully reasonable that when persons are worried they should have access to someone qualified to answer their concerns. Indeed, this is what physicians and public health practitioners have been urging the public to do for decades.

Providing ready access to a practitioner is not particularly expensive. What makes access expensive is the decisions the physician makes, once the patient arrives. Because physicians are gatekeepers of an elaborate technological system, they have considerable choice in the measures they take to detect illness, to provide care, and to maintain surveillance. And it is these decisions that make care costly. Costs are high partly because of the nature of medical technology and the types of diagnostic strategies used by physicians, and partly because determining whether the patient is "really sick" is no easy matter. But an informed decision is more sensible than an uninformed one, and if cost controls are to be imposed, they ought to be rational controls. It is more rational to encourage physicians to establish controls on the basis of established knowledge over unnecessary diagnostic and therapeutic decisions than it is to encourage patients to be their own doctors. In short, we need an approach to primary medical care that is responsive to patients' concerns but that also is based on sound principles of scientific medical care.

Rational Controls over Medical Demand

I believe that a rational system to control costs must involve incentives affecting how physician decisions are made. It must do this in a way that does not elaborate medical bureaucracy or interfere seriously with the morale, judgement, or flexibility of the physician. Thus the system must be structured to facilitate patients entering primary care, and limitations on the elaboration of medical care must follow in some fashion from physician decision making. In my view, the best mechanism to do this is to develop a situation where physicians work with a specified budget and must establish priorities within economic limits. Also, by holding health professionals responsible for the health needs of a specified population, it is more possible to plan reasonably, to monitor needs and performance, and to deal with special problems that arise. A health service, organized in terms of population areas, also is the most reasonable way to provide services that are responsive to the entire population.

Any model of organizing health systems involves difficulties. As long as physicians are paid agents of individual patients and as long as third parties pay the costs of care, physicians are unlikely to limit expensive decisions which in their judgement yield any benefits to the patient. One way of getting around the issue is to make it personally costly for physicians to provide marginal increments of care, as some HMO proposals would allegedly do.[8] But putting the patient's interests in conflict with those of the physician might produce pressures toward insufficient care and unwillingness to undertake expensive lifesaving measures, and may increase suspiciousness between doctor and patient as well as the patient's insecurities.

The rationing of services through planning can be an uncertain process and, without proper protections, can lead to the failure to meet patients' needs; or the structure of priorities can come to reflect professional in contrast to clients' interests. Thus, it is essential that planning and allocation of resources follow certain guidelines that take into account the possible conflicts between the needs of patients and professionals. Such systems, however structured, should insure every person in the defined area a minimal but reasonable guaranteed level of services including ready access to the system.

The priorities established by professionals should focus on the allocation of resources for care beyond initial access. The guidelines that govern or restrain such decisions should be based on medical knowledge on which there is considerable medical consensus. Rational guidelines would control the performance of procedures that are of dubious value and may be dangerous as well. These guidelines should set broad standards, allowing for considerable professional discretion; and, within situations where proper management remains uncertain, professional judgement should be very extensive. Limits might include dangerous therapies that are of unknown or questionnable effect. Evaluations of important but uncertain therapies should be performed through well-controlled and rigorous investigations amply funded, but budgeted separately from service programs.

I could elaborate on how such guidelines might be developed, but it seems more appropriate that they develop from within the medical community itself. Presently, there are limited restrictions on how physicians treat patients or few mechanisms to intervene even when there is widespread belief that the physician is behaving irresponsibly. Such mechanisms are necessary, but they must be constructed carefully so that attempts to regulate the small number of irresponsible professionals do not impede the profession as a whole. In short, guidelines are necessary, but they must not overly bureaucratize professional practice or impose petty restrictions and controls over the doctor's practice. Before a guideline is imposed, it must be weighed—like any other intervention —in terms of its potential gains and costs. Petty restrictions can be seriously damaging to morale, innovation, and to responsible professional behavior.

The idea of a fixed budget is attractive to many observers because it offers a potential opportunity to control the trend of increasing medical care costs. The English National Health Service, to some extent, has controlled costs in this way, although they too have not been able to avoid rising investments in medical care. But a certain caution is necessary, since it is highly likely that Americans would insist on a relatively high level of minimal service, and I doubt that they would find acceptable the average level of services and amenities available to the English population through the National Health Service.

I think that it is the responsibility of government to insure a reasonable minimal level of health care service and to see that essential services reach all people in need. What is "minimal" and "essential" to one may not be to another and, in any case, coverage is an issue that must be openly debated. But the principle of working to establish a floor of services directs our thinking and provides a criterion to evaluate various proposals for extending services to the American population.

In an affluent country like the United States one can anticipate that many people will seek amenities above and beyond a reasonable minimal floor. Thus I assume that whatever national system develops, there will continue to be substantial private investment in the purchase of health services. Assuming that the national system provided a reasonable level of care—acceptable to the average American—private competition could be constructive in maintaining quality incentives within the system. In all probability, Americans would be quite demanding of medical services and would be very critical of a system that departed too much from competing alternatives. Moreover, the system of care must be of sufficient quality to attract middle-class consumers, or we face the danger of institutionalizing two levels of medical care. An important function of establishing budgetary priorities is that it carries incentives to develop a more appropriate allocation of tasks among the specialties and between physicians and other health workers, and it offers an opportunity to provide more continuous and comprehensive care.

Organization in terms of a fixed budgetary allowance is only one of many conditions necessary to achieve balanced priorities and rational and efficient forms of organization. We are all aware of how stifling and incompetent bureaucratic organizations can be and how they can be bogged down in petty and burdensome rules and lack of initiative. We know from various experiences that, without adequate additional incentives, persons working on salaried systems may not put forth the effort or responsiveness characteristic of persons whose payment is more closely tied to performance. Specifically, studies of physicians and organized practice suggest that physicians on other than fee-for-service arrangements may be less responsive to patients and their feelings, and may tend to work shorter hours.[9-11] It is also true, however, that rewards only tied specifically to physician responsiveness may encourage unnecessary and dangerous work with the physician catering to patients' desires rather than to high standards of technical care.[12] Thus we seek some kind of optimal balance.

It would not be very difficult to develop mechanisms to reward salaried physicians for working longer hours or performing one or another activity. Modifications of remuneration schedules can achieve these ends. From my standpoint, the quality of service and the impersonality of patient care are more significant problems, and we must devote greater attention toward these problems. Salaried systems in noncompetitive service organizations significantly diminish any semblance of client control and encourage physicians and hospitals to treat patients in an uncaring and impersonal way. To correct such abuses it is necessary to define appropriate standards of demeanor and behavior, and make clear to personnel that they will be evaluated by these criteria in the determination of remuneration and other rewards. Moreover, efforts must be made to facilitate the expression of consumers' feelings concerning improper and unsympathetic care and to provide feedback to professional personnel.

For example, some component of physicians' remuneration, as well as that of other personnel, might be determined by merit evaluations made by supervisors, peers, and clients. The formula for remuneration might be based on the evaluations of varying groups—each applying criteria within their competence. Thus supervisors and peers might evaluate on the criteria of knowledge, technical quality of care, and cooperation in team efforts; while clients might evaluate on the basis of interest, consideration, and responsiveness. The exact features of these evaluations are not crucial, but it is reasonably clear that remuneration should probably include incentive features, at least in some part. Such incentive systems may be based on money, rank, prestige, honors, and the like. They may include features like the merit remuneration scheme used in England to reward outstanding medical consultants[13] or those used in distinguished universities to keep tenured professors active. But they must also include significant consumer input because, without such input, the system of rewards comes to maintain a set of professional standards that may not be equivalent to the public's definition of a high level of performance. It is essential, however, that patients' input be in relation to criteria that they are capable of judging, and whatever system we develop should not assume their ability to judge in areas where they lack competence. While consumers should have an important voice in determining the nature of the formula by which rewards are distributed, each criterion should be applied by persons best qualified to make the judgment.

Whatever internal reward systems are developed in the aggregate to encourage effective and responsive behavior, they may not fit the needs of a particular patient. A medical care system that fails to offer significant choice to both professionals and patients is likely to be a stagnant one and one with many unhappy recipients. Thus, no matter how medical care is organized, and under whatever authorities, it must be sufficiently diversified to offer choices to patients and professionals who may have different needs and orientations. We must develop a structured form of competition that encourages different ways of achieving goals within limitations that protect against the more gross abuses of the competitive process and tightly organized centralization. Some have maintained that there is no fundamental difference between nonprofit and profit-oriented organizations in that personnel in both pursue their self-interest. Although it is quite possible for organizational participants to pursue personal goals at the expense of public goals in nonprofit organizations, these organizations allow greater direction over the nature of the competitive process and thus, if they develop incentives carefully, can facilitate a more constructive form of competition.

In discussing various approaches to developing a national system of health care, I have purposely evaded specific proposals now receiving public attention. In reading the various legislation put before the Congress I am impressed by how difficult it is to responsibly project what the administration, quality, and costs would be in practice. Experience tells us that what may appear impressive on paper is frequently disappointing in reality. Obviously judgments must be made, but I have chosen not to deal with these issues here. However, certain clear principles emerge from this discussion that have bearing on any proposal for developing a national system of health care. First, the national government has responsibility for insuring entitlement for all Americans to a reasonable minimum of services. The development of coverage must, in my view, reflect this responsibility, and comprehensiveness must be built from a floor of services for all Americans. Thus, in constructing any program of coverage, the issue should be the essential services people need and not population categories or particular diseases and disabilities. Second, the basic budget for providing essential services must be developed relative to defined populations, and competing priorities for any population must be resolved within the context of known and available resources. The basic priorities in reference to any defined population must be decided jointly by providers and consumers, but the system must be structured to avoid petty restrictions and interference with professional discretion, and incentives must be developed that insure both technical quality and responsiveness. The distribution of professional and other personnel must be based on realistic assessment of need for varying specialties and types of manpower, and financing for education must take into account the various shortages and excesses. Finally, the system must be structured to allow ready primary access to persons who are worried, uncertain, and sick, but rational controls must be established in relation to the decision-making process, once the patient is in the system. Various criteria may seem to be in conflict. We obviously cannot maximize each of these aspects simultaneously. What we seek is a realistic balance that reflects the goals for which we strive.

As I write this, future support for the basic sciences in health, health care, and government-financed health programs looks bleak. I emphasize that much of medical activity remains uncertain, and we still know relatively little, compared to what it is possible to know about relieving distress and curing disease. In the long range it is shortsighted to deemphasize efforts that will determine the effectiveness of health services in the future, since the product delivered is only as good as the knowledge on which it is based. In seeking solutions, it is essential to balance both short-range and long-term considerations. Here I refer not only to research in the basic biological sciences and in medical technology but also to the behavioral factors that affect the morbidity of populations and use of health services.

In the last analysis, the work of health professionals is determined largely by the problems people present and the conceptions they have of medical services. There are persons who will contest my thesis that basic access to the system of health care must be open to those who are worried and feel in need of assistance. They discredit such persons by designating them as hypochondriacs, crocks, malingerers, and neurotics. But we must remain constantly aware that medicine is a sustaining profession in a context where our social institutions are becoming more and more bureaucratized and impersonal. The use of physicians stems from many needs and varying motives. The fact that the form basic primary services take may not, in the long run, make much difference to objective health status and longevity is not crucial because the consequences flow from what men define as reality, not reality itself. Obviously, we seek to apply our skills and knowledge in the most useful and effective way we can. But if we fail to appreciate the larger functions of medicine in society and to structure health institutions to nurture these functions, medical care will be mediocre, no matter how impressive its technical virtues.

Notes

1. Lave, J., and L. Lave (1970). "Medical Care and Its Delivery: An Economic Appraisal." *Law and Contemporary Problems*, **35**:252–266.
2. Fuchs, V. (1972). "Health Care and the United States Economic System: An Essay in Abnormal Physiology." *Milbank Memorial Fund Quarterly*, **50**:211–237.

3. For an illustration of increased demand generated by physicians, see Fuchs, V., and M. Kramer (1972). *Determinants of Expenditures for Physicians' Services in the United States, 1948-68.* Washington, D.C.: National Center for Health Services Research and Development, DHEW Publication No. HSM 73-3013. Also see Fuchs, V. (ed.) (1972). *Essays in the Economics of Health and Medical Care.* New York: National Bureau of Economic Research, Columbia University Press.

4. Mechanic, D. (1968). *Medical Sociology: A Selective View.* New York: Free Press.

5. Donabedian, A. (1965). *A Review of Some Experiences with Prepaid Group Practice.* School of Public Health, Ann Arbor, Michigan, Research Series No. 12.

6. Donabedian, A., *ibid.*

7. Schwartz, H. (1972). *The Case for American Medicine.* New York: McKay.

8. See Mechanic, D. (1972). *Public Expectations and Health Care.* New York: Wiley-Interscience, pp. 102-111.

9. Bailey, R. (1970). "Economics of Scale in Medical Practice." In H. E. Klarman (ed.), *Empirical Studies in Health Economics.* Baltimore: Johns Hopkins Press. And "Philosophy, Faith and Fiction in the Production of Medical Services." *Inquiry,* 7:37-53.

10. Mechanic, D. (1971). "Physician Satisfaction in Varying Settings." Manpower Conference, National Center for Health Services Research and Development, Chicago, Ill.

11. Enterline, P., et al. (1973). "Effects of 'Free' Medical Care on Medical Practice—The Quebec Experience." *New England Journal of Medicine.* **288:**1152-1155.

12. Freidson, E. (1963). "Medical Care and the Public: Case Study of a Medical Group." *Annals of the American Academy of Political and Social Science,* **346:**57-66.

13. Stevens, R. (1966). *Medical Pradtice in Modern England.* New Haven: Yale University Press.

Index

293

British Medical Guild, 92, 96, 103
British Medical Journal, 141
Brown, F., 128, 134
Brown, G. W., 216
Brucellosis, 134
Bryce Hospital, 233
Buchenwald, 169
Bureaucracy, 14, 51, 206, 218, 240, 246, 251, 285, 287, 290
  and organization of medicine, 14, 118
  procedures of, 209, 214, 223
  sponsorship of, 13
  Weber's concept of, 206

Canada, 37, 41, 43, 94
Cancer, 14
Capetown, 31
Capitation payments, 119–120
Careers in medicine, 274
Cartwright, A., 142, 145
Case-finding, 184–185
Catastrophic services, 4
Categorical programs, 4
Catholics, 77
Centralized systems, 281
Certification of illness, 102, 160
"Charter for the Family Doctor Service," 93
Child development, 267
Child guidance movement, 230
Children, 60, 136, 181
China, 3, 37, 38–39, 41
Chronic complainer, 134–137
Civil commitment of the mentally ill, 183, 234, 243
Clausen, J., 183
Client control, 120, 255
Clinical interview, 172
Clinical judgments, 13
Clinical research, 180
Co-insurance, 4, 51, 284
Coleman, J., 105
Collective action, 170
Collective bargaining, 170
College of General Practitioners, 106, 153, 156, 158
Colombotos, J., 69
Commercial advertising, 268
Commitment of organizational personnel, 208, 214, 217, 219, 222–223

Commitment of the mentally ill, 183, 234, 243
Commitments to serve in underdoctored areas, 273–274
Communication, 15, 136, 280
Communication appeals, 135–136, 267–268
Community care facilities, 241
Community care movement, 231
Community care of the mentally ill, 190, 193, 215, 231–232
Community control, 213
Community expectations, 211
Community "institutionalism," 232
Community leaders, 185–186
Community mental health centers, 193, 203, 209, 211, 215, 217, 223, 231, 234
Community networks, 185
Community psychiatry ideology, 231, 246
Community representation, 56
Compensation, 176
Competence to stand trial, 243
Competition, 175, 280–282, 287, 289
Complaints, bodily, 123–137
  social acceptability of, 131–132
  timing of, 115
  trivial, 14, 51, 102, 116, 142, 146
Compliance structures, 206
Comprehensive services, 51, 287
Concentration camps, 168, 170
Conflicting interests, 47
Conformity with medical advice, 252, 254
Congress, 256, 289
Constitutional rights, 227, 233
Constitutional standards, 233–234
Consultants in the National Health Service, 90–91, 94
Consulting specialties, 38, 48
Consumers, decisions of, 283–284
  expression of feelings by, 288
  knowledge of, 263–264
  middle-class, 287
Contraceptives, 10
Convalescence, 134
Cooperation, 168, 170
  with physicians, 65–66
Coping, 128–129, 132, 137, 166, 168, 170–172, 183–184, 189, 190, 195, 216, 222
  among doctors, 161
  capabilities, 166

Hypothesis of convergence, 37
Hysterectomy, 131
Hysteria, 131

Iatrogenic disease, 14
"Ideal types," 206
Identification, 127–128
Ideology, 1, 3, 37–44, 208
Idiopathic endomyocardial fibrosis in South Africa, 23
Illness, attributional processes in, 123–137
emotional factors in, 101, 116
reactive component in, 134
subjective aspects of, 119
Illness-avoiding behaviors, 266
Illness behavior, 11–13, 183–184, 191
Illness-detection behaviors, 267
Imboden, J. B., 134
Immunization, 263
in South Africa, 26
Inactivity, 15, 189–190, 193, 215–216
physical, 264
Incentives, 4–5, 42, 48, 53, 119–120, 281, 284–285, 287–288
for change in organizations, 3–5
financial, 51
quality, 287
societal, 189
in treatment of alcoholics, 195
Incentive systems, 166
Incidence, 191
Income, inequalities of in South Africa, 25
of physicians, 77, 93
redistribution of, 3
Incompetency to stand trial, 183
Indentured service in South Africa, 25
Indicators of general well-being, 185
Individualism, 228
Individualized treatment plans, 233, 240–241
Industrialization, 229
Industrial medicine, 2
Industrial work groups, 209
Infant mortality, 16, 40
in South Africa, 14, 26, 28
Inflatable air-bag, 262
Influence processes, 182, 196
Influenza, 134
Informal networks, 211–212
Informal structure, 208–214

Informal work groups, 205
Information programs, 265
Information systems, 54
"Informed consent," 64–65
Ingelfinger, F., 62–64
Innovations, 218, 240, 257–258
adoption of, 258, 281
diffusion of, 265
in the effective use of manpower, 251
receptivity to, 69–87
Insanity plea, 239
Insomnia, 135, 192
Instructions in medical care, 136–137
Interagency relationships, 205, 211–213
Interest groups, 48, 53
Intergenerational conflict, 196
Internists, 49, 69–87, 271
Intervening processes, 190–191
Interview studies, response biases in, 186
Involuntary hospitalization, 227, 232–233, 237, 239, 243–245
reform of, 244–246
Irish, 130, 258
Italians, 130, 134, 258

Jacksonian society, 228
Jews, 78, 130–131, 258
Johannesburg, 23, 25, 27, 30–31
Judicial action, 227–246

Kennedy, Senator Edward, 42
Kenyon, F. E., 126
Kerckhoff, A. C., 131
Kidney disease, 4
Knowledge, about disease, 11
uncertainty of, 55
Kogon, E., 169
Kwashiorkor, 27

Labeling theory, 189
Laboratory studies, 175
Labor government in England, 93
Labor party in England, 92
Ladee, G. A., 128
Lancet, The, 106
Langlie, J., 266
Lay therapists, 195
Leadership groups, 221
Learning theories, 182
Leeuwkop Prison, 31–32

"Legal insanity," 243
Legislatures, 53, 234, 245–246
Lemert, E., 182
Length of stay in hospitals, 44, 136, 193
Leonard, R., 60, 62, 136, 173
Licensing, 16
Life changes, 189
Life stress, 282
List size among English general practitioners, 152, 158
Loan forgiveness programs, 272, 275
London, 39
Loneliness, 132, 174
Loyalty, 208, 210, 218

Males, 130, 196
Malingerers, 117
Malnutrition in South Africa, 23–24, 25–27
Management, of health care systems, 3
of the patient, 15
Manpower, 4, 14, 290
allocation of, 38
redistribution of, 52, 277
roles of, 251
Marijuana, 265
Market mechanisms, 283
Mason, H., 272
Matching programs, 236
Measles in South Africa, 26
Mechanic, D., 132
Medicaid, 4, 41, 69, 236
Medical care, accessibility of, 4–5, 12–13, 39, 47–49, 120, 121, 264, 271, 275, 286, 290
and social values, 9–10
as a "nonsystem," 279
as a right, 235
consumers' views of, 283
controls over, 286
convergences in organization, 41
coordination of, 4, 16, 39, 42, 280
costs of, 39–41, 43–44, 51–52, 66, 170, 262, 281–282, 285, 287
curative system of, 261
demand for, 281–282
distribution of, 3, 14–15, 17, 40, 47, 287
diversification of, 289
effectiveness of, 43–44
efficiency of, 43–44, 240, 251

fragmentation of, 39
functions of, 5, 290
guidelines for, 286–287
impersonality of, 288
inequalities in, 41, 280
influence on quality of health, 17
in South Africa, 23, 27–31
investments in, 287
legislation, 54
organizations, 12, 17, 37–44, 55–56
planning, 52–55
preventive services, 4, 11–13, 136, 262–263, 266
preventive services in South Africa, 26, 28, 30
primary, see Primary care
private investment in, 287
quality of, 5, 47, 49, 118, 143, 159, 279–280, 283–284, 288
rationing of, 286
regulation of, 282
responsiveness of, 14–15, 118, 286
use of pharmacists, 253–254
utilization of, 11–13, 130–131, 174, 281, 283–284
Medical care research, 59–67
Medical colleagues, consultation with, 102, 104
Medical College Admission Test, 272
Medical demand, generation of, 282, 285
rational controls over, 285–290
Medical education, 16–17, 37–38, 63, 66, 79, 82, 274
in Britain, 95
postgraduate, 48, 79, 86, 149, 156
public financing of, 52
Medical errors, 118
Medical facilities, inclination to use, 132
Medical functions, distribution of, 48–49
Medical history, 117
Medical judgments, 13
Medical knowledge, uncertainty of, 161
Medical labeling, consequences of, 13–15
Medical model, 180–181, 209, 244
Medical monopoly, 240
Medical organization in South Africa, 22–27
Medical politics, 50
Medical practice, controls over, 240–241
educational models of, 276

Social workers, 14, 118, 210, 251
Societal reactions, 182, 189
Socioeconomic factors, 11–13, 131, 184
Sociological research in medicine, 64–66
Solo practice of medicine, 251, 253
South Africa, 21–35
    Asians in, 21
    birth control programs in, 28
    curative clinics in, 28
    dehydrated infants in, 29
    discriminatory wage, 25
    disregard of human factors in, 32–33
    distribution of physicians in, 22
    distribution of wealth in, 14
    economic status in, 21
    fertility in, 28
    health status in, 21–35
    immunization in, 26
    indentured service in, 25
    infant mortality in, 14, 26, 28
    malnutrition in, 23–27
    medical care in, 22–31
    medical schools in, 22, 31
    mission hospitals in, 29
    nutritional status in, 23
    pass laws in, 24, 32
    patterns of disease in, 14
    physical and mental growth in, 23, 26
    police in, 24
    political intimidation in, 30
    poverty in, 33–34
    preventive service in, 26, 28, 30
    primary care in, 30
    prisons in, 31–32
    protein-calorie deficiency disease in, 25
    reserves in, 23–24, 26
    resettlement areas in, 26
    segregation in, 22–23
    social services in, 25, 28
    tuberculosis in, 26–27
    wage gap in, 24–25
Soviet Union, 2, 37–39, 41
Soweto, 23, 25, 27, 32
Specialization, 14, 16, 37–39, 48–49, 118, 141, 271–272, 280
Specialty boards, 79, 85–86
Standard of living, 17
Standards, 4–5, 233, 237–242
State government, 232
Status, 91, 141, 176

Stereotypes, 56
Stevens, R., 48, 91
Stigma, 180, 189
Stoicism, 130, 282
Storms, M. D., 135
Strength of association, 190
Stress, 15, 60, 65, 124–127, 129–130, 132–134, 136, 165–177, 189–191, 195, 284
Strikes, 141
Subordinate personnel, power of, 169
Suggestibility, 135
Support, emotional, 136
Supportive care, 158
Surgery, 38, 44, 49, 60, 133, 136, 259, 271, 282–283
Sweden, 38–39, 41
Symptoms, gastrointestinal, 126
    and genetics, 186
    headache, 126
    indicators measuring, 186
    musculoskeletal, 126
    natural history of, 188
    neurotic, 184, 186
    normalization of, 183
    and pain, 133–134
    perception of, 13, 123–124, 129, 136
    psychophysiological, 185
    psychotic, 185
    social undesirability of, 186
    transitory, 188
    trivial, 14, 51, 102, 116, 132
Szasz, T., 183, 194, 237

Targeted audiences, 268
Tasks, allocation of, 240, 280, 287
    delegation, 15–16
    performance, 211
Team research, 170
Technical development of medicine, 17
Technical skills, 16
Technical solutions to individual behavior problems, 262
Technological change, 14, 167
"Technological imperative," 40
Technology, 1, 52, 60, 141, 170, 190, 208
Tendencies to respond, 174
Thalidomide tragedy, 258
Thomas, W. I., 171
Thompson, J., 205